Geriatric Emergency Medicine

Christian Nickel
Abdelouahab Bellou · Simon Conroy
Editors

Geriatric Emergency Medicine

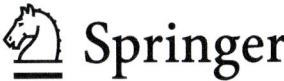

Editors
Christian Nickel
Emergency Department
University Hospital Basel
Basel, Switzerland

Abdelouahab Bellou
Department of Emergency Medicine
Beth Israel Deaconess Medical Center
Harvard Medical School
Boston, MA, USA

Simon Conroy
Department of Health Sciences
University of Leicester
Leicester, United Kingdom

ISBN 978-3-319-19317-5   ISBN 978-3-319-19318-2   (eBook)
https://doi.org/10.1007/978-3-319-19318-2

Library of Congress Control Number: 2017960903

© Springer International Publishing Switzerland 2018
This work is subject to copyright. All rights are reserved by the Publisher, whether the whole or part of the material is concerned, specifically the rights of translation, reprinting, reuse of illustrations, recitation, broadcasting, reproduction on microfilms or in any other physical way, and transmission or information storage and retrieval, electronic adaptation, computer software, or by similar or dissimilar methodology now known or hereafter developed.
The use of general descriptive names, registered names, trademarks, service marks, etc. in this publication does not imply, even in the absence of a specific statement, that such names are exempt from the relevant protective laws and regulations and therefore free for general use.
The publisher, the authors and the editors are safe to assume that the advice and information in this book are believed to be true and accurate at the date of publication. Neither the publisher nor the authors or the editors give a warranty, express or implied, with respect to the material contained herein or for any errors or omissions that may have been made. The publisher remains neutral with regard to jurisdictional claims in published maps and institutional affiliations.

Printed on acid-free paper

This Springer imprint is published by Springer Nature
The registered company is Springer International Publishing AG
The registered company address is: Gewerbestrasse 11, 6330 Cham, Switzerland

Foreword I

As EUSEM President and immediate Past-President, and EUGMS President and President-Elect, we congratulate the authors of this excellent textbook on geriatric emergency medicine. This book will help physicians to provide emergency care of the highest standard in a difficult sector that has a rapidly growing number of patients.

Geriatric emergency medicine is an ever more important specialist medical sector in every European country. The number of European emergency patients is growing. Statistically, every year the number of patients in emergency departments in many European states is equivalent to a quarter of the population of those countries. If these patients bring only one relative or friend with them, then half of the population of many European countries has contact with an emergency department.

In Europe with the further development of medical and social care, the average age of patients has reached a high level never seen in the past. This naturally also means the number of older patients seeking care every day in emergency departments is constantly rising. Older people need special treatment, which does not always correspond to the general guidelines we normally use for other patients. This specialist care may encompass social, psychological, behavioural and end-of-life aspects of treatment. Illness presentations in older patients may be different and sometimes difficult. Critical decisions on their treatment and case management must often be taken considering specific problems related to age such as the impact of falls, loneliness and lack of compliance.

This book will help provide structured and timely answers to the questions raised about illnesses and symptoms affecting these patients and how to manage them.

The EUSEM executive and council have strongly supported this project, which was undertaken jointly with the European Union Geriatric Medicine Society (EUGMS).

EUSEM's definition of emergency medicine declares that this is a medical specialty involving the prevention, diagnosis, treatment and management of acute illnesses and injuries needing immediate treatment. Emergency care involves patients **of all ages** and covers the entire body and also psychiatric illnesses. Rapid provision of treatment plays a key role in emergency medicine and places great demands on both in-hospital and pre-hospital care.

A recent conference of European health ministers about the future requirements of Europe's health care systems made an important comment:

There will be changing demands on health care. This is especially seen in the important sectors geriatrics and emergency medicine. We must identify the needs of the future today and decide how best these challenges can be met, not only nationally but also on a European level.

We believe this new textbook will provide excellent support to physicians working to meet this challenge. This book provides the answers to many questions that are posed every day when geriatric medicine and emergency medicine come together in emergency departments.

Roberta Petrino
Emergency Medicine Unite at S. Andrea Hospital of Vercelli and
S. Pietro and Paolo Hospital of Borgosesia, Italy
President of the European Society for Emergency Medicine (EuSEM)

Barbara Hogan
Emergency Departments at Mühlenkreiskliniken Hospital Group, Germany
Immediate Past-President EuSEM

Stefania Maggi
Aging Branch, CNR-Neuroscience Institute, Padua, Italy
President of the European Union Geriatric Medicine Society (EUGMS)

Finbarr C. Martin
Dept. of Aging and Health, St. Thomas Hospital Dept. of Aging and Health
London, UK
President-Elect EUGMS

Foreword II

The ageing of the population is slowly transforming the practice of emergency medicine. Improvements in public health, medical technology and therapy have resulted in longer and healthier lives but at the cost of growth in the medical needs of the population. During the twentieth century, the percentage of patients older than 65 grew from 4% to 14%. This growth is expected to continue and reach 20% by 2026. Furthermore, older emergency patients have had disproportionally higher use of the emergency department (ED) than the rest of the population because they are more likely to develop life-threatening conditions.

Emergency medicine, the youngest primary specialty, came into existence because of the need to provide a unique approach to patients presenting to ED. The importance of timely interventions in emergency conditions resulted from significant dramatic improvements in diagnostics and therapeutic options from the dramatic improvements in healthcare in the twentieth century. The combined social pressures resulting from the need to provide high-quality healthcare and the desire to provide access to everyone, at any time, for any problem required the development of a new specialty. The same pressures that created the specialty are now pushing for the development of expertise specific for geriatric emergencies. Because older patients will need access to all emergency departments, it remains to be determined if this expertise should be used to create a subspecialty or an expectation of all emergency providers.

Older patients now account for more than a quarter of emergency visits in the USA. This developing change in the emergency patient population is also creating a strain on the resources available for emergency care. Emergency crowding particularly impacts older patients who are often among the first groups affected by the shortage of inpatient capacity.

The dichotomous nature of the emergency management of older patients presents a dilemma in terms of patient management. On one hand, frailty, blunted inflammatory response and cognitive disabilities vastly complicate the assessment of these patients. With age, a different and broader spectrum of emergency conditions develops. Life threats are more common and clinical presentations are often atypical or occult. Safely ensuring a timely diagnosis often requires prolonged investigations. On the other hand, there is a recognised mismatch between the services traditionally provided by the emergency department and the desires of the patients. Rather than the highly aggressive approach to diagnosis and therapy traditionally used in emergencies, what most patients at the end of life want are supportive services and a focus on improving the quality of life rather than simply prolonging it.

Until recently, the evidence base for geriatric emergency medicine (GEM) has been somewhat neglected. Besides the challenges of delivering care, there is also the need to understand the biology of GEM: the unique aspects of ageing and how these affect a patient's ability to respond to a physical or psychological crisis. How can we measure frailty and immunologic impairment? How does ageing affect the endothelium, the cell, or the mitochondrion? What are the implications of these changes on resuscitation? There is a need for basic and clinical science in GEM to add new knowledge to acquire the evidence, which will help in improving management and outcome. The complexity of acute care of older patients in emergency medicine settings will require a multidisciplinary approach from researchers and a wide range of specialties with a close partnership between emergency physicians and geriatricians.

This book is an important step in disseminating knowledge, standardising care and setting a direction for future work on how to address the challenges of GEM. By providing medical providers with the information needed to improve the emergency care for older patients, we can begin to deliver a high-quality approach geared towards the needs of this vulnerable population.

Richard Wolfe
Associate Professor of Emergency Medicine
Chair of the Department of Emergency Medicine
Beth Israel Deaconess Medical Center a Teaching Hospital
of Harvard Medical School, Boston, MA, USA

Contents

Part I Pre-hospital Care and Initial Assessment

1 **Prehospital Management of Older Patients** 3
   Eric Revue, James Wallace, and Shuja Punekar

2 **Triage of Older ED Patients**................................ 17
   Florian F. Grossmann and Christian Nickel

3 **Primary Assessment and Stabilization of Life-Threatening
   Conditions in Older Patients** 23
   Mehmet Akif Karamercan, Abdelouahab Bellou, and Hubert Blain

4 **Secondary Assessment of Life-Threatening Conditions
   of Older Patients** 49
   Hubert Blain, Abdelouahab Bellou, Mehmet Akif Karamercan, and
   Jacques Boddaert

5 **Clinical Assessment and Management of Older People:
   What's Different?** 75
   Gertrude Chikura, Simon Conroy, and Fabio Salvi

6 **Comprehensive Geriatric Assessment in the Emergency
   Department** 91
   Els Devriendt and Simon Conroy

Part II Management of Common Conditions

7 **Pitfalls in the Management of Older Patients
   in the Emergency Department**................................. 111
   Fredrik Sjöstrand and Christian Nickel

8 **Nonspecific Disease Presentation: The Emergency
   Department Perspective** 127
   Alexandra Malinovska, Christian Nickel, and Roland Bingisser

9	**Falls Presenting in the Emergency Department**.................	137
	Jay Banerjee and Anna Björg Jónsdóttir	
10	**Syncope in Older People in the Emergency Department**..........	147
	Nissa J. Ali, Laure Joly, and Shamai A. Grossman	
11	**Trauma in Older People**.......................................	163
	Nicolas Bless	
12	**Management of Sepsis in Older Patients in the Emergency Department**..	177
	Abdelouahab Bellou and Hubert Blain	
13	**Cognitive Impairment in Older People Presenting to ED**.........	199
	Chris Miller, Elizabeth Teale, and Jay Banerjee	
14	**Depression in Acute Geriatric Care**	209
	R. Prettyman and J. Banerjee	
15	**Abdominal Pain in Older Patients**............................	217
	Zerrin Defne Dündar, A. Bulent Dogrul, Mehmet Ergin, and R. Tuna Dogrul	
16	**Urinary Tract Infections in Older Patients**....................	235
	Roberta Petrino, Aldo Tua, and Fabio Salvi	
17	**Management of Acute Chest Pain in Older Patients**.............	247
	Tim Arnold, Ursula Müller-Werdan, and Martin Möckel	
18	**Dyspnoea in Older People in the Emergency Department**.........	261
	F. Javier Martín-Sánchez and Juan González del Castillo	
19	**Management of Back Pain in Older Patients**....................	275
	Jennifer Truchot and Jean Laganier	

Part III Special Considerations in Frail Older People

20	**Medicine in Older Patients: Evidence Based?**...................	291
	Simon P. Mooijaart	
21	**Prescribing for Older Patients**...............................	299
	Paul Gallagher, Amanda Lavan, and Denis O'Mahony	
22	**Pain in Older People Attending Emergency Departments**	315
	Sophie Pautex	
23	**Transitions of Care and Disposition**	329
	Sarah Turpin and Sarah Vince	
24	**Principles of Rehabilitation in Geriatric Emergency Medicine**.....	345
	Ebby Sigmund	

25 **Palliative and End of Life Care for Dementia Patients in the Emergency Department**.............................. 353
Jo James

26 **Palliative and End of Life Care for the Older Person in the Emergency Department**.............................. 361
Mary Dawood

27 **Ethical Issues of Emergency Medical Care for Older Patients**...... 369
Helen Askitopoulou, Katrin Singler, Thomas Frühwald, and Monique Weissenberger-Leduc

Index.. 397

Part I
Pre-hospital Care and Initial Assessment

Prehospital Management of Older Patients

Eric Revue, James Wallace, and Shuja Punekar

1.1 Background

The number of older inpatients has been steadily increasing worldwide. Changing global demography is resulting in increasing numbers of older people presenting to emergency departments (EDs) and also being more likely to be admitted to hospital; in 2014–2015 in England, the percentage of older patients admitted from EDs was 50% compared to 16% for those under 65 [1]. Older patients account for the most rapidly growing segment of the European and US populations [2]; in 2016 persons over 65 years old represented greater than 13% of the worldwide population, with the population over 75 in France growing by 0.2% every year, whilst in England between 2001 and 2011, the population of people over 85 increased at a rate three and a half times higher than the rest of the population [3]. The percentage of older patients is projected to increase over the next decade with more than 25% of ED visits generated by this age group by 2030 [2, 4].

E. Revue, MD (✉)
Emergency Department, Louis Pasteur Hospital, Chartres, France
e-mail: eric.revue@yahoo.fr

J. Wallace, MD
Emergency Department, Warrington and Halton Hospitals NHS Foundation Trust, Warrington, UK
e-mail: j.m.wallace@doctors.org.uk

S. Punekar, MD
Geriatric Department, Warrington and Halton Hospitals NHS Foundation Trust, Warrington, UK

© Springer International Publishing Switzerland 2018
C. Nickel et al. (eds.), *Geriatric Emergency Medicine*,
https://doi.org/10.1007/978-3-319-19318-2_1

1.1.1 The Impact on Services

Older adults (age ≥ 65) in the USA comprise 38% of emergency medical services (EMS) patients and use EMS services almost four times more frequently than younger patients [5, 6]. In the United Kingdom (UK), about one third of attendances are due to trauma and falls, with the remainder being due to a medical illness [7], but approximately one fifth of admissions are for conditions which could be managed by primary, community or social care [1]. UK ambulance services cost around £1.9 billion or 2% of the National Health Service (NHS) spend per year, but have an impact on over £20 billion or 20% of the subsequent NHS spend [8].

In the 1990s, a multicentre study demonstrated that 15% of 100 million emergency department (ED) visits were made by older patients and that these patients were more likely to be brought in by ambulance, consume more ED resources, have a more serious illness or injury and were more likely to require surgery or admission [9].

Older patients are known to experience longer waits for care and suffer poorer health outcomes after ED attendance, with higher mortality rates, greater dependence in activities and higher rates of admission to nursing homes [10–14]. Mann et al. found that older patients have multiple undiagnosed pathologies across several organ systems, highlighting the need for a systematic approach of prehospital services towards their patients and respective pathologies [15]. Considering the potential impact older patients have on hospital and prehospital systems and conversely the EMS providers have on patient outcomes both pre- and inhospital, it is important to understand the health-care needs of older patients to ensure they are triaged, treated and managed appropriately.

1.1.2 Prehospital Personnel Training

EMS providers must be able to adjust for the changes that occur in patients at extremes of age, but unfortunately, most EMS providers get little geriatric education during their initial training [16, 17]. The curriculum for emergency Medical Technician (EMT) training does not include any dedicated sections that specifically teach EMT about physiological or psychological changes with ageing patients [18, 19]. Specific geriatric focus education can improve the basic knowledge of EMS personnel, but patient outcomes from targeted education have not been studied.

In 2014, the UK Association of Ambulance Chief Executives (AACE) recognised that, as part of a future national priority in improving clinical care, prehospital personnel require more training around the assessment and management of frail older patients [20]. The emphasis would be on clinical decision-making, psychosocial context, attitudinal aspects of care, communication barriers and techniques, assessment of capacity as well as training in ethics and law [20].

The British Geriatrics Society identified in their campaign "The Silver Book" that paramedics (EMS personnel) face unique challenges when responding to older patients, especially those that are alone or cognitively impaired. They identified that polypharmacy, complex comorbidities and lack of information make the assessment of conditions and decisions to manage the patient at home more difficult [3].

1.2 The Prehospital Geriatric Patient

1.2.1 Anatomical and Physiological Differences

The anatomy and physiology of the older patients differ from that of younger adult patients. Although some of these differences may appear to be inconsequential, they can significantly affect the treatment that is provided in the prehospital situation.

With increasing age, blood flow to the brain decreases, leading to a decrease in cerebral perfusion and oxygenation [21]. Peripheral nerve conduction also slows and may be further impaired by the chronic use of analgesics [22]. When these factors are combined, older patients' ability to "sense" that they have been injured may be reduced. Thermoregulatory mechanisms may also be impaired, leading to hypothermia [23, 24]. The ability of an older patient to react to an adverse environment may be reduced due to limitations in their sensory perception of surroundings [25, 26], which can negatively impact the patient's recovery from injury and even their final health outcome. These factors not only increase the risk of falls and peripheral injuries but also increase the risk of exposure and pressure-related illnesses [21, 25]. Recognising the risk of these injuries is key in the prehospital field, especially with long transfers to hospital care. Requiring prolonged immobilisation further increases the risk of pressure-related injuries and physical deconditioning [27, 28].

1.2.2 Disability and Function

Physical disability of older patients manifests as the loss of ability to complete basic needs without assistance, such as bathing, dressing, rising from a bed or chair, using the toilet and eating. Frail, cognitively impaired or disabled people can become rapidly immobile or confused, suffer increased falls and deteriorate from coping to a state of acopia with minor acute illnesses or worsening of a pre-existing condition [29–31]. Ideally, older inpatients with disability and reduced function are rehabilitated by a physiotherapist with the aim of improving the patient's functional capacity and outcome during the hospital stay, to then be discharged safely back to their homes.

Although several functional scores exist in the ED for individual conditions, and individual risk factors are known to predict outcome, [32] there is still a paucity of risk stratification tools for undifferentiated older patient presenting complaints [33]. Likewise, several specific prehospital predictors exist for outcomes in major trauma [34], stroke diagnosis [35] and sepsis [36]. However, even fever studies exist in the prehospital field to predict functional outcome across the general aspects of care [37].

1.2.3 The Patient as a Whole

Epidemiology has demonstrated that with increases in age, the number of identifiable diseases or pathologies also increases [38]. However, the clinical relevance of this polypathology varies according to the main reason for calling and requiring EMS and that not all underlying pathologies are necessarily implicated in all prehospital encounters [38].

Whereas the younger patient typically presents to EMS and EDs with a symptom-based chief complaint, geriatric adults more commonly report atypical or non-specific symptoms that prompted the patient to seek medical care [39, 40]. Although these symptoms can be the manifestation of an acute and reversible life-threatening illness, more often, the symptoms are a result of a complex mix of chronic disease processes [39].

Carpenter and Platts-Mills also state that assessing and treating the patient as a whole involves looking at aspects of their presentation to medical services which are not traditionally part of ED or prehospital emergency care [39]. The holistic approach incorporates evaluation of cognition, falls risk, adequacy of social circumstances, potential abuse or neglect and mental health.

1.3 Pathologies in Older Patients

1.3.1 Recognition of Pathology

The main presenting complaints of older patients calling for EMS and then attending EDs have been well recognized for decades; they include:

1. Pain [41–43]
2. Falls [44]
3. Walking disabilities [45]
4. Trauma [46]
5. Confusion or delirium [47–49]
6. Neurologic weakness [50]
7. Depression
8. Chest pain [51, 52]

The optimal way to identify and treat the majority of these pathologies before an ED attendance, with the outcome of improved health, minimal iatrogenic effects and reduced risk of deterioration during hospitalisation has not yet been discovered or studied robustly.

1.3.2 Time Critical Pathologies

There are certain pathologies in older patients in which prehospital service personnel can significantly improve patient outcomes by identifying the time critical nature of the presenting complaint. Recognition of these pathologies and having an understanding of the time critical treatment involved can assist personnel with stabilisation and appropriate transfer to specialist centres for definitive care [53].

Examples include:

Condition	Outcome
Acute cerebrovascular accident (CVA) [54, 55]	Reduction in disability from major stroke if fibrinolytic therapy can be administered within 3 h of onset of symptoms
Acute myocardial infarct (MI) [51, 52, 56, 57]	Reduced morbidity/mortality from ST-segment elevation MI if reperfusion can be restored via PTCA or fibrinolysis, if within 6 h; PTCA preferred if available
Multiple trauma [34, 58]	Rapid transport to trauma centre favours recovery due to aggressive early management
Pneumonia [59]	Early institution of antibiotics enhances recovery
Surgical abdomen [60]	Older patients have higher incidence of surgical abdomen including cholecystitis, bowel obstruction, mesenteric ischemia, aortic disruption and appendicitis. Early operation reduces likelihood of perforation and peritonitis

1.3.3 Pain

Twenty to fifty percent of older patients in the community suffer from pain, which in 20–40% of individuals occurs on most days in 1 month [3]. Sixty to seventy percent of older patients living at home have self-reported pain, with a prevalence of 65% among people living in nursing home [61]. Multiple pain aetiologies that occur in older patients may be due to multiple chronic diseases. Pain is also a morbid condition in older individuals and associated with poor physical function, falls and mortality [62].

Pain has a significant impact on an older person's cognitive state and mental health, yet older patients with acute pain are less likely to receive pain medication than younger patients during emergency department (ED) care [63–65]. However, the epidemiology of acute pain treatment for older adults is not completely understood, as are the causes for observed differences between older and younger adults [65]. A substantial portion of older ED patients with pain are transported to the ED by ambulance [4, 6] which provides an early opportunity for pain treatment under different conditions.

1.3.4 Prehospital Older Patients' Trauma

Trauma in older patients differs from younger patients due to associated physiological changes that occur with normal ageing, multiple comorbidities and polypharmacy; therefore, relatively minor accidents can have devastating consequences. This can be attributed mostly to the response to bleeding, injury and shock differing from 18-year-old trauma counterparts. Skaga et al found that pre-injury comorbidity, score according to the American Society of Anaesthesiologists (ASA) classification system, was an independent predictor of trauma mortality [66].

Older trauma patients are five times more likely to die from trauma than a younger patient with a similar mechanism of injury, with almost 25% of traumatic injuries from motor vehicle/road traffic collisions (MVCs/RTCs) and 4% from penetrating trauma [67]. MVCs have almost double the mortality for geriatric patients, with about 25% suffering rib fractures and flail segments [68]. Precipitating medical events can cause trauma; therefore, it is crucial for EMS to determine what may have caused the trauma, obtaining pre-event status and conditions which may alter treatment and transfer decisions.

Assessing the older trauma patient in the prehospital setting using a structured ABC technique may be challenging. They may have altered mental status due to dementia or have difficulty in communicating due to movement disorders or functional deficits from neurological disorders.

The airway of an older patient may have foreign bodies such as partial plates or dental appliances which have implications for instrumentation and ventilation. Limitation in the movement of the neck due to arthritis may limit the view using conventional airway techniques. Rapid sequence induction may require a reduction in standard doses of induction and paralysing agents, especially as the older may have a higher incidence of hyperkalaemia and neuromuscular disorders.

Older adults have less pulmonary reserve; therefore, application of oxygen will help avoid hypoxia; however, care must be given in the chronic pulmonary disease patient to prevent hypercarbia. End-tidal carbon dioxide concentration (ETCO2) does correlate with outcome in trauma, and with outcome 20 minutes after intubation [69].

Crystalloid fluid resuscitation in trauma has been shown to be harmful in trauma, especially when large volumes are given to older patients [70]. Permissive hypotension is a technique that can be used in the older trauma patient to avoid fluid overload but does not affect outcomes of surgery [71].

Due to the normal ageing process, skin and other collagen-based structures lose elasticity, which increases the risk of skin tears and subcutaneous bruising, which in the presence of anticoagulants can cause significant loss of blood, potentially affecting perfusion. Immobilisation should take consideration of extremities, with application of pressure devices to control bleeding and even avoid skin to skin taping.

1.4 Models of Care

With the increasing number of older patients, and increase in hospital attendances, alternative models of care have been explored across the globe and various healthcare systems. Alternative management methods are essential to ensure high-quality and efficient emergency care for the growing number of older adults worldwide [39].

With the emphasis on improved outcomes in the care of older patients, the following models or changes to care have been identified:

1. Geriatric trained personnel
2. Integration of prehospital and community services

3. Improved communication between prehospital, EDs and inpatient and outpatient services
4. Validated protocols for the treatment of geriatric and frail patients
5. Specifically designed geriatric departments and infrastructure

1.4.1 The Emergency Department (ED)

The emergency department is a key link in the geriatric network and allows us to offer a suitable orientation and initiation of an older person's care. In the case of hospitalisation, the choice of ward would be the short-stay geriatric inpatient unit, ideally reducing the length of stay to minimise deconditioning and limit the iatrogenic effects of hospitalisation [3, 39, 72, 73].

This is especially the case as 10–20% of hospitalisations are linked to iatrogenic adverse events [74]. The prevalence of adverse drug reactions is about 10% in hospitalised patients, and over 10% of hospitalised older patients have no adherence to their community treatment [75].

1.4.2 Acute Geriatric Units

Fox et al. compared the effectiveness of acute geriatric unit care, based on all or part of the Acute Care for Elders (ACE) model and introduced in the acute phase of illness or injury, with that of usual care [72]. Eleven meta-analyses were performed on data from papers that studied functional decline between baseline 2-week prehospital admission status and discharge, length of hospital stay [9, 76], mortality [77] and costs [78, 79]. Acute geriatric unit care was associated with significantly fewer falls and non-significantly fewer pressure ulcers in acutely ill or injured older adults than usual care [72].

1.4.3 Traditional Inpatient Management Models

During hospitalisation for an acute event such as illness or injury, older adults are at risk of experiencing functional decline and iatrogenic complications, including falls, pressure ulcers and delirium, which further contribute to functional decline [39]. Hospital-acquired functional decline is associated with institutionalisation and mortality in older adults [72, 80]. Therefore, geriatric targeted intervention is critical because of the short length of time during which older persons can recover functional losses, resume their former lives and avoid institutionalisation [10, 78, 79].

1.4.4 Community and Primary Care

The BGS "Silver Book" identifies that more community-based services with a quicker response time may reduce the need for hospitalisation [3]. Very rarely is the urgent care need in the patients first 24 h entirely dependent on health services, yet a slight deterioration in a chronic disease impairing their functional ability traditionally results in a hospital admission. In the UK, there is variation in response times for urgent health-care needs; the ambulance service has a response time in minutes, but even in normal working hours, there is a greater variability in the response from community general practitioners and social care across the nation [3].

The authors also found that that a 1% decrease in primary care response to a crisis can lead to a 20% increase in demand for secondary care [3]. Bankart et al. found in 2006/2007 that for a 5% increase of patients being able to access their primary doctor, there is a 3.5% decrease in admissions [81].

Single clinician case management was looked at in a meta-analysis by Purdy [73], in which 4/5 randomised control trials showed no advantage of a single nurse clinician to manage patients in care home health outcome vs usual team approach (0.05 95% CI −0.04, 0.15); however, one RCT did show a small non-significant reduction in the relative risk of unplanned hospital admissions, based upon a GP leading a multidisciplinary team for patients already in a care home environment.

1.4.5 Out of Hours' Care

Caring for older people out of hours is known to have its own set of challenges, especially as the clinician will not be familiar with the individual's history or understand all the local services available [3]. The British Geriatrics Society state that a 34 hour, 7 days a week single point of access with multidisciplinary response within 2 hours (14 overnight) should be commissioned, coupled to a live directory of services with consistent clinical content [3]. Conversely, they also stated that discharge to an older person's normal residence should be possible within 24 h, 7 days a week.

1.4.6 Hospital at Home

Hospital at home describes services in which traditional hospital-based care is provided in the patient's own home, thus avoiding an acute admission. Patients can be referred by their primary care team, secondary care or even the EMS/ambulance service.

A Cochrane review in 2011 [82] looked at seven eligible RCTs, finding that there was not a significant reduction in mortality at 3 months for the hospital at home group (adjusted HR 0.77 (95% CI 0.54–1.09)), but at 6 months, there was a significant reduction in mortality (adjusted HR 0.62 (95% CI 0.45–0.87)). However, there was a non-significant increase in admissions from patients in the hospital at home group (adjusted HR 1.49 (95% CI 0.96–2.33)), with minimal differences in functional ability. Hospital at home was less expensive and patients had increased satisfaction staying at home [83].

A more recent meta-analysis in Australia included 61 papers [84] and, contrarily to the Cochrane review, found hospital at home care led to a reduced mortality (OR 0.81 [95% CI 0.69–0.95]), reduced admission rates (OR 0.75 [95% CI 0.59–0.95]) and reduced cost. The authors also stated that the number needed to treat at home to prevent one death was 50, and patient satisfaction was higher in 21 out of 22 studies [84].

National bodies in the UK [1, 3, 8, 20] state in their reviews that more home-based care should be provided by primary care teams and specialist teams such as heart failure, dementia and respiratory diseases, in conjunction with specialist secondary care teams outreaching to give support and prevent admissions.

1.4.7 EMS/EMT/Ambulance Care

The UK ambulance service has been identified by the BGS to play a key role in changing the prehospital management of older patients, for example, by referring non-conveyed patients to urgent care, community and primary care services and falls services [3].

In 2011, ambulance services were managing between 30 and 50% of all emergency call-outs without taking a person to secondary care, but by providing advice (hear and treat) referring to an appropriate alternative service (see and refer) or by treating the person on scene (see and treat) [8].

Malson et al. showed that trained paramedic interventions did have some effect on unplanned hospital admissions at 28 days (RR 0.87 (95%CI 0.81, 0.94)), and those patients were less likely to attend an ED (RR 0.72% (95%CI 0.68, 0.75)) [85]. The intervention studied was extended paramedic skills in assessing, treating and discharging older patients with minor acute conditions in the community.

A more recent randomised control trial of 656 older patients by Vicente et al. in 2014 showed that a nurse dispatcher in EMS appropriately triaged 93.3% of the participants to a community geriatric hospital avoiding an ED visit or admission [86].

Falls being one of the commonest presentations to EMS, Logan et al showed that a referral by prehospital personnel to a community falls prevention team versus standard medical and social care had less falls over 12 months [87]. The incidence of falls was 3.45 in the intervention group and 7.68 in the control group (rate ratio 0.45 [95% CI 0.35–0.59]). Secondary outcomes showed that the intervention group had higher scores on the Barthel index and Nottingham extended activities of daily living and lower scores on the falls efficacy scale.

Conclusion

The world's population is getting older, combined with higher rates of admission to hospital, and is putting a strain on most countries' health economies. Emergency medical services traditionally have not had specific training on how to recognise or manage geriatric-specific pathologies, yet there is recognition at the national service level for the need to improve knowledge and integrate care services with the ultimate goal of reducing unplanned admissions to hospital or attendances to emergency departments.

Older persons are more likely to fall and have multiple complicating pathologies, but also are at increased risk of iatrogenicity from prehospital transport and immobilisation. They have altered physiology, meaning trauma care is having to develop new standards of care for physiological stabilisation, and are more likely to have a medical cause for their trauma.

Models of care in the prehospital field have been tried and studied worldwide with varying degrees of success. Hospital at home, integrated care, better access to primary care, increased skills of prehospital personnel, facilitated discharges and alternative pathways of care have been studied individually, yet there is still no perfect answer for the management of undifferentiated prehospital geriatric patients.

References

1. A Morse, National Audit Office (2016) Discharging older patients from hospital. In: Health DO (ed) London. https://www.nao.org.uk/wp-content/uploads/2015/12/Discharging-older-patients-from-hospital.pdf
2. Medicine IO (2008) Retooling for an aging America: building the health care workforce. The National Academies Press, Washington
3. Society BG (2012) Quality care for older people with urgent and emergency care needs. The British Geriatrics Society, Leicester
4. Platts-Mills TF, Leacock B, Cabanas JG, Shofer FS, Mclean SA (2010) Emergency medical services use by the elderly: analysis of a statewide database. Prehosp Emerg Care 14:329–333
5. Shah MN, Bazarian JJ, Lerner EB, Fairbanks RJ, Barker WH, Auinger P, Friedman B (2007) The epidemiology of emergency medical services use by older adults: an analysis of the National Hospital Ambulatory Medical Care Survey. Acad Emerg Med 14:441–447
6. Wofford JL, Moran WP, Heuser MD, Schwartz E, Velez R, Mittelmark MB (1995) Emergency medical transport of the elderly: a population-based study. Am J Emerg Med 13:297–300
7. Downing A, Wilson R (2005) Older people's use of accident and emergency services. Age Ageing 34:24–30
8. A Mrse, National Audit Office (2017) NHS ambulance services. https://www.nao.org.uk/wp-content/uploads/2017/01/NHS-Ambulance-Services.pdf
9. Strange GR, Chen EH (1998) Use of emergency departments by elder patients: a five-year follow-up study. Acad Emerg Med 5:1157–1162
10. Aminzadeh F, Dalziel WB (2002) Older adults in the emergency department: a systematic review of patterns of use, adverse outcomes, and effectiveness of interventions. Ann Emerg Med 39:238–247
11. Fernandez HM, Callahan KE, Likourezos A, Leipzig RM (2008) House staff member awareness of older inpatients' risks for hazards of hospitalization. Arch Int Med 168:390–396
12. Gill TM, Allore HG, Holford TR, Guo Z (2004) Hospitalization, restricted activity, and the development of disability among older persons. JAMA 292:2115–2124
13. Hastings SN, Heflin MT (2005) A systematic review of interventions to improve outcomes for elders discharged from the emergency department. Acad Emerg Med 12:978–986
14. Hastings SN, Oddone EZ, Fillenbaum G, Sloane RJ, Schmader KE (2008) Frequency and predictors of adverse health outcomes in older Medicare beneficiaries discharged from the emergency department. Med Care 46:771–777
15. Mann E, Koller M, Mann C, Van Der Cammen T, Steurer J (2004) Comprehensive geriatric assessment (CGA) in general practice: results from a pilot study in Vorarlberg, Austria. BMC Geriatr 4:4
16. DJ Samuels, HC. Bock, United States Department of Transportation National Highway Traffic Safety Administration (NHTSA) EMT-Basic: National Standard Curriculum (1996). https://www.ems.gov/pdf/education/Emergency-Medical-Technician/EMT_Basic_1996.pdf
17. National EMS Education Standards (2009). https://www.ems.gov/pdf/education/EMS-Education-for-the-Future-A-Systems-Approach/National_EMS_Education_Standards.pdf

18. Peterson LK, Fairbanks RJ, Hettinger AZ, Shah MN (2009) Emergency medical service attitudes toward geriatric prehospital care and continuing medical education in geriatrics. J Am Geriatr Soc 57:530–535
19. Shah MN, Rajasekaran K, Sheahan WD, Wimbush T, Karuza J (2008) The effect of the geriatrics education for emergency medical services training program in a rural community. J Am Geriatr Soc 56:1134–1139
20. Directors NASM (2014) Future national clinical priorities for ambulance services in England. Association of Ambulance Chief Executives, London
21. Walston J, Hadley EC, Ferrucci L, Guralnik JM, Newman AB, Studenski SA, Ershler WB, Harris T, Fried LP (2006) Research agenda for frailty in older adults: toward a better understanding of physiology and etiology: summary from the American Geriatrics Society/National Institute on Aging research conference on frailty in older adults. J Am Geriatr Soc 54:991–1001
22. Ward RE, Caserotti P, Cauley JA, Boudreau RM, Goodpaster BH, Vinik AI, Newman AB, Strotmeyer ES (2016) Mobility-related consequences of reduced lower-extremity peripheral nerve function with age: a systematic review. Aging Dis 7:466–478
23. Ballester JM, Harchelroad FP (1999) Hypothermia: an easy-to-miss, dangerous disorder in winter weather. Geriatrics 54(51–2):55–57
24. Harchelroad F (1993) Acute thermoregulatory disorders. Clin Geriatr Med 9:621–639
25. Perrin PP, Jeandel C, Perrin CA, Bene MC (1997) Influence of visual control, conduction, and central integration on static and dynamic balance in healthy older adults. Gerontology 43:223–231
26. Whipple R, Wolfson L, Derby C, Singh D, Tobin J (1993) Altered sensory function and balance in older persons. J Gerontol 48(Special Issue):71–76
27. Convertino VA, Bloomfield SA, Greenleaf JE (1997) An overview of the issues: physiological effects of bed rest and restricted physical activity. Med Sci Sports Exerc 29:187–190
28. Ham HW, Schoonhoven LL, Schuurmans MM, Leenen LL (2016) Pressure ulcer development in trauma patients with suspected spinal injury; the influence of risk factors present in the emergency department. Int Emerg Nurs 30:13–19
29. Clegg AP, Barber SE, Young JB, Forster A, Iliffe SJ (2012) Do home-based exercise interventions improve outcomes for frail older people? Findings from a systematic review. Rev Clin Gerontol 22:68–78
30. Covinsky KE, Palmer RM, Fortinsky RH, Counsell SR, Stewart AL, Kresevic D, Burant CJ, Landefeld CS (2003) Loss of independence in activities of daily living in older adults hospitalized with medical illnesses: increased vulnerability with age. J Am Geriatr Soc 51:451–458
31. Zisberg A, Shadmi E, Sinoff G, Gur-Yaish N, Srulovici E, Admi H (2011) Low mobility during hospitalization and functional decline in older adults. J Am Geriatr Soc 59:266–273
32. Gill TM, Gahbauer EA, Han L, Allore HG (2009) Factors associated with recovery of prehospital function among older persons admitted to a nursing home with disability after an acute hospitalization. J Gerontol A Biol Sci Med Sci 64:1296–1303
33. Carpenter CR, Shelton E, Fowler S, Suffoletto B, Platts-Mills TF, Rothman RE, Hogan TM (2015) Risk factors and screening instruments to predict adverse outcomes for undifferentiated older emergency department patients: a systematic review and meta-analysis. Acad Emerg Med 22:1–21
34. Bala M, Willner D, Klauzni D, Bdolah-Abram T, Rivkind AI, Gazala MA, Elazary R, Almogy G (2013) Pre-hospital and admission parameters predict in-hospital mortality among patients 60 years and older following severe trauma. Scand J Trauma Resusc Emerg Med 21:91
35. Evenson KR, Foraker RE, Morris DL, Rosamond WD (2009) A comprehensive review of prehospital and in-hospital delay times in acute stroke care. Int J Stroke 4:187–199
36. Williams TA, Tohira H, Finn J, Perkins GD, Ho KM (2016) The ability of early warning scores (EWS) to detect critical illness in the prehospital setting: a systematic review. Resuscitation 102:35–43
37. Goldstein JP, Andrew MK, Travers A (2012) Frailty in older adults using pre-hospital care and the emergency department: a narrative review. Can Geriatr J 15:16–22
38. Saint-Jean O, Berigaud S, Bouchon JP (1991) Polypathology and co-morbidity: a dynamic way for describing morbidity in aged patients. Study of 100 patients, aged 80 and over, in a short-stay geriatric internal medicine unit. Ann Med Interne (Paris) 142:563–569

39. Carpenter CR, Platts-Mills TF (2013) Evolving prehospital, emergency department, and "inpatient" management models for geriatric emergencies. Clin Geriatr Med 29:31–47
40. Hogan TM, Losman ED, Carpenter CR, Sauvigne K, Irmiter C, Emanuel L, Leipzig RM (2010) Development of geriatric competencies for emergency medicine residents using an expert consensus process. Acad Emerg Med 17:316–324
41. Heft MW, Gracely RH, Dubner R, Mcgrath PA (1980) A validation model for verbal description scaling of human clinical pain. Pain 9:363–373
42. Hicks CL, Von Baeyer CL, Spafford PA, Van Korlaar I, Goodenough B (2001) The faces pain scale-revised: toward a common metric in pediatric pain measurement. Pain 93:173–183
43. Jensen MP, Karoly P, Braver S (1986) The measurement of clinical pain intensity: a comparison of six methods. Pain 27:117–126
44. Perell KL, Nelson A, Goldman RL, Luther SL, Prieto-Lewis N, Rubenstein LZ (2001) Fall risk assessment measures: an analytic review. J Gerontol A Biol Sci Med Sci 56:M761–M766
45. Mathias S, Nayak US, Isaacs B (1986) Balance in elderly patients: the "get-up and go" test. Arch Phys Med Rehabil 67:387–389
46. Mandavia D, Newton K (1998) Geriatric trauma. Emerg Med Clin North Am 16:257–274
47. Inouye SK, Van Dyck CH, Alessi CA, Balkin S, Siegal AP, Horwitz RI (1990) Clarifying confusion: the confusion assessment method. A new method for detection of delirium. Ann Intern Med 113:941–948
48. Manckoundia P, Mourey F, Perennou D, Pfitzenmeyer P (2008) Backward disequilibrium in elderly subjects. Clin Interv Aging 3:667–672
49. Siddiqi N, House AO, Holmes JD (2006) Occurrence and outcome of delirium in medical inpatients: a systematic literature review. Age Ageing 35:350–364
50. Brott T, Adams HP Jr, Olinger CP, Marler JR, Barsan WG, Biller J, Spilker J, Holleran R, Eberle R, Hertzberg V et al (1989) Measurements of acute cerebral infarction: a clinical examination scale. Stroke 20:864–870
51. Gottwalles Y, Dangelser G, De Poli F, Mathien C, Levai L, Boulenc JM, Monassier JP, Jacquemin L, El Belghiti R, Couppie P, Hanssen M (2004) Acute STEMI in old and very old patients. The real life. Ann Cardiol Angeiol (Paris) 53:305–313
52. Wroblewski M, Mikulowski P, Steen B (1986) Symptoms of myocardial infarction in old age: clinical case, retrospective and prospective studies. Age Ageing 15:99–104
53. Hogan TM, Geriatric Emergencies: an EMT teaching manual. Medicalert Foundation Retirement Research Foundation (RRF) (1994). https://www.medicalert.org/sites/default/files/document/geriatric_manual%5B1%5D.pdf
54. Adams HP, Del Zoppo G, Alberts MJ, Bhatt DL, Brass L, Furlan A, Grubb RL, Higashida RT, Jauch EC, Kidwell C, Lyden PD, Morgenstern LB, Qureshi AI, Rosenwasser RH, Scott PA, Wijdicks EFM (2007) Guidelines for the early management of adults with ischemic stroke. Guideline from the American Heart Association/American Stroke Association Stroke Council. Stroke 115:e478–e534
55. Hill MD, Buchan AM (2005) Thrombolysis for acute ischemic stroke: results of the Canadian Alteplase for stroke effectiveness study. CMAJ 172:1307–1312
56. Dangelser G, Gottwalles Y, Huk M, De Poli F, Levai L, Boulenc JM, Monassier JP, Jacquemin L, Couppie P, Hanssen M (2005) Acute ST-elevation myocardial infarction in the elderly (>75 years). Results from a regional multicenter study. Presse Med 34:983–989
57. Makam RP, Erskine N, Yarzebski J, Lessard D, Lau J, Allison J, Gore JM, Gurwitz J, Mcmanus DD, Goldberg RJ (2016) Decade long trends (2001–2011) in duration of pre-hospital delay among elderly patients hospitalized for an acute myocardial infarction. J Am Heart Assoc 5(4):e002664
58. Hashmi A, Ibrahim-Zada I, Rhee P, Aziz H, Fain MJ, Friese RS, Joseph B (2014) Predictors of mortality in geriatric trauma patients: a systematic review and meta-analysis. J Trauma Acute Care Surg 76:894–901
59. Phua J, Dean NC, Guo Q, Kuan WS, Lim HF, Lim TK (2016) Severe community-acquired pneumonia: timely management measures in the first 24 hours. Crit Care 20:237

60. Al-Qurayshi Z, Srivastav S, Kandil E (2016) Postoperative outcomes in patients with perforated bowel: early versus late intervention. J Surg Res 203:75–81
61. Leveau P 2009 La personne agee aux urgences. EM Consulte 1–8
62. Vadivelu N, Hines RL (2008) Management of chronic pain in the elderly: focus on transdermal buprenorphine. Clin Interv Aging 3:421–430
63. Jennings PA, Cameron P, Bernard S (2012) Determinants of clinically important pain severity reduction in the prehospital setting. Emerg Med J 29:333–334
64. Jones JS, Johnson K, Mcninch M (1996) Age as a risk factor for inadequate emergency department analgesia. Am J Emerg Med 14:157–160
65. Platts-Mills TF, Esserman DA, Brown DL, Bortsov AV, Sloane PD, Mclean SA (2012) Older US emergency department patients are less likely to receive pain medication than younger patients: results from a national survey. Ann Emerg Med 60:199–206
66. Skaga NO, Eken T, Sovik S, Jones JM, Steen PA (2007) Pre-injury ASA physical status classification is an independent predictor of mortality after trauma. J Trauma 63:972–978
67. Labib N, Nouh T, Winocour S, Deckelbaum D, Banici L, Fata P, Razek T, Khwaja K (2011) Severely injured geriatric population: morbidity, mortality, and risk factors. J Trauma 71:1908–1914
68. Lee WY, Cameron PA, Bailey MJ (2006) Road traffic injuries in the elderly. Emerg Med J 23:42–46
69. Deakin CD, Sado DM, Coats TJ, Davies G (2004) Prehospital end-tidal carbon dioxide concentration and outcome in major trauma. J Trauma 57:65–68
70. Ley EJ, Clond MA, Srour MK, Barnajian M, Mirocha J, Margulies DR, Salim A (2011) Emergency department crystalloid resuscitation of 1.5 L or more is associated with increased mortality in elderly and nonelderly trauma patients. J Trauma 70:398–400
71. Bridges LC, Waibel BH, Newell MA (2015) Permissive hypotension: potentially harmful in the elderly? A national trauma data bank analysis. Am Surg 81:770–777
72. Fox MT, Persaud M, Maimets I, O'Brien K, Brooks D, Tregunno D, Schraa E (2012) Effectiveness of acute geriatric unit care using acute care for elders components: a systematic review and meta-analysis. J Am Geriatr Soc 60:2237–2245
73. Purdy S, Paranjothy S, Huntley A, Thomas R, Mann M, Huws D, Brindle P, Elwyn G (2012) Interventions to reduce unplanned hospital admission. Bristol University, Bristol
74. Medicine IO (2000) To err is human: building a safer health system. The National Academies Press, Washington
75. Maher RL, Hanlon J, Hajjar ER (2014) Clinical consequences of polypharmacy in elderly. Expert Opin Drug Saf 13:57–65
76. Covinsky KE, King JT Jr, Quinn LM, Siddique R, Palmer R, Kresevic DM, Fortinsky RH, Kowal J, Landefeld CS (1997) Do acute care for elders units increase hospital costs? A cost analysis using the hospital perspective. J Am Geriatr Soc 45:729–734
77. Somme D, Andrieux N, Guerot E, Lahjibi-Paulet H, Lazarovici C, Gisselbrecht M, Fagon JY, Saint-Jean O (2010) Loss of autonomy among elderly patients after a stay in a medical intensive care unit (ICU): a randomized study of the benefit of transfer to a geriatric ward. Arch Gerontol Geriatr 50:e36–e40
78. Barnes DE, Palmer RM, Kresevic DM, Fortinsky RH, Kowal J, Chren MM, Landefeld CS (2012) Acute care for elders units produced shorter hospital stays at lower cost while maintaining patients' functional status. Health Aff (Millwood) 31:1227–1236
79. Counsell SR, Holder CM, Liebenauer LL, Palmer RM, Fortinsky RH, Kresevic DM, Quinn LM, Allen KR, Covinsky KE, Landefeld CS (2000) Effects of a multicomponent intervention on functional outcomes and process of care in hospitalized older patients: a randomized controlled trial of Acute Care for Elders (ACE) in a community hospital. J Am Geriatr Soc 48:1572–1581
80. Brown CJ, Friedkin RJ, Inouye SK (2004) Prevalence and outcomes of low mobility in hospitalized older patients. J Am Geriatr Soc 52:1263–1270
81. Bankart MJ, Baker R, Rashid A, Habiba M, Banerjee J, Hsu R, Conroy S, Agarwal S, Wilson A (2011) Characteristics of general practices associated with emergency admission rates to hospital: a cross-sectional study. Emerg Med J 28:558–563

82. Shepperd S, Doll H, Angus RM, Clarke MJ, Iliffe S, Kalra L, Ricauda NA, Wilson AD (2008) Admission avoidance hospital at home. Cochrane Database Syst Rev Cd007491
83. Shepperd S, Doll H, Angus RM, Clarke MJ, Iliffe S, Kalra L, Ricauda NA, Tibaldi V, Wilson AD (2009) Avoiding hospital admission through provision of hospital care at home: a systematic review and meta-analysis of individual patient data. CMAJ 180:175–182
84. Caplan GA, Sulaiman NS, Mangin DA, Aimonino Ricauda N, Wilson AD, Barclay L (2012) A meta-analysis of "hospital in the home". Med J Aust 197:512–519
85. Mason S, Knowles E, Colwell B, Dixon S, Wardrope J, Gorringe R, Snooks H, Perrin J, Nicholl J (2007) Effectiveness of paramedic practitioners in attending 999 calls from elderly people in the community: cluster randomised controlled trial. BMJ 335:919
86. Vicente V, Svensson L, Wireklint Sundstrom B, Sjostrand F, Castren M (2014) Randomized controlled trial of a prehospital decision system by emergency medical services to ensure optimal treatment for older adults in Sweden. J Am Geriatr Soc 62:1281–1287
87. Logan PA, Coupland CA, Gladman JR, Sahota O, Stoner-Hobbs V, Robertson K, Tomlinson V, Ward M, Sach T, Avery AJ (2010) Community falls prevention for people who call an emergency ambulance after a fall: randomised controlled trial. BMJ 340:c2102

Triage of Older ED Patients

2

Florian F. Grossmann and Christian Nickel

ED triage is the process of quickly sorting patients to determine the priority for further evaluation and care at the time of patient arrival in the emergency department [1]. This definition of ED triage by the ACEP/ENA Five-level Triage Task Force is universally applicable for all ED patients irrespective of their complaint or age. However, adherence to all aspects of this definition often becomes challenging when older ED patients present at the ED front door.

To establish a process that allows triage to be performed quickly is essential. However, this is not always possible in older ED patients. This may be due to sensory or cognitive impairment affecting history taking. Nevertheless, the process of triage needs to be quick and effective, because otherwise patients would have to wait to be triaged, which takes the whole concept ad absurdum (waiting for triage).

Patients with complex conditions particularly benefit from processes that guarantee continuity of care and information and that minimise interruptions. Therefore, traditional concepts of triage processes have to be challenged. However, identifying patients who benefit from immediate interventions by determining priorities according to the acuity of a situation remains one of the core tasks of ED staff in order to increase safety of all ED patients. This is especially true in situations where the demand exceeds the available resources, such as ED crowding.

Correct determination of priorities is especially difficult in older patients. Usually, health histories become more complex with advanced age, and health-care professionals need more time to get an overview on relevant comorbidities,

---

F.F. Grossmann, MSc
Department of Emergency Medicine, University Hospital Basel,
Petersgraben 2, CH-4032 Basel, Switzerland

C. Nickel, MD (✉)
Emergency Department, University Hospital Basel,
Petersgraben 2, CH-4032 Basel, Switzerland
e-mail: christian.nickel@usb.ch

© Springer International Publishing Switzerland 2018
C. Nickel et al. (eds.), *Geriatric Emergency Medicine*,
https://doi.org/10.1007/978-3-319-19318-2_2

medication lists and actual complaints to reach a triage decision. Phenomena like high prevalence of non-specific complaints [2, 3], altered physiological response (vital signs) relating to ageing physiology, comorbidities and medication and higher vulnerability in the case of trauma, but also factors like (unconscious) bias towards older people by health-care professionals might play a role.

Thus, two issues deserve attention in order to warrant accurate and safe triage of older ED patients: First, the triage environment should enable smooth processes and provide adequate resources including a triage tool that is suited for older patients. Second, triage clinicians have to be skilled to address the special care needs of older ED patients and to deal with challenges in triage of this patient group.

2.1 Triage Environment

2.1.1 Design of Processes

It is worth noting that triage ideally begins in the moment when the patient enters the door. Initial relevant information can be gathered by observing the patient approaching the registration desk. Otherwise, if a helpful person places the patient in a wheelchair at the front door, the patient may be sitting in this chair during triage or even during the whole treatment process. In this scenario, valuable information on mobility has to be gathered with much more effort or, more probably, will simply be lost. This however implies that the triage area is located near the front door and, in other words, that the entrance area is staffed with clinicians who are capable of including this information into their decision-making. The next implication is that, consequent to clinicians beginning the process of care at the front door, a personalised health record has to be available from the start. Thus, registration has to be easy and should be limited to the data that are absolutely necessary to unambiguously identify the patient (given name, surname, sex and date of birth). This is also true for situations where identification is necessary for application of life-saving interventions, such as blood transfusion. Information from previous ED visits or prior hospitalisations that include diagnoses or medications may affect triage decisions. Therefore, access to electronic health records might ease triage decision-making in patients with complex conditions such as many older patients. Comprehensive registration can be completed after the triage process by administrative staff.

2.1.2 Triage Tools

Importantly, a triage tool should be used that is suitable to quickly identify older ED patients at risk. On a conceptual level, it is critical that the triage tool is applicable to older patients presenting with non-specific complaints such as weakness or to patients with atypical symptoms, as these presentations are highly prevalent in the older age group [3, 4]. For example, older patients with sepsis or myocardial infarction may present with delirium. A study from the late 1980s showed that confusion (13%) as the chief complaint is almost as prevalent as classic chest pain (19%) in a sample of patients aged 85 or older with myocardial infarction [5]. Therefore, triage tools that rely on predefined (typical) symptoms or diagnoses may not be suitable for this patient group. Further, older ED patients often have multiple comorbidities, polypharmacy and functional and cognitive impairment. To deal with this complexity, a triage tool should, besides providing standardisation that allows reliable analytical decision-making, allow enough flexibility. This means, for example, that routine collection of a past medical history or a detailed reconciliation of current medication is not reasonable due to time constraints at triage, but rather focusing on recent history and relevant medication. In this context, a triage tool should allow clinicians to make so-called type 1 decisions, which come from intuition and experience, because they are fast and usually effective. However, they are prone to bias [6]. Vital signs should not play an overly dominant role in triage, as abnormal initial vital signs have been shown to be a poor predictor for severe illness in older persons [7]. However, if they are abnormal, they should be considered as a warning sign [8].

The Manchester Triage System (MTS) [9] is a five-level triage tool which consists of 50 flow charts, each representing a chief complaint. Every flow chart depicts six general discriminators. However, as the MTS is based on symptoms and diagnoses, its usefulness in older ED patients might be questionable. As an example, no flow chart exists for patients presenting with weakness. Studies that investigated the performance of the MTS in older ED patients do not exist to date, and therefore it should be used with caution [10].

A triage tool of which performance criteria are well investigated, also in older ED patients [11, 12], is the Emergency Severity Index (ESI), originally developed in the USA, but spreading more and more all over the world, including Europe [13]. Because the authors believe that the ESI is well suited for triage of older persons, this tool is described in more detail. The ESI is a five-level triage tool that consists of one single algorithm with four decision points (A–D). At decision point A, patients who are in need of an immediate life-saving intervention are identified. Examples are patients with cardiac arrest, unconsciousness, or severe dyspnoea requiring breathing support. These patients are assigned ESI level 1; all other patients are evaluated at decision point B if they should not wait. Situations that require immediate treatment can be high-risk situations (such as chest pain, dyspnoea, but also suicidal patients), patients with new onset of confusion, disorientation and lethargy or patients with severe pain or distress. Patients who do not meet one of these criteria are further evaluated at decision point C. Here, the anticipated number of resources (briefly, all interventions that are beyond a physical examination and history taking) is used as a proxy for complexity. The more resources, the more complex is the underlying condition and the higher the acuity. Patients requiring no resources are assigned ESI level 5; one resource ESI level 4 and all other patients are further evaluated. At decision point D, the patient's vital signs are assessed. If heart rate, respiratory rate and oxygen saturation are out of predefined limits, the triage clinician has to consider "upgrading" the patient to ESI level 2. For the ESI, reliability and validity for older ED patients were shown. However, performance was not as good as for younger patients [12].

The ESI has several features that make it superior to other triage tools with respect to older ED patients. First, patients with confusion, disorientation and lethargy are assigned ESI level 2. These patients often have delirium. By including "lethargy" into this decision point, it is even possible to identify patients with hypoactive delirium. Second, because triage decision-making happens at a more conceptual level instead of using distinct symptoms, the ESI can be easily applied to patients with non-specific presentations. At decision point B, intuition can be used to identify patients with high-risk situations. This is helpful especially in complex patient situations. Third, the ESI does not rely solely on vital signs, but vitals are used as a "safety feature" for patients with complex conditions at decision point D.

2.2 Essential Triage Skills and Knowledge

To date, it is not well understood whether experience or factual knowledge is more important in triage decision-making, as the evidence is scarce. But it is a common sense that triage clinicians should possess both. The Emergency Nurses Association [14] recommends triage staff to be registered nurses with additional education in emergency nursing. Additionally, triage clinicians should have passed a comprehensive triage training focusing on the accurate use of the triage tool. However, it is unclear how triage competency is assessed reliably [15]. We do know that several issues make triage (and care) of older ED patients more challenging.

Only identifying a chief complaint often is the first challenge in older patients. Even identifying patient in life-threatening condition may be difficult [16]. Multimorbidity and chronic illness may render acute conditions less obvious.

Second, vital signs as an indicator of physiological responses to illness or trauma have to be interpreted with caution in older ED patients. Due to physiological changes in advanced age, and due to complicated polypharmacy, vital signs can be misleading in triage of older patients. This was shown in several studies in (preclinical) trauma triage [17, 18]. Also in the clinical setting, vital signs at triage lack predictive ability to detect severe illness or injury [7]. This affects primarily blood pressure and heart rate. Therefore, triage staff should attach special importance to the patient's respiratory rate [8]. Even if respiratory rate cannot currently be measured with electronic devices at triage, it is predictive for illness severity and patient outcomes in multiple conditions [19–21]. However, even respiratory rate may be affected by medications such as opioids which make even this vital sign to be interpreted with caution.

A third issue relates to cognitive impairment. Because delirium is a highly prevalent condition that may indicate severe illness, it should result in a high priority at triage. However, delirium detection is a challenge. A key feature that can be used as a triage criterion for probable delirium is acute onset of mental status changes or disorientation. In the case of hypoactive delirium, which is often missed by ED clinicians, lethargy or impaired level of consciousness may be present. At triage, these conditions need special attention.

Fourth, functional decline makes triage of older patients challenging, as older patients are not always able to move as quickly as desired by the triage staff. However, by observing gait speed/walking abilities, important information can be captured without the need for additional tests. This information, captured with a simple four-item scale, was shown to be a good predictor of severe illness predictive for patient outcomes in an acute care setting [22]. Thus, the patient's mobility at triage should influence not only triage decision-making but can also guide the team which patients need special attention, e.g. geriatric assessments. Capturing this information early in the ED treatment course is essential for discharge planning. If a risk for dependency is identified early at triage, nurses may approach primary care providers and family members early to secure the patient's safety after discharge. Otherwise, this may result in unsafe discharge or unnecessary hospitalisation.

Lastly, triage clinicians must be aware of the vulnerability of the older ED population, which becomes obvious in a greater risk for undertriage compared to younger patients. In our study, undertriage rates remained stable, even after efforts to reduce it [23]. Reasons for this phenomenon are probably multifactorial, and its occurrence seems to be unrelated to the triage tool used, as undertriage is also a pattern in the MTS [10]. Because reasons can be considered to be multifactorial, the importance of adherence to the triage tool should be emphasised.

Older patients are often accompanied by family members or other close persons. These persons should be integrated into the triage process for several reasons. First and foremost, they can often give relevant information about the patient's condition especially if the patient's mental status or ability to communicate is impaired. Others can also help patients to orient themselves in a busy ED, which reduces the risk of anxiety or delirium. Finally, family members can help patients to address their needs and to complete the registration and can assist in discharge planning.

To improve patient flow and to improve triage performance for triage of older ED patients, clinicians might consider the following hands-on recommendations:

- Have wheelchairs available if necessary, but observe gait and assist patients in taking off their coat before placing them in a chair.
- Do not lay patients on stretchers at triage if they can sit or stand.
- Pain management should be started already at triage, especially in older persons as pain is a major risk factor for delirium.
- Assess respiratory rate.
- Talk to the patient and give orientation.

In summary, triage professionals need to combine profound history taking, observation, clinical assessment and communication skills with adherence to the triage tool used. Clinical reasoning is essential to combine history, observation and clinical assessment in order to focus quickly on relevant conditions even in highly complex situations.

References

1. Fernandes CM et al (2005) Five-level triage: a report from the ACEP/ENA five-level triage task force. J Emerg Nurs 31(1):39–50
2. Safwenberg U, Terent A, Lind L (2007) The emergency department presenting complaint as predictor of in-hospital fatality. Eur J Emerg Med 14(6):324–331
3. Bhalla MC et al (2014) Weakness and fatigue in older ED patients in the United States. Am J Emerg Med 32(11):1395–1398
4. Bingisser R, Nickel CH (2013) The last century of symptom-oriented research in emergency presentations - have we made any progress? Swiss Med Wkly 143:w13829
5. Day JJ et al (1987) Acute myocardial infarction: diagnostic difficulties and outcome in advanced old age. Age Ageing 16(4):239–243
6. Croskerry P, Singhal G, Mamede S (2013) Cognitive debiasing 1: origins of bias and theory of debiasing. BMJ Qual Saf 22(Suppl 2):ii58–ii64
7. Lamantia MA et al (2013) Predictive value of initial triage vital signs for critically ill older adults. West J Emerg Med 14(5):453–460
8. Buist M et al (2004) Association between clinically abnormal observations and subsequent in-hospital mortality: a prospective study. Resuscitation 62(2):137–141
9. Manchester Triage Group, et al (eds) (2006) Emergency triage, 2nd edn. Blackwell Publishing Ltd
10. Parenti N et al (2014) A systematic review on the validity and reliability of an emergency department triage scale, the Manchester triage system. Int J Nurs Stud 51(7):1062–1069
11. Baumann MR, Strout TD (2007) Triage of geriatric patients in the emergency department: validity and survival with the emergency severity index. Ann Emerg Med 49(2):234–240
12. Grossmann FF et al (2012) At risk of undertriage? Testing the performance and accuracy of the emergency severity index in elderly ED patients. Ann Emerg Med 60(3):317–325
13. Grossmann FF et al (2011) Transporting clinical tools to new settings: cultural adaptation and validation of the emergency severity index in german. Ann Emerg Med 57(3):257–264
14. Emergency Nurses Association (2011) Triage qualifications - position statement. Available from: https://www.ena.org/SiteCollectionDocuments/Position%20Statements/TriageQualifications.pdf
15. Jordi K et al (2015) Nurses' accuracy and self-perceived ability using the emergency severity index triage tool: a cross-sectional study in four Swiss hospitals. Scand J Trauma Resusc Emerg Med 23(1):62
16. Platts-Mills TF et al (2010) Accuracy of the emergency severity index triage instrument for identifying elder emergency department patients receiving an immediate life-saving intervention. Acad Emerg Med 17(3):238–243
17. Phillips S et al (1996) The failure of triage criteria to identify geriatric patients with trauma: results from the Florida trauma triage study. J Trauma 40(2):278–283
18. Lehmann R et al (2009) The impact of advanced age on trauma triage decisions and outcomes: a statewide analysis. Am J Surg 197(5):571–574. discussion 574-5
19. Subbe CP et al (2003) Effect of introducing the modified early warning score on clinical outcomes, cardio-pulmonary arrests and intensive care utilisation in acute medical admissions. Anaesthesia 58(8):797–802
20. Fine MJ et al (1997) A prediction rule to identify low-risk patients with community-acquired pneumonia. N Engl J Med 336(4):243–250
21. Egermayer P et al (1998) Usefulness of D-dimer, blood gas, and respiratory rate measurements for excluding pulmonary embolism. Thorax 53(10):830–834
22. Kellett J et al (2014) A four item scale based on gait for the immediate global assessment of acutely ill medical patients – one look is more than 1000 words. Eur Geriatr Med 5(2):92–96
23. Grossmann FF et al (2014) Undertriage in older emergency department patients--tilting against windmills? PLoS One 9(8):e106203

Primary Assessment and Stabilization of Life-Threatening Conditions in Older Patients

3

Mehmet Akif Karamercan, Abdelouahab Bellou, and Hubert Blain

3.1 Introduction

Life-threatening conditions are defined as an acute disease or chronic illness expected to cause death in the immediate or near future without ongoing and life-supporting healthcare treatment directly provided by a healthcare professional [1], the technique of advanced cardiovascular life support is not specifically different for older patients, and the primary assessment and stabilization should follow the European and international resuscitation guidelines [2]. However, specific consideration to physiologic reserve of older patients coping with life-threatening condition in this specific population mainly depends on underlying chronic conditions [3].

If a patient has a life-threatening condition, the assessment and treatment should start immediately, and in this situation, the diagnostic procedures should go simultaneously with the treatment modalities unless there is a clear Do Not Attempt Resuscitation (DNAR) document. This situation is frequently encountered in pre-hospital settings. Except in this specific situation, the resuscitation must start immediately with a simultaneous call to the emergency medical services (EMS) dispatching center asking for help.

In older patients, chronic diseases and medication effects superimpose on age-related physiologic changes and may conceal a critical illness. Compared with the

---

M.A. Karamercan (✉)
Gazi University School of Medicine Emergency Medicine Department, Ankara, Turkey
e-mail: makaramercan@gazi.edu.tr

A. Bellou, MD, PhD
Department of Emergency Medicine, Beth Israel Deaconess Medical Center,
Harvard Medical School, Boston, MA, USA
e-mail: abellou@bidmc.harvard.edu

H. Blain
Department of Geriatrics, University Hospital of Montpellier, University of Montpellier,
Montpellier, France
e-mail: h-blain@chu-montpellier.fr

general population, older patients are more acutely ill, more frequently admitted to the hospital (especially to the intensive care units), and more likely to suffer a cardiac arrest [2]. Emergency physicians (EPs) or nonmedical professionals are frequently confronted with the question whether resuscitation is an appropriate treatment for older people. For physicians, patients, and relatives, it is important to know the chance of survival and the functional outcome after resuscitation in order to make an informed decision.

This chapter outlines the main characteristics of primary assessment and stabilization of the life-threatening conditions, including common pitfalls and priorities in older patients with special challenges to facilitate the emergency care of the critically ill older patient.

3.2 General Approach

Aging is an inevitable and extremely complex, multifactorial process, which is characterized by the progressive degeneration of organ systems and tissues. It is largely determined by genetics, and influenced by a wide range of environmental factors, such as diet, exercise, and exposure to microorganisms and pollutants [4]. The physiological changes of various organ systems in older patients (Table 3.1) affect their functional ability and must be taken into account in the primary assessment and management of these patients which is extremely important in case of life-threatening conditions [5]. In old people, dementia is frequently seen and can wherret the assessment of the mental status. If possible, family members and caregivers will help to determine change in comparison to baseline status.

The airway, breathing, circulation (ABC) approach in the primary survey is a systematic approach used in immediate assessment and lifesaving management of critically ill or injured patients and should be applied in critical emergencies whatever the age [6]. However, due to changes of the cardiorespiratory system, older

Table 3.1 Structural and physiologic changes in older adults regarding ABCs

Airway changes (A)	*Respiratory changes (B)*
• ↑ cervical and temporomandibular joint rigidity	• ↓ in number of alveoli, lung capillaries, and parenchymal elastic fibers
• ↑ dental loss, dental protrusion, and irregular dentition	• ↓ cough and mucociliary clearance
• ↓ thyromental distance and submandibular compliance	• ↓ in forced expiratory volume and forced vital capacity
• ↑ prevalence of macroglossia and microstomia	• ↑ residual volume
	• ↓ ventilatory response to hypoxemia and hypercarbia
	• ↑ stiffness of the chest wall
Cardiovascular (C) changes	*Neurological changes*
• ↑ thickness of left ventricular wall	• ↓ weight and cerebral blood flow of the brain
• ↓ in maximal heart rate, cardiac output, and cardiac index	• ↓ in number and functioning nerve cells
• ↓ of pacemaker cells	• ↓ in motor nerve blood flow
• ↑ in dilatation, elasticity, and rigidity of arterial walls	• ↓ in vibratory and thermal sensation, sensory perception
	• ↓ autonomic nervous system responsiveness

persons have increased risk of developing respiratory and cardiac failure and should be taken into account (Table 3.1). Indeed, these changes explain that older patients may have less likely obvious signs and symptoms of life-threatening injuries, which can make the airway management difficult. Older patients may require more aggressive, goal-directed, and prompt therapy, often associated with a worse prognosis [5, 7, 8].

3.3 Primary Assessment of Life-Threatening Emergencies

The primary evaluation is designed to detect and manage all life-threatening injuries or illness and determines the patient's triage priority. The initial assessment follows the sequence of patient response/mental status, airway, breathing, and circulation.

The goals of the primary assessment for critically ill patients are to rapidly and systematically identify life threats and provide simultaneous treatment of all life threats identified.

3.3.1 Patient Response/Mental Status Assessment

The initial observation will help to decide whether the patient's condition is stable or unstable, based on the level of distress and mental status. Initially, the patient responsiveness is determined using the AVPU scale (which is used in many early-warning scores in the general ward setting) [9]:

A—Alert. The patient is awake, oriented, responsive, and able to communicate.
V—Verbal. The patient appears to be unresponsive initially, but will respond to a loud verbal stimulus (patient may speak, grunt, groan, or simply look at you).
P—Painful. The patient does not respond to verbal stimuli and may respond to painful stimuli such as compressing the fingernail bed or pinching the web between the thumb and index finger or a sternal rub.
U—Unresponsive. The patient doesn't show any kind of response to both verbal and painful stimuli.

At this point, more accurate and detailed scores such as Glasgow Coma Scale (GCS) and/or Richmond Agitation Sedation Scale (RASS) could also be use to determine mental status of the patients [9]. But for easiness to remember and simplicity, AVPU scale would be enough.

If the patient is unresponsive to painful stimuli or does not exhibit signs of life, it should be assumed he/she is in cardiac arrest until proven otherwise, and medical professionals should check carotid pulse for less than 10 s while simultaneously observing respiratory effort. If at the end of the 10 s, it is not certain that the patient has a pulse, cardiopulmonary resuscitation in line with Advanced Cardiac Life Support guidelines must be started [10].

If the patient exhibits signs of life but has an abnormal RASS, the process of assessment should proceed with identification of causes involved in the life-threatening situation. Examples of situations might be central nervous system infections, stroke, drug overdose (especially sedative-hypnotics), or alcohol/drug abuse. In these cases, a brief past history and history of the illness should be taken as soon as possible including previous medications, chronic illness (related to cardiovascular and neurologic system), and acuteness of the hemodynamic compromise. At this point, patients should generally be managed according to the worst clinical scenario and should be overlooked carefully. More importantly, the physician should be aware that the clock is working against him/her [11, 12]. In general, all vital signs should be taken promptly and monitored continuously. Curable causes of the altered mental status (such as hypoglycemia, intoxication, hypercapnia, carbon monoxide intoxication, etc.) should be taken into consideration and managed promptly [11].

After the assessment of the patient's mental status, the critical situation is frequently complex, and the systematic approach helps breaking down issues into manageable parts as described below.

3.3.2 Airway Assessment and Management (A)

3.3.2.1 Airway Assessment

There are significant physiologic, structural, and functional changes induced by aging (see Table 3.1), such as decreased pulmonary reserves, cardiac index, an edentulous mouth, and decreased neck range of motion that may make the airway management difficult [13, 14].

It is important to distinguish between changes due to the physiology of aging and pathologic changes brought on by chronic disease. Despite the contributory role played by the physiologic factors given in Table 3.1, data suggest that comorbid conditions and frailty play the most important role in determining patient outcome after respiratory failure in older patients [14]. For example, a vigorous 80-year-old patient who exercises daily has far more physiologic reserve and will tolerate the stress of acute illness far better than another old patient with cerebrovascular or cardiovascular disease. Chronic illness (such as chronic obstructive lung disease, diabetes mellitus, heart failure, renal failure, etc.) and disability are more common in older patients. These chronic conditions often exhaust the patient's limited cardiopulmonary reserve, leading to respiratory distress or failure and the need for intubation [15]. Such patients may not tolerate the greater work of breathing, leading to respiratory failure much earlier than in their healthier or younger counterparts. In addition, acquired illnesses, such as community- or hospital-acquired pneumonia or urinary tract infection, can progress to sepsis and rapidly deplete physiologic reserves in susceptible older patients.

The ability to speak is generally accepted as the single most important indicator of airway patency. If the patient is able to communicate verbally, the airway is likely to be compromised. However, repeated assessment of airway patency is recommended.

When the patient is unable to communicate verbally, the possible causes must be immediately determined, and assume that there is a potential serious airway

Table 3.2 Some conditions that can lead to progressive airway compromise

Foreign body
- Food particles and aspiration
- Dentures and dental fillings
- Pills and caustic medications

Infection
- Bacterial tracheitis
- Diphtheria
- Epiglottis
- Ludwig's angina
- Laryngotracheitis
- Retropharyngeal abscess
- Tetanus

Immune
- Angioedema
- Anaphylaxis

Trauma
- Neck hematoma (e.g., trauma, bleeding diathesis, anticoagulants)
- Laryngeal fracture
- Burns
- Postoperative complications

Tumor
- Laryngeal
- Tracheobronchial
- Mediastinal

Poisoning and toxic exposures
- Caustic ingestion
- Smoke inhalation
- Carbon monoxide poisoning
- Strychnine poisoning
- Ingestion of poisonous plants

Laryngospasm
- Drug induced (e.g., acute dystonic reactions, ketamine, etc.)
- Physical or chemical stimuli

Other
- Altered level of consciousness
- Cranial nerve palsies
- Hysterical stridor
- Paralysis
- Myoedema

compromise till rule out. In addition, if there is an altered level of consciousness with airway severely compromised, an endotracheal intubation must be decided to maintain and secure the airway patency, especially in cases of trauma and poisoning [16, 17]. The finding of non-purposeful motor responses and patient with history of stroke strongly suggests the need for definitive airway management. Although every speechless patient cannot be accepted as having a compromised airway, the patency of airway should be questioned immediately. On the other hand, equally important is the necessity to recognize the potential for progressive airway loss and deterioration. In these instances, frequent reevaluation of airway patency is essential to identify and treat patients who are losing the ability to maintain an adequate airway.

Airway obstruction can be complete or incomplete (partial) (see Table 3.2). Signs of a partial airway obstruction are correlated with the level and degree of obstruction, including change in voice, high-pitched breathing noises (e.g., stridor), gasping for air, difficulty in breathing, and even agitation or reduced consciousness. With a completely obstructed airway, the patient cannot talk, cough, or breathe. Apnea and paradoxical respirations (no respiration despite great effort) may be noted. Cyanosis should not be used as a feature in identifying the obstructed airway because it is a very late preterminal sign.

The following signs on rapid physical examination may help to identify the obstructed airway:

Look—Look externally for cyanosis, retractions, use of accessory muscles of respiration, and swelling of the tongue, lips, or neck. Look inside the mouth for foreign bodies, dental appliance, loose teeth, food, vomitus, or secretions.

Listen—Listen to abnormal breath sounds with naked ear (gurgling, snoring, stridor, crackles) and stethoscope. Stridor is a high-pitched sound usually heard on inspiration that suggests high-grade upper airway obstruction, which is almost always an emergency. Asymmetrical breath sounds together with tachypnea suggests inadequate airway.

Feel—Feel the neck for tracheal deviation, swelling or masses—can be a sign of tracheolaryngeal injury, and feel the upper chest for crepitus (subcutaneous emphysema)—can be a sign of pneumothorax.

If there is any or combination of the above signs present, the patient should be presumed to have a partial or complete airway obstruction and needed to have immediate management. Even if there is no sign, critical patients (e.g., burns, history of smoke inhalation, angioedema), those that may rapidly progress to compromised airway, should be identified and intubated in a timely manner before the patient loses their airway patency.

3.3.2.2 Airway Management

Although an untreated airway obstruction leads to cardiac arrest rapidly, not every patient with compromised airway or breathing requires intubation. Many patients with hypoxia and/or respiratory problems can be managed conservatively (positioning or nasopharyngeal airway placement) and can be stabilized with supplemental oxygen or respiratory therapies. Simple maneuvers (head-tilt/chin-lift or jaw-thrust) in a compromised patient may help to improve the patency of the airway, and all EM providers should be trained to do them (Fig. 3.1). The oropharyngeal and nasopharyngeal airways are simple adjuncts and relieve backward displacement of the tongue. The airways must be suctioned with proper equipment as soon as possible. If the patient becomes unconscious, cardiopulmonary resuscitation must be started immediately according to guidelines [10].

The following are the main indications for tracheal intubation but not limited to:

- Persistant apnea
- High-grade airway obstruction of any etiology
- Suspected imminent airway obstruction of any etiology
- Absence of airway protective reflexes
- Severe hypoxia and/or hypercarbia refractory to less invasive treatment
- Coma with a risk of increased intracranial pressure
- Cardiopulmonary arrest

The next critical aspect of airway management is recognizing a potentially difficult airway and planning management strategies accordingly. A methodological stepwise plan should be made to assess difficult intubation. BONES and LEMON mnemonic can be used to remember the signs of a potential difficult airway [18, 19]:

Fig. 3.1 (**a**) Head-tilt-chin-lift maneuver. (**b**) Jaw-thrust maneuver

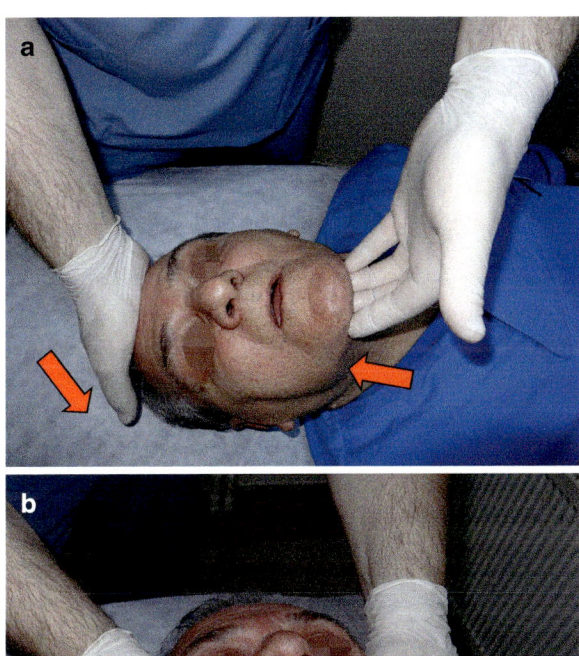

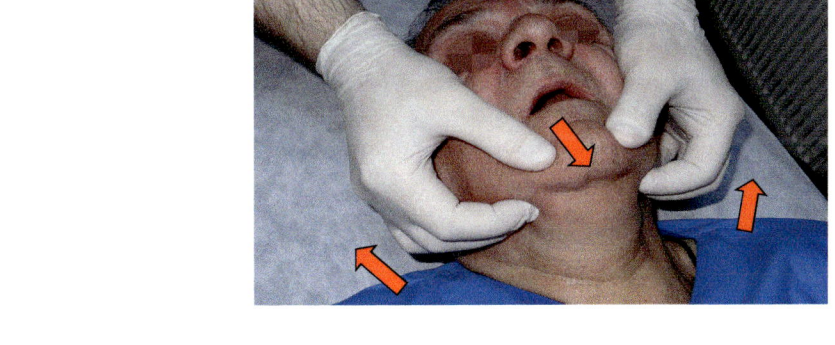

BONES mnemonic for assessment of difficult mask ventilation (if ≥2 following parameters present):

B for beard, O for obesity (body mass index more than 26 kg/m^2), N for no teeth, E for older patient (over 65 years old), S for sleep apnea/snorer.

LEMON mnemonic for assessment of difficult intubation [18];

Look: Externally look for characteristics that are known to cause difficult intubation or ventilation: facial or neck trauma/swelling, facial dysmporphism (particularly micrognathia), and dental abnormalities, short or thick neck.

Evaluate 3/3/2 rule: Refers to the normal facial and neck anatomy in terms of the patient's finger breadths—if the distance between the patient's incisor teeth is less than three-finger breadths, the distance between the hyoid bone and the chin is less than three-finger breadths; the distance between hyoid bone and thyroid notch is less than two-finger breadths which suggest difficult intubation.

Mallampati score: The hypopharynx should be visualized adequately. This is a great tool for cooperative patients in the preoperative setting, but is less useful for critically ill patients in the ED or in a prehospital setting. The patient sits up straight, opens mouth widely, and protrudes the tongue. The score is mainly based on visibility of the uvula, posterior pharynx, and hard and soft palate.

Obstruction: The possible conditions leading to airway obstruction should be assessed as stated above.

Neck mobility: Assess range of motion of the neck after a deep C-spine assessment to detect any injury with a risk of spine damage, as placing the patient's chin down onto his chest and extend his neck. Poor neck mobility can make limitations for positioning of intubation.

For patients with difficult airways, it is essential to expect that standard intubation will fail and to prepare backup plans including surgical cricothyrotomy.

Patients with difficult airways should never receive sedative or paralytic agents until all necessary equipment and personnel required to implement backup plans for a failed airway are present and available.

Both bag-mask ventilation and intubation are more likely to be difficult in older patients, and edentulous patients are harder to ventilate with a bag-valve mask [20]. The loss of upper airway, muscle tone, and loose lips unsupported by teeth make mask seal and maintenance of a patent airway more difficult [21]. A stiffer chest wall also increases the difficulty of ventilation with a bag-valve mask or a rescue airway (e.g., laryngeal mask airway). Baseline oxygen saturation is often low in older patients, and adequate preoxygenation may be difficult or impossible. In addition, older patients desaturate more rapidly than healthy, younger patients [2]. Thus, the safe apnea period is decreased despite best attempts at preoxygenation compared with routine intubations in younger, healthy adults [22]. Older patients are more susceptible to hypoxic insults. Even brief periods of oxygen desaturation can result in permanent cardiac and neurologic damage in older patients. Whenever possible, the emergency physician should maintain the oxyhemoglobin saturation at or above 90% in patients without chronic obstructive lung disease, even if this requires aborting an attempt at laryngoscopy in order to oxygenate by bag and mask or with an extraglottic device. When difficult airway assessment indicates that the patient is unlikely to be successfully intubated by direct laryngoscopy, an awake approach to intubation is recommended. Video laryngoscopes improve the rate of successful laryngoscopy and so may permit rapid sequence intubation in patients for whom direct laryngoscopy with a conventional laryngoscope is not likely to provide an adequate glottic view. These new devices may significantly improve the management of difficult intubation in older patients [23–25].

Despite the higher incidence of difficult airways in older patients, most are appropriate candidates for rapid sequence intubation (RSI). When performing RSI, drug selection and drug dosing are of great importance. The medications used for

RSI cause more pronounced hypopnea and hypotension in older patients than in younger, healthy patients [26–28]. Therefore, it is generally best to reduce the doses of short-acting opioids (e.g., fentanyl) used for pretreatment and induction agents by approximately 30–50% to a dose of 1–1.5 μg/kg because older patients are more susceptible to adverse effects from both hypotension and respiratory depression [26, 27]. Pretreatment doses of non-depolarizing neuromuscular blockers (typically one-tenth the full paralytic dose) are of no proven benefit, can sometimes cause complete paralysis (and apnea) in older patients, and therefore are not recommended. Short-acting opioids (e.g., fentanyl) may be given to older patients at risk from the hypertension caused by the sympathetic response stimulated by laryngoscopy and intubation. However, careful assessment of the risks and benefits is important because of the increased sensitivity of older patients to the hypoventilatory effects of opioids [2]. Examples of patients who may benefit from opioids include those with cardiovascular disease or cerebral vascular disease with hypertension or intracranial hemorrhage. Etomidate might be the preferred induction agent for older patients undergoing RSI which maintains hemodynamic stability and has a rapid and reliable onset of action and a short duration of effect [29].

Special considerations for older patients:

- Foreign body aspiration in older patients is more common than in younger patients since risk factors including the use of sedatives, abnormal mental status, stroke, Parkinson's syndromes, and polypharmacy are the main risk factors of choking [30]. Clinical diagnosis of foreign body aspiration in older patients requires a high degree of suspicion, which is critical for timely diagnosis and prevention of serious complications including death [31].
- Less dentition can interfere with achieving a proper seal of the face mask. Well-fitting intact dentures should be left in place to help better seal of the face mask (Table 3.1).
- Due to these numerous anatomic changes in older patients, the emergency physician often must use alternative strategies and techniques in securing airway. In critically ill older patients, intubation and mechanical ventilation often become necessary, and it should not be withheld because of the patient's age. If intubation is necessary, it is important to be wary of anatomical features in older people, and preoxygenation becomes an even more critical component in older patients due to their low physiologic respiratory reserves [32].
- Care must be taken when placing nasogastric and nasotracheal tubes because nasopharyngeal friability, especially around the turbinates, is a risk factor of profound bleeding [33].
- The oral cavity may be compromised by either macroglossia, associated with amyloidosis or acromegaly, or microstomia, such as the constricted, birdlike mouth of progressive systemic sclerosis (Table 3.1) [34].
- Arthritis of the temporomandibular joints and the cervical spine, commonly seen in older patients, might result in difficult endotracheal intubation. It should not be forgotten that manipulation of the osteoarthritic spine increases the risk of spinal cord injury [34].

3.3.3 Breathing Assessment and Management (B)

3.3.3.1 Breathing Assessment

Once the patient's airway is opened, the adequacy of ventilation and oxygenation should be evaluated. The first and most important step in the assessment of breathing is to determine if the patient is apneic or not. The apneic patient's ventilation should be assisted immediately to prevent any further life-threatening deterioration due to hypoxia and hypercapnia.

If the patient is breathing, adequacy and sufficiency of the respiration should be assessed. Normal breathing is characterized as almost imperceptible rise and fall of the abdomen and chest wall, and the accessory muscles of breathing should not be used. To identify respiratory failure, the EM providers should specifically evaluate the patient's general appearance for respiratory distress such as pale, cool, or cyanotic skin, diaphoresis, retractions, and nasal flaring or sitting up in a "tripod position" (patient sits upright to breathe or lean forward) [35]. Patient's breathing should be assessed for tachypnea, tachycardia, stridor, and use of the accessory respiratory muscles (especially sternocleidomastoid, sternoclavicular, pectoralis, and intercostal). Other signs and symptoms of approaching respiratory failure are hypoxia-induced agitation or lethargy, breathlessness-induced speechless, hypercapnia-induced depressed consciousness, and paradoxical abdominal wall movements (abdominal wall retracts inward with inspiration, indicating diaphragmatic fatigue).

For determination of the adequacy of the respiration, respiratory rate, SaO2, and the quality of breathing sounds should also be evaluated. Arterial blood pressure, heart rate, and mental status must also be monitored continuously. The normal rate of breathing is about 12–20 breaths/min for an adult and the rhythm should be regular. Rapid or slow and deep or shallow breathing indicates respiratory distress. Auscultation should be done over all quadrants of the anterior and posterior thorax moving side to side. Unilateral absence of sounds may indicate a tension pneumothorax or hemothorax, which needs immediate drainage. Breathing sounds may also provide additional clues in differential diagnosis of cardiac or pulmonary ethiology [35]. Sometimes breathing sounds might be difficult to evaluate especially in noisy or distracting environments.

The goal of respiratory assessment for a critical patient is to determine whether the patient has respiratory distress or failure. Patients with respiratory distress are trying to compensate for an underlying pathology by increasing their effort of respiration. If they cannot overcome, they start to get tired together with increased metabolic rate. Increased metabolic rate results in more hypercapnia and hypoxia, which starts viscous cycle, and respiratory failure can evolve over minutes. These patients are exhausted and no longer able to compensate for their underlying pathology.

3.3.3.2 Management of Respiratory Emergencies

Apnea and Irregular Respirations

If the patient is apneic or the respiration is inadequate, the ventilation should be assisted immediately. Bag-valve-mask device (BVMD) is the most common mechanical aid used in emergency care to initially administer positive-pressure

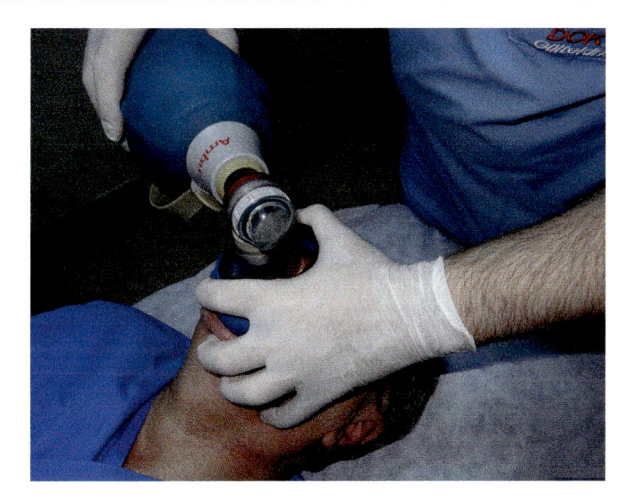

Fig. 3.2 "C/E" technique

ventilation [36]. BVMD should not be used in spontaneously breathing patient, which can result in worsening of the hypoxia. While administering positive-pressure ventilation, the patient should be closely monitored for chest rise because delivery of low tidal volumes is a common complication when the mask is inadequately sealed to the patient's face. If the patient's chest does not rise and/or the abdomen is rising, repositioning of your hands, ensuring properly, applying "C/E" technique (Fig. 3.2), and taking the patient in "sniffing position" (35° neck flexion and 15° head extension) will usually overcome this situation [37]. If the chest still does not rise, airway obstruction must be excluded. Always consider the use of oropharyngeal or nasopharyngeal airways to help keeping the airway open. Ultimately, intubation can be decided if indicated, but in the initial phase of resuscitation, BVMD is enough for the vast majority of patients.

Respiratory Distress

Every patient with respiratory distress should receive oxygen therapy. The choice of delivery devices depends on the patient's oxygen requirement and patient acceptance. The first-line options are "nasal cannula" and "venturi mask" those which can deliver an inspiratory oxygen fraction (FI O_2) of 24–40% and mostly appropriate for mild and moderate level of respiratory distressed patients. The second-line options for oxygen delivery are "simple face mask" and "Nonrebreathing Face Mask with Reservoir and One-Way Valve" which can deliver FI O_2 of 40–60% and FI O_2 of up to 90% and appropriate for severe respiratory-distressed patients [38].

Oxygen therapy is initially appropriate for every patient with respiratory distress. However, prolonged and high concentration use of oxygen can be detrimental (due to oxygen toxicity) and should be titrated to the lowest flow rate appropriate for the patient [39].

Noninvasive positive-pressure ventilation (NIPPV) is a helpful treatment for some common causes of respiratory distress commonly found in older patients, including asthma, chronic obstructive pulmonary disease (COPD), acute congestive heart failure (without myocardial infarction), and pulmonary edema [40, 41]. NIPPV increases alveolar ventilation without significant modifications in the alveolar ventilation/perfusion mismatching, reduces work of breathing, and redistributes fluid from alveoli back into the vasculature. In patients with COPD and pulmonary edema, NIPPV has been shown to significantly decrease both the need for intubation and overall patient mortality and to generate significant improvements in pH, pCO2, and respiratory rate [42]. NIPPV is absolutely contraindicated in patients with impaired mental status and cardiovascular instability (e.g., arrhythmias, myocardial infarction) frequently encountered in older patients. The use of NIPPV as a first-line supportive therapy for acute respiratory failure (ARF) is increasing [43]. In patients aged 65 years or more, complications during mechanical ventilation increase hospital mortality [44]. This suggests that avoiding invasive procedures might be particularly helpful in decreasing mortality in older patients. Increasing longevity in many populations makes it common to find older patients (most often on long-term oxygen therapy) with severe ARF presenting to the emergency department (ED) [45].

"Do Not Intubate" cannot be considered as an indication for NIPPV; however, the use of NIPPV as a palliative measure is increasing. In a recent study, Nava et al. showed that patients with hypercapnic respiratory failure had better outcomes when treated with NIPPV in ICU [46]. The success of NIPPV is inversely related to the number and the severity of comorbidities and level of consciousness and directly related to the early resolution of the respiratory distress.

A randomized, controlled study showed that the use of NIPPV to treat acute respiratory failure (ARF) in older patients reduces the need for intubation, improves survival, and induces a faster resolution of respiratory distress compared with standard medical therapy (SMT). Rescue therapy with NIPPV has been very successful (75%) [46]. NIPPV improves the survival rate, but also reduces tachypnea and dyspnea, the major symptoms of respiratory distress. A recent Italian study involving individuals aged 80 years and older who underwent NIPPV in a pneumogeriatric unit showed that NIPPV is effective and safe in very old hospitalized adults in a non-ICU setting followed by multidisciplinary medical staff; in particular, NIPPV is well tolerated when concomitant dementia is present [47]. NIPPV not only treats the cardiorespiratory problem but also decreases the risk of delirium and malnutrition [48, 49]. Segrelles Calvo et al. provided an important assessment of the effectiveness of NIPPV in older patients, but showed some limiting factors: severe comorbidities and frequent readmission [50].

There is a broad differential diagnosis for respiratory distress, including pulmonary, cardiac, neurologic, and metabolic conditions, and other treatments apart from oxygen therapy depend on the etiology and disease specific. Clues to the underlying cause of respiratory distress can be obtained through history, physical examination, and ancillary tests like chest imaging and laboratory studies.

Respiratory Failure

Patients in respiratory failure are no longer able to compensate for their underlying disease process and require respiratory support. Hypoxemia is the most important

3 Primary Assessment and Stabilization

and immediate expression of acute respiratory failure. The specific treatment depends on the etiology of respiratory failure. In some cases, ventilator support can be accomplished with NIPPV, but usually intubation and mechanical ventilation will be required. General and initial approach to respiratory failure is summarized in Fig. 3.3.

Some of the important causes of respiratory failure are summarized in Table 3.3. *Special considerations for older patients*:

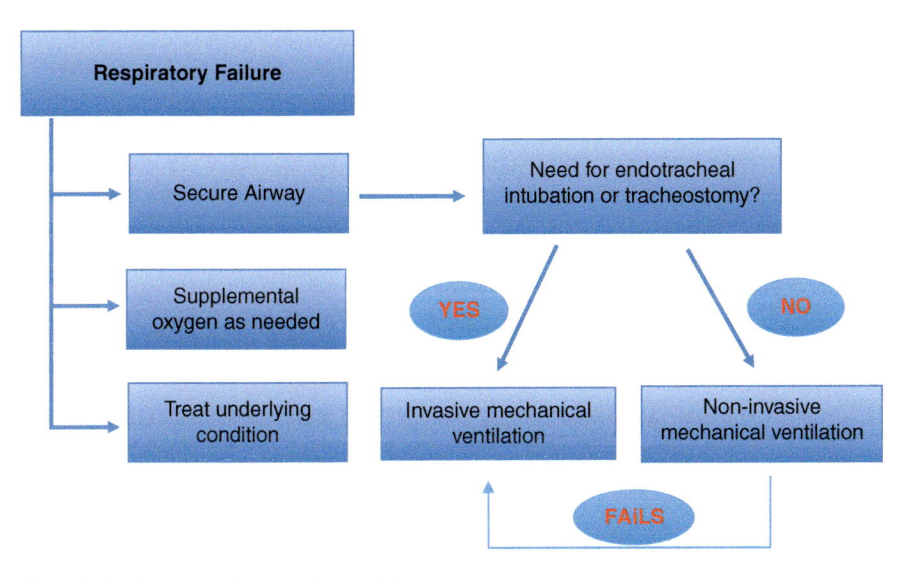

Fig. 3.3 Initial approach to respiratory failure

Table 3.3 Important conditions causing respiratory distress and respiratory failure

Conditions that affect the areas of the brain that control breathing	*Conditions that affect the flow of blood into the lungs*
• Stroke	• Pulmonary embolism
• Drug/alcohol overdose	• Myocardial infarction
Conditions that affect gas exchange in the alveoli (air sacs)	*Conditions that affect the nerves and muscles that control breathing*
• Acute respiratory distress syndromes	• Muscular dystrophy
• Pneumonia	• Amyotrophic lateral sclerosis
• Pulmonary edema	• Spinal cord injuries
Conditions that affect the flow of air in and out of the lung	*Other*
• Chronic obstructive lung disease	• Tension pneumothorax
• Asthma	• Metabolic acidosis

- In patients who have profound dyspnea and tachypnea, their primary problem is usually related to an inadequate airway. However, if the ventilation problem is caused by a pneumothorax or tension pneumothorax, which is much more common in older patients, intubation with vigorous bag-mask ventilation and forthcoming mechanical ventilation can rapidly lead to further deterioration of the patient. Patient's chest must be reevaluated, and chest X-ray should be obtained as soon as possible after intubation.
- Older patients have decreased respiratory reserves due to effects of aging and chronic cardiopulmonary diseases, together with respiratory response to hypoxia and hypercapnia decreases about fifty percent [51, 52]. Critically ill older patients should be carefully monitored even if they are stable, and to decrease the threshold level for ventilatory support is a safer approach. Admission to the hospital is usually necessary, even with apparently mild respiratory distress.
- Administration of supplemental oxygen is mandatory for most of critically ill patients. However, physicians should have kept in mind that some older patients rely on hypoxic drive to maintain ventilation, and supplemental oxygen can cause carbon dioxide retention and respiratory acidosis in COPD.
- Secondary to neurologic disorders, the loss of cough reflex and swallowing dysfunctions are much more common in older patients, which predispose to aspiration resulting in increased frequency and severity of pneumonia in older patients. Prevention and early identifying of aspirations in older patients are essential.
- Impaired mental status is more common in critically ill older patients than younger patients. Because of that, although NIPPV decreases the rate of intubation, mortality, and nosocomial pneumonia, it should be used cautiously in older patients.

3.3.4 Circulation Assessment and Management (C)

3.3.4.1 Circulation Assessment

The goal of circulation assessment in critically ill older patients is ultimately to determine whether the patient has adequate end-organ perfusion or the patient is in shock state. Determination of the adequacy of end-organ perfusion involves a measurement of patient's heart rate, blood pressure, extremity pulses, nail bed capillary refill, and the skin.

First of all, assess the general appearance and the temperature of the skin of the patient especially on the hands and digits. Pallor or bluish discoloration of the skin or mucous membranes and/or cold extremities indicate poor perfusion. Then, measure the nail bed capillary refill time, which has the normal value of less than 2 s, and if it is prolonged, it suggests poor peripheral perfusion. Pulse rate should be counted preferably by heart auscultation. Tachycardia is one of the first compensatory responses to shock. But bradycardia or irregular pulse indicates more severe and critical state of shock. Weak/thread pulses suggest poor perfusion. Blood pressure of the patient is the most objective and informative sign in the assessment of circulation, is a sign of uncompensated shock, and occurs when compensatory mechanisms are no longer adequate to support perfusion. Hypotension is a late sign of shock, and shock may be present in the absence of hypotension especially if the patients' baseline blood pressure is high. Pulse pressure defined as the difference between systolic and diastolic blood pressure is useful in shock conditions where decreased pulse pressure is a sign of early (compensated) shock. Mean arterial blood pressure is a more reliable parameter in assessing the end-organ perfusion due to its close association with sufficient perfusion, and mean arterial blood pressure goal is a target for the initial resuscitation of shock [53]. There are four main types of shock: hypovolemic (e.g., hemorrhagic), cardiogenic, distributive or vasodilatory (e.g., septic, anaphylaxis), and obstructive (e.g., cardiac tamponade, tension pneumothorax). Appropriate management is dependent on correct identification of the cause of the decompensation.

3.3.4.2 Management of Circulatory Emergencies

Hypovolemic shock is due to a decrease in the volume of blood due to bleeding (internal or external), loss of plasma, or dehydration. Restoration of the blood volume by intravenous fluids and blood stands for the main point of the initial treatment of hypovolemic shock.

Cardiogenic shock is due to decreased ventricular dysfunction by any cause. Identifying right- versus left-sided cardiogenic shock is imperative because treatment strategies differ accordingly.

Distributive or vasodilatory shock results from decreased vascular tone and/or redistribution of the blood. The most common cause is sepsis. Initial treatment is fluid resuscitation and vasopressors (preferably norepinephrine but caution must be taken in patients with severe peripheral vascular disease) and prompt administration of early, appropriate antibiotics (see Chap. 12). Rarely in older patients, it might be caused by anaphylaxis treated with epinephrine and airway protection in case of laryngeal angioedema.

Obstructive shock is caused by an extra-cardiac obstruction to blood flow like cardiac tamponade or tension pneumothorax. It is one of the most severe types of the shock, and initial treatment consists of prompt relief of the obstruction.

Whatever the cause of shock, every patient must have adequate vascular access preferably large-bore peripheral intravenous line. Although the treatment of shock varies according to the cause, intravenous crystalloids are generally helpful in the initial stabilization of the patient except for cardiogenic shock. In cardiogenic shock, volume replacement usually results in worsening of the respiratory and circulatory status. Cardiogenic shock should be ruled out in the initial assessment of the circulation. Echocardiography is the best test for the diagnosis of cardiogenic shock in emergency settings.

Special considerations for older patients:

- The number of CPR-related skeletal chest injury increased with age which is much more prominent with the increased duration of the CPR [54]. Because of that, the rescuers and postresuscitation care physicians should be aware of the risk of both sternal and rib fractures in older people [2].

- In older patients, cardiac output is maintained with increased ventricular filling (preload) and stroke volume instead of increasing rate, which is not the case for younger patients. Because of this dependence on preload, even mild hypovolemia can result in significant cardiac failure and deteriorate older patients within seconds.
- Myocardial infarction in older patients is more frequently suspected with atypical symptoms such as syncope, shortness of breath, and abdominal pain, and this should be detected during the primary assessment of the unstable older patient [2, 55].
- Although the resting heart rate may vary, the maximum tachycardic response decreases with age, which is more prominent under inotropic drug treatment. Hypovolemic shock in older patients can be asymptomatic until the terminal stage [5].
- All kinds of dysrhythmias more easily develop in aged heart especially under stress [56]. Atrial fibrillation is the most common supraventricular arrhythmia in the older people. It often causes cardiovascular compromise due to loss of the atrial contribution for diastolic filling, particularly in the older patient who has reduced ventricular compliance. Hypotension and an increased heart rate may reduce coronary perfusion and precipitate cardiac ischemia, which is more likely in an older population [2]. Because of all these, older patients should be closely monitored, and repeated electrocardiographic evaluation should be performed systematically in older patient.
- There is a significant decrease in renal functions with age. In addition, older critically ill patients are often hypovolemic due to a reduction of both fluid intake and urine-concentrating ability [2]. As a result, creatinine clearance decreases in older patients, and older patients are more susceptible to kidney failure due to hypovolemia, medications, and other nephrotoxins. Because of this, if it is possible, creatine clearance must be calculated, and treatments should be adapted to renal function.

3.4 Special Considerations

3.4.1 Trauma

When trauma-injured patients present with shock, there is a more limited differential diagnosis, and specific treatments must be provided. Here, specific considerations and detailed characteristics of older trauma patients will not be discussed, whereas the main points on stabilization process of unstable older trauma patients will be described.

Although advanced age clearly correlates with increased morbidity and mortality in trauma, studies indicate that undertriage in older trauma patients is twofold in younger patients [57]. Prehospital trauma triage guidelines developed for use with a general adult population may not be sensitive enough to detect covert injuries in older trauma patients, and these guidelines should include age as a decision point to avoid placing older persons at risk for undertriage [58].

In the older trauma patient, special attention should be focused on vital signs. A common pitfall in the assessment of older trauma patients is the mistaken impression that normal blood pressure indicates normovolemia. The normal blood pressure tends to increase with age. Thus, a normal systolic blood pressure may indicate hypotension in older patients whose basal value is high. The onset of hypotension might also be delayed and might indicate pre-arrest condition.

Older patients should be resuscitated in the same process as the younger patients keeping in mind that they are more sensitive not only to over-resuscitation but also to the under-resuscitation [59]. Although securing airway in older trauma patients is more challenging, early endotracheal intubation should be considered if there are signs of shock, chest trauma, or changes in mental status. Because older patients have limited cardiac reserves, all sources of blood loss should be identified and controlled as soon as possible. More aggressive testing and interventions might be considered accordingly. All operative and nonoperative management of older patients must be done by experienced (preferably trauma) surgeons in collaboration with emergency physicians.

This loss of brain volume allows more brain movement during acceleration-deceleration injuries (especially in dehydrated cases) increases the incidence of subdural hematoma, and allows more blood collection before overt symptoms become apparent. Because of this, in older patient's brain, CT scan threshold should be lowered. Furthermore, preexisting medical conditions (such as dementia) or psychotropic drugs make more difficult to assess mental status. Spinal injuries are also more common, due to osteoporosis, and may be occult and difficult to diagnose in older patients due to osteoarthritis. Because of this, older patients with suspected spinal injuries should be carefully evaluated, and investigation with CT scan or MRI should be done even if the plain radiographs do not show any evidence of fracture.

The mortality risk of trauma patients rises dramatically with age. A six times greater mortality rate has been reported in older patients compared to the younger trauma patients when controlling for the degree of injury [60]. Nevertheless, because older trauma patients are more challenging due to comorbidities, decreased physiological reserves, and occult presentation, they get more benefit from aggressive monitoring and early resuscitative approach than younger patients who have similar degree of traumatic injury.

3.4.2 Abuse

Abused older patients are at high risk of death, and mortality is three times higher than non-abused patients [61]. Although primary assessment and stabilization of the abused older patients do not differ from others, special attention should be given to detect these patients due to their poor prognosis.

After stabilization of life-threatening conditions, it is crucial that all medical practitioners should conduct a detailed history and physical examination, to identify and prevent abuse in older patients, including the following factors:

- Apparent delays in seeking medical help for significant injuries or illnesses
- Functionally impaired older patients with life-threatening conditions who arrive without their main caregivers
- Differing case histories from the patient and the caregivers
- Unexplained signs of injury (such as contusions, bruises, scars, broken bones, dislocations) especially when they are symmetrical
- Report of drug overdose or overmedication/undermedication
- Refusal of caregivers to allow physical examination of the patient alone
- Unexplained genital or anal bleeding/injury
- Inconceivable or doubtful explanations for injuries or illness, from either the patient or caregivers
- Laboratory findings that are incompatible with the history provided by caregivers and the patient's condition

These findings are suspect geriatric abuse. During the assessment of the critically ill older patients, it should never be forgotten that most abusers are family members (about 89% of all), those that usually give the main medical history of the critical patients [62].

3.4.3 Intoxications

Intoxication is a significant problem in older patients. Although the majority of the intoxication cases in older patients are unintentional (due to dementia, confusion, improper use, and storage), they might also be due to suicidal attempt, which are more likely to be successful in older patients [63].

General assessment and management procedures of intoxicated older patients differ from younger ones by the importance to take care of underlying medical condition and concurrent medications. After the initial ABC assessment of the poisoned patient, the physician should determine the causative substance and the entrance route and time of the poison to the body. If the substance is a volatile or toxic chemical agent, the decontamination of the patient and preventive measures must start together with the primary assessment and initial stabilization procedures. At least the patient should be isolated until decontamination can be set up which is vitally important in mass casualties. The goal is to prevent rescuers from becoming victims and extension of the contamination to others. For any substance affecting the skin, clothing removal and irrigation of the skin are essential. Antidotes and early hemodialysis-hemoperfusion should be considered for unstable patients. While specific indications for antidotes are identical for all age groups, the dosage alterations and precautions should be considered in older patients [64]. Aggressive initial management is crucial for older intoxicated patients due to high susceptibility of toxic effects of the drugs. The physicians providing medical care of older patients must keep in mind that cardiovascular and neurological toxicities occur with overdoses of drugs more frequently and severely in older patients.

In older trauma patients (especially injuries due to falls), drug intoxications and adverse effects should be considered in the differential diagnosis of the primary cause of trauma. If intoxication is suspected as the primary cause of trauma, toxicologic treatments (e.g., activated charcoal, hemodialysis, drug antidotes) should be given while stabilizing the presenting trauma condition.

3.4.4 Hypothermia

Hypothermia is defined as a body core temperature below 35.0°C, and it is well known that older adults are more vulnerable to hypothermia for many reasons including, but not limited to, decreased metabolic rate, ability to detect changes in the temperature, shivering, and increased incidence of chronic medical conditions (such as diabetes, stoke, Parkinson's disease, etc.) and medications (such as antidepressants and sedatives) [65]. On the other hand, signs of hypothermia in older people are easy to miss which could have serious consequences if not dealt with swiftly and effectively [66].

Assessment and identification of hypothermia in older people could be difficult, and tympanic membrane measurements are often offered over axilla measurements [67]. In case of severe hypothermia, invasive core active rewarming techniques, such as administration of warmed intravenous fluids, should be used, and the speed of recovery should depend on how long the patient was exposed to the cold and the state of his general health status.

3.4.5 Whom to Resuscitate/Ethics of Resuscitation

Given the fact that the increase in the presentation of critically ill older patients is more challenging for physicians to make decisions with regard to CPR on these patients who are at high risk of death in the near future or have terminal illnesses, it is clear that physicians must take into account DNAR orders, which is usually not present in emergency circumstances.

Advanced age is frequently mentioned as a negative predictor for outcome of CPR, and there is scattered data on the long-term outcomes of CPR in older patients. In a recent systematic review of 29 including 417,190 patients over 70 years of age that were investigated for the survival rates after in-hospital CPR, almost 40% of patients had successful CPR or "return of spontaneous circulation," but more than half of those patients ultimately died in the hospital [68]. In general, patients who are highly functional with fewer chronic illnesses, hospitalized for a cardiac etiology, and closely monitored before the arrest were more likely to benefit from CPR. In this case, older patients benefited from the CPR as much as younger patients [69].

Immediate short- and long-term prognosis of in-hospital CPR seems independent of age, or at least age alone might not be a limiting factor, whereas pre-arrest factors such as independent function level and normal mental status are significant prognostic factors [2, 70, 71].

Survival rates of older patients following an out-of-hospital arrest depend also on witnessed status, resuscitation times, and the presenting rhythm (better survival rates in ventricular fibrillation or arrhythmia compared to asystole or electromechanical dissociation) [2, 32].

Even though advanced age might be a predictor of mortality in older patient's cardiac arrest, there are still survival rates of more than 10% in different subsets of old population [72]. Outcomes of patients with initial shockable rhythms (ventricular fibrillation and pulseless ventricular tachycardia) are often excellent, but outcomes in patients with non-shockable rhythms (PEA and asystole) are generally poor. A recent Japanese study of patients with initial non-shockable rhythm showed that the 1-month survival rate is lower in older patients aged 85 and more (1.7%) as compared to old patients aged 65–74 (2.4%) and 75–84 (3.3%) [73]. In patients aged ≥75 years, rhythm conversion and subsequent shock delivery are not associated or negatively associated with 1-month Cerebral Performance Category scale 1 (good cerebral performance)–2 (moderate cerebral disability).

Van de Glind et al. showed that, in general, patients aged over 70 years had less chance of surviving to discharge after an out-of-hospital cardiac arrest (4.1%) than the patients of all age groups (pooled survival 7.6%) [71].

Furthermore, the factors of nursing home residency [74–78] and pre-arrest comorbidity [79] were associated with decreased chances of survival.

Evidence for the predictive value of comorbidities and for the predictive value of age on quality of life of survivors is scarce [71]. Although the available evidence on the effect of pre-arrest factors on survival is limited, it is important to accurately inform older people of their limited chances of survival following out-of-hospital CPR.

Adams et al. showed that older patients' beliefs regarding the chances of survival after CPR are overly optimistic. Similarly, physicians' expectations of the likelihood of survival are not realistic [80]. However, older people understand prognostic information, and such information may alter their preferences with respect to resuscitation [81]. This kind of treatment decisions should be based on both scientific evidence and doctor's and patient's preferences.

However, the outcomes of older patients seemed to be exceptionally poor in frail individuals and need to be considered in order to reduce unnecessary treatment decisions [82]. Frailty was directly associated with mortality, showing a 30-day survival of 5.6% and a favorable neurological outcome of 1.1% among older individuals. Quantifying the risk of dying and frailty in acute care setting is very difficult [83]. Decisions need to be based on evidence (discussion with the patient, a preexisting advance directive, or discussions with family or informed others if the patient lacks capacity). When the individual has capacity, the doctor must provide choices and guidance to facilitate choice. Current guidelines require staff to involve patients and their families in resuscitation decisions in accordance with local policies [84]. At the bedside, ultrasonography may play a significant role in guidance of the management decisions in the resuscitation of older patients, as well as in determining the etiologies such as undifferentiated shock states, aortic aneurysm, cardiac tamponade, and massive pulmonary embolism [85].

Even if medical professionals believe CPR is futile, they are expected to respect patients' wishes. On the other hand, medical professionals should balance compassion with appropriate care focused on functional and cognitive outcome [86]. It is clear that physicians may not be expected to attempt to resuscitate a patient who is in the terminal phase of an illness, or the burden associated with the treatment clearly outweighs the benefit [87].

In some instances, death can be a respectful alternative to CPR without any chance of recovery, especially in critically ill older patients. Because of all these, recognizing prognostic factors in CPR of older patients has absolute importance [88].

Although physicians in the ED usually possess a reflexive instinct toward saving life of a cardiopulmonary arrest case on arrival, they should take into account patient's pre-arrest functional and cognitive condition as well as their chronic or terminal illnesses which has more importance in older patients. Aggressive resuscitation of older patients with metastatic neoplasms, chronic liver/renal disease, chronic obstructive lung disease, organ failure (especially respiratory or cardiac), and nursing home residence is futile and might be devastating not only for the patient but also for their relatives [2].

Emergency physicians should acknowledge and respect their patient's needs for end-of-life care which requires searching for previous or working on current advance directives/DNAR orders and the underlying medical futility. Even though emergency physicians may feel that these procedures are difficult and/or time-consuming, to have more patient-centric and humanistic approach, these should be taken into account. If there is doubt about the validity of the advance directives/DNAR orders, or the families or healthcare proxy insists on resuscitation, it is reasonable to resuscitate the patient and then discuss these issues in more detail. Emergency physicians should actively engage primary care providers, specialists, prehospital providers, patients, and families in this process.

Conclusion

The primary assessment including the "ABC approach" and stabilization procedures of life-threatening conditions in older patients follows the principles recommended by the guidelines but represents a challenge for EM care providers in the ED and in the prehospital setting since age-related physiologic changes in vital organ systems and frailty reduce the physiological reserves to cope with life-threatening conditions, which necessitate aggressive, goal-directed, and prompt therapy. Age alone is not a factor for non-resuscitation, but EM care providers have to carefully assess whether resuscitation is futile or not in very frail older patients.

Caution and a high index of suspicion for older trauma patients require optimal primary assessment and stabilization. Comorbidities and medications may not only cause but also complicate injuries in older patients.

Abuse and neglect in older patients continue to be underrecognized and underreported. Special attention should be given to detect abuse and intoxication conditions during the assessment of critically ill older patients, which should lead to earlier diagnosis and improved outcomes.

As quality of life, frailty, cognitive, and functional status are even more important at older age than survival per se, these outcomes should be reported too in future resuscitation studies in older patients. This would help both doctors and patients in decision-making about the desirability of cardiopulmonary resuscitation. It will also help to identify older patients that will benefit or not from resuscitation.

References

1. Camilloni L, Farchi S, Giorgi Rossi P, Chini F, Borgia P (2008) Mortality in older injured patients: the role of comorbidities. Int J Inj Control Saf Promot 15(1):25–31. doi:10.1080/17457300701800118
2. Truhlar A, Deakin CD, Soar J, Khalifa GE, Alfonzo A, Bierens JJ et al (2015) European resuscitation council guidelines for resuscitation 2015: section 4. Cardiac arrest in special circumstances. Resuscitation 95:148–201. doi:10.1016/j.resuscitation.2015.07.017
3. Thim T, Krarup NH, Grove EL, Rohde CV, Lofgren B (2012) Initial assessment and treatment with the airway, breathing, circulation, disability, exposure (ABCDE) approach. Int J Gen Med 5:117–121. doi:10.2147/ijgm.s28478
4. Nigam Y, Knight J, Bhattacharya S, Bayer A (2012) Physiological changes associated with aging and immobility. J Aging Res 2012:1–2. doi:10.1155/2012/468469
5. Priebe HJ (2000) The aged cardiovascular risk patient. Br J Anaesth 85(5):763–778
6. Thim T, Krarup NH, Grove EL, Lofgren B (2010) ABCDE—a systematic approach to critically ill patients. Ugeskr Laeger 172(47):3264–3266
7. Menaker J, Scalea TM (2010) Geriatric care in the surgical intensive care unit. Crit Care Med 38(9 Suppl):S452–S459. doi:10.1097/CCM.0b013e3181ec5697
8. Shinmura K (2016) Cardiac senescence, heart failure, and frailty: a triangle in elderly people. Keio J Med 65:25–32. doi:10.2302/kjm.2015-0015-IR
9. Zadravecz FJ, Tien L, Robertson-Dick BJ, Yuen TC, Twu NM, Churpek MM et al (2015) Comparison of mental-status scales for predicting mortality on the general wards. J Hosp Med 10(10):658–663. doi:10.1002/jhm.2415
10. Link MS, Berkow LC, Kudenchuk PJ, Halperin HR, Hess EP, Moitra VK et al (2015) Part 7: adult advanced cardiovascular life support: 2015 American Heart Association guidelines update for cardiopulmonary resuscitation and emergency cardiovascular care. Circulation 132(18 Suppl 2):S444–S464. doi:10.1161/cir.0000000000000261
11. Kern JW, Shoemaker WC (2002) Meta-analysis of hemodynamic optimization in high-risk patients. Crit Care Med 30(8):1686–1692
12. Sox HC Jr, Woloshin S (2000) How many deaths are due to medical error? Getting the number right. Eff Clin Pract 3(6):277–283
13. Johnson KN, Botros DB, Groban L, Bryan YF (2015) Anatomic and physiopathologic changes affecting the airway of the elderly patient: implications for geriatric-focused airway management. Clin Interv Aging 10:1925–1934. doi:10.2147/cia.s93796

14. Sevransky JE, Haponik EF (2003) Respiratory failure in elderly patients. Clin Geriatr Med 19(1):205–224
15. Hasegawa K, Hagiwara Y, Imamura T, Chiba T, Watase H, Brown CA 3rd et al (2013) Increased incidence of hypotension in elderly patients who underwent emergency airway management: an analysis of a multi-centre prospective observational study. Int J Emerg Med 6:12. doi:10.1186/1865-1380-6-12
16. Cosgrove JF, Gascoigne AD (1999) Inadequate assessment of the airway and ventilation in acute poisoning. A need for improved education? Resuscitation 40(3):161–164
17. Khan RM, Sharma PK, Kaul N (2011) Airway management in trauma. Ind J Anaesth 55(5):463–469. doi:10.4103/0019-5049.89870
18. Overbeck MC (2016) Airway management of respiratory failure. Emerg Med Clin North Am 34(1):97–127. doi:10.1016/j.emc.2015.08.007
19. Reed MJ, Rennie LM, Dunn MJ, Gray AJ, Robertson CE, McKeown DW (2004) Is the 'LEMON' method an easily applied emergency airway assessment tool? Eur J Emerg Med 11(3):154–157
20. Racine SX, Solis A, Hamou NA, Letoumelin P, Hepner DL, Beloucif S et al (2010) Face mask ventilation in edentulous patients: a comparison of mandibular groove and lower lip placement. Anesthesiology 112(5):1190–1193. doi:10.1097/ALN.0b013e3181d5dfea
21. Langeron O, Masso E, Huraux C, Guggiari M, Bianchi A, Coriat P et al (2000) Prediction of difficult mask ventilation. Anesthesiology 92(5):1229–1236
22. Benumof JL, Dagg R, Benumof R (1997) Critical hemoglobin desaturation will occur before return to an unparalyzed state following 1 mg/kg intravenous succinylcholine. Anesthesiology 87(4):979–982
23. Aziz MF, Abrons RO, Cattano D, Bayman EO, Swanson DE, Hagberg CA et al (2016) First-attempt intubation success of video laryngoscopy in patients with anticipated difficult direct laryngoscopy: a multicenter randomized controlled trial comparing the C-MAC D-blade versus the glidescope in a mixed provider and diverse patient population. Anesth Analg 122(3):740–750. doi:10.1213/ane.0000000000001084
24. Shirgoska B, Netkovski J (2012) New techniques and devices for difficult airway management. Acta Clin Croat 51(3):457–461
25. Vassiliadis J, Tzannes A, Hitos K, Brimble J, Fogg T (2015) Comparison of the C-MAC video laryngoscope with direct Macintosh laryngoscopy in the emergency department. EMA 27(2):119–125. doi:10.1111/1742-6723.12358
26. Cressey DM, Claydon P, Bhaskaran NC, Reilly CS (2001) Effect of midazolam pretreatment on induction dose requirements of propofol in combination with fentanyl in younger and older adults. Anaesthesia 56:108
27. Jones NA, Elliott S, Knight J (2002) A comparison between midazolam co-induction and propofol predosing for the induction of anaesthesia in the elderly. Anaesthesia 57:649
28. Martin G, Glass PS, Breslin DS et al (2003) A study of anesthetic drug utilization in different age groups. J Clin Anesth 15:194
29. Benson M, Junger A, Fuchs C, Quinzio L, Bottger S, Hempelmann G (2000) Use of an anesthesia information management system (AIMS) to evaluate the physiologic effects of hypnotic agents used to induce anesthesia. J Clin Monit Comput 16(3):183–190
30. Folch E, Majid A (2015) Foreign body aspiration in the elderly patient. Curr Geriatr Rep 4(2):192–201. doi:10.1007/s13670-015-0131-z
31. Lin L, Lv L, Wang Y, Zha X, Tang F, Liu X (2014) The clinical features of foreign body aspiration into the lower airway in geriatric patients. Clin Interv Aging 9:1613–1618. doi:10.2147/cia.s70924
32. Narang AT, Sikka R (2006) Resuscitation of the elderly. Emerg Med Clin North Am 24(2):261–272. doi:10.1016/j.emc.2006.01.001
33. Nelson R, Tse B, Edwards S (2005) Systematic review of prophylactic nasogastric decompression after abdominal operations. Br J Surg 92(6):673–680. doi:10.1002/bjs.5090
34. ATLS Subcommittee, American College of Surgeons' Committee on Trauma, International ATLS Working Group (2013) Advanced trauma life support (ATLS®): the ninth edition. J Trauma Acute Care Surg 74(5):1363–1366. doi:10.1097/TA.0b013e31828b82f5

35. De Vos E, Jacobson L (2016) Approach to adult patients with acute dyspnea. Emerg Med Clin North Am 34(1):129–149. doi:10.1016/j.emc.2015.08.008
36. Groombridge C, Chin CW, Hanrahan B, Holdgate A (2016) Assessment of common preoxygenation strategies outside of the operating room environment. Acad Emerg Med 23(3):342–346. doi:10.1111/acem.12889
37. El-Orbany M, Woehlck H, Salem MR (2011) Head and neck position for direct laryngoscopy. Anesth Analg 113(1):103–109. doi:10.1213/ANE.0b013e31821c7e9c
38. Hodgkin JE (1997) Respiratory care—a guide to clinical practice. Philidelphia, Lippincott-Raven Publication and Co
39. Kane B, Decalmer S, Ronan O'Driscoll B (2013) Emergency oxygen therapy: from guideline to implementation. Breathe 9(4):246–253. doi:10.1183/20734735.025212
40. Kida Y, Minakata Y, Yamada Y, Ichinose M (2012) Efficacy of noninvasive positive pressure ventilation in elderly patients with acute hypercapnic respiratory failure. Respiration 83(5):377–382. doi:10.1159/000328399
41. Yeow ME, Santanilla JI (2008) Noninvasive positive pressure ventilation in the emergency department. Emerg Med Clin North Am 26(3):835–847. doi:10.1016/j.emc.2008.04.005
42. Ram FS, Picot J, Lightowler J, Wedzicha JA (2004) Non-invasive positive pressure ventilation for treatment of respiratory failure due to exacerbations of chronic obstructive pulmonary disease. Cochrane Database Syst Rev 3:CD004104. doi:10.1002/14651858.CD004104.pub3
43. Piroddi IMG, Barlascini C, Esquinas A, Braido F, Banfi P, Nicolini A (2017) Non-invasive mechanical ventilation in elderly patients: A narrative review. Geriatr Gerontol Int 17(5):689–696. doi:10.1111/ggi.12810. Epub 2016 May 23
44. Esteban A, Anzueto A, Frutos-Vivar F, Alía I, Ely EW, Brochard L, Stewart TE, Apezteguía C, Tobin MJ, Nightingale P, Matamis D, Pimentel J (2004) Abroug F; Mechanical Ventilation International Study Group. Outcome of older patients receiving mechanical ventilation. Intensive Care Med 30(4):639–646. Epub 2004 Feb 28
45. Scarpazza P, Incorvaia C, di Franco G, Raschi S, Usai P, Bernareggi M, Bonacina C, Melacini C, Vanni S, Bencini S, Pravettoni C, Di Cara G, Yacoub MR, Riario-Sforza GG, Guffanti E, Casali W (2008) Effect of noninvasive mechanical ventilation in elderly patients with hypercapnic acute-on-chronic respiratory failure and a do-not-intubate order. Int J Chron Obstruct Pulmon Dis 3(4):797–801
46. Nava S, Grassi M, Fanfulla F, Domenighetti G, Carlucci A, Perren A, Dell'Orso D, Vitacca M, Ceriana P, Karakurt Z, Clini E (2011) Non-invasive ventilation in elderly patients with acute hypercapnic respiratory failure: a randomised controlled trial. Age Ageing 40(4):444–450. doi:10.1093/ageing/afr003. Epub 2011 Feb 22
47. Lunghar L, D'Ambrosio CM (2007) Noninvasive ventilation in the older patient who has acute respiratory failure. Clin Chest Med 28(4):793–800
48. Tate JA, Sereika S, Divirgilio D, Nilsen M, Demerci J, Campbell G, Happ MB (2013) Symptom communication during critical illness: the impact of age, delirium, and delirium presentation. J Gerontol Nurs 39(8):28–38. doi:10.3928/00989134-20130530-03. Epub 2013 Jun 10
49. Soguel L, Revelly JP, Schaller MD, Longchamp C, Berger MM (2012) Energy deficit and length of hospital stay can be reduced by a two-step quality improvement of nutrition therapy: the intensive care unit dietitian can make the difference. Crit Care Med 40(2):412–419. doi:10.1097/CCM.0b013e31822f0ad7
50. Segrelles Calvo G, Zamora García E, Girón Moreno R, Vázquez Espinosa E, Gómez Punter RM, Fernandes Vasconcelos G, Valenzuela C, Ancochea BJ (2012) Non-invasive ventilation in an elderly population admitted to a respiratory monitoring unit: causes, complications and one-year evolution. Arch Bronconeumol 48(10):349–354. doi:10.1016/j.arbres.2012.05.001. Epub 2012 Jun 15
51. Krumpe PE, Knudson RJ, Parsons G, Reiser K (1985) The aging respiratory system. Clin Geriatr Med 1(1):143–175
52. Rosenthal RA, Kavic SM (2004) Assessment and management of the geriatric patient. Crit Care Med 32(4 Suppl):S92–105
53. Asfar P, Meziani F, Hamel JF, Grelon F, Megarbane B, Anguel N et al (2014) High versus low blood-pressure target in patients with septic shock. N Engl J Med 370(17):1583–1593. doi:10.1056/NEJMoa1312173

54. Kralj E, Podbregar M, Kejžar N, Balažic J (2015) Frequency and number of resuscitation related rib and sternum fractures are higher than generally considered. Resuscitation 93:136–141. doi:10.1016/j.resuscitation.2015.02.034
55. Grosmaitre P, Le Vavasseur O, Yachouh E, Courtial Y, Jacob X, Meyran S et al (2013) Significance of atypical symptoms for the diagnosis and management of myocardial infarction in elderly patients admitted to emergency departments. Arch Cardiovasc Dis 106(11):586–592. doi:10.1016/j.acvd.2013.04.010
56. Chow GV, Marine JE, Fleg JL (2012) Epidemiology of arrhythmias and conduction disorders in older adults. Clin Geriatr Med 28(4):539–553. doi:10.1016/j.cger.2012.07.003
57. Callaway DW, Wolfe R (2007) Geriatric trauma. Emerg Med Clin North Am 25(3):837–860. doi:10.1016/j.emc.2007.06.005
58. O'Connor RE (2006) Trauma triage: concepts in prehospital trauma care. Prehosp Emerg Care 10(3):307–310. doi:10.1080/10903120600723947
59. Salottolo KM, Mains CW, Offner PJ, Bourg PW, Bar-Or D (2013) A retrospective analysis of geriatric trauma patients: venous lactate is a better predictor of mortality than traditional vital signs. Scand J Trauma Resusc Emerg Med 21:7. doi:10.1186/1757-7241-21-7
60. Dimitriou R, Calori GM, Giannoudis PV (2011) Polytrauma in the elderly: specific considerations and current concepts of management. Eur J Trauma Emerg Surg 37(6):539–548. doi:10.1007/s00068-011-0137-y
61. Bond MC, Butler KH (2013) Elder abuse and neglect: definitions, epidemiology, and approaches to emergency department screening. Clin Geriatr Med 29(1):257–273. doi:10.1016/j.cger.2012.09.004
62. Abbey L (2009) Elder abuse and neglect: when home is not safe. Clin Geriatr Med 25(1):47–60. doi:10.1016/j.cger.2008.10.003
63. Klein-Schwartz W, Oderda GM (1991) Poisoning in the elderly. Epidemiological, clinical and management considerations. Drugs Aging 1(1):67–89
64. Haselberger MB, Kroner BA (1995) Drug poisoning in older patients. Preventative and management strategies. Drugs Aging 7(4):292–297
65. Pedley DK, Paterson B, Morrison W (2002) Hypothermia in elderly patients presenting to accident & emergency during the onset of winter. Scott Med J 47(1):10-1. doi:10.1177/003693300204700105
66. Neno R (2005) Hypothermia: assessment, treatment and prevention. Nurs Stand 19(20):47–52. doi:10.7748/ns2005.01.19.20.47.c3792
67. Gallimore D (2004) Reviewing the effectiveness of tympanic thermometers. Nurs Times 100(32):32–34
68. van Gijn MS, Frijns D, van de Glind EMM, van Munster BC, Hamaker ME (2014) The chance of survival and the functional outcome after in-hospital cardiopulmonary resuscitation in older people: a systematic review. Age Ageing 43:456–463. doi:10.1093/ageing/afu035
69. Tresch D, Heudebert G, Kutty K, Ohlert J, Van Beek K, Masi A (1994) Cardiopulmonary resuscitation in elderly patients hospitalized in the 1990s: a favorable outcome. J Am Geriatr Soc 42(2):137–141
70. Di Bari M, Chiarlone M, Fumagalli S, Boncinelli L, Tarantini F, Ungar A et al (2000) Cardiopulmonary resuscitation of older, inhospital patients: immediate efficacy and long-term outcome. Crit Care Med 28(7):2320–2325
71. van de Glind EM, van Munster BC, van de Wetering FT, van Delden JJ, Scholten RJ, Hooft L (2013) Pre-arrest predictors of survival after resuscitation from out-of-hospital cardiac arrest in the elderly a systematic review. BMC Geriatr 13:68. doi:10.1186/1471-2318-13-68
72. Libungan B, Lindqvist J, Stromsoe A, Nordberg P, Hollenberg J, Albertsson P et al (2015) Out-of-hospital cardiac arrest in the elderly: a large-scale population-based study. Resuscitation 94:28–32. doi:10.1016/j.resuscitation.2015.05.031
73. Funada A, Goto Y, Tada H, Teramoto R, Shimojima M, Hayashi K, Yamagishi M (2016) Age-specific differences in prognostic significance of rhythm conversion from initial non-shockable to shockable rhythm and subsequent shock delivery in out-of-hospital cardiac arrest. Resuscitation 108:61–67. doi:10.1016/j.resuscitation.2016.09.013. Epub 2016 Sep 21
74. Applebaum GE, King JE, Finucane TE (1990) The outcome of CPR initiated in nursing homes. J Am Geriatr Soc 38(3):197–200

75. Awoke S, Mouton CP, Parrott M (1992) Outcomes of skilled cardiopulmonary resuscitation in a long-term-care facility: futile therapy? J Am Geriatr Soc 40(6):593–595
76. Deasy C, Bray JE, Smith K, Harriss LR, Bernard SA, Cameron P, VACAR Steering Committee (2011) Out-of-hospital cardiac arrests in the older age groups in Melbourne, Australia. Resuscitation 82(4):398–403. doi:10.1016/j.resuscitation.2010.12.016. Epub 2011 Feb 1
77. Kim HK, Hisata M, Kai I, Lee SK (2000) Social support exchange and quality of life among the Korean elderly. J Cross Cult Gerontol 15(4):331–347
78. Iwami T, Hiraide A, Nakanishi N, Hayashi Y, Nishiuchi T, Uejima T, Morita H, Shigemoto T, Ikeuchi H, Matsusaka M, Shinya H, Yukioka H, Sugimoto H (2006) Outcome and characteristics of out-of-hospital cardiac arrest according to location of arrest: a report from a large-scale, population-based study in Osaka, Japan. Resuscitation 69(2):221–228. Epub 2006 Mar 6
79. Fabbri A, Marchesini G, Spada M, Iervese T, Dente M, Galvani M, Vandelli A (2006) Monitoring intervention programmes for out-of-hospital cardiac arrest in a mixed urban and rural setting. Resuscitation 71(2):180–187. Epub 2006 Sep 18
80. Adams DH, Snedden DP (2006) How misconceptions among elderly patients regarding survival outcomes of inpatient cardiopulmonary resuscitation affect do-not-resuscitate orders. J Am Osteopath Assoc 106:402–404
81. Murphy DJ, Burrows D, Santilli S, Kemp AW, Tenner S, Kreling B, Teno J (1994) The influence of the probability of survival on patients' preferences regarding cardiopulmonary resuscitation. N Engl J Med 330(8):545–549
82. Sulzgruber P, Sterz F, Poppe M, Schober A, Lobmeyr E, Datler P, Keferböck M, Zeiner S, Nürnberger A, Hubner P, Stratil P, Wallmueller C, Weiser C, Warenits AM, van Tulder R, Zajicek A, Buchinger A, Testori C (2017) Age-specific prognostication after out-of-hospital cardiac arrest - the ethical dilemma between 'life-sustaining treatment' and 'the right to die' in the elderly. Eur Heart J Acute Cardiovasc Care 6(2):112–120. doi:10.1177/2048872616672076. Epub 2016 Sep 27
83. Evans SJ, Sayers M, Mitnitski A, Rockwood K (2014) The risk of adverse outcomes in hospitalized older patients in relation to a frailty index based on a comprehensive geriatric assessment. Age Ageing 43(1):127–132. doi:10.1093/ageing/aft156
84. Conroy SP, Luxton T, Dingwall R, Harwood RH, Gladman JR (2006) Cardiopulmonary resuscitation in continuing care settings: time for a rethink? BMJ 332(7539):479–482. doi:10.1136/bmj.332.7539.479
85. Byrne MW, Hwang JQ (2011) Ultrasound in the critically ill. Ultrasound Clin 6(2):235–259. doi:10.1016/j.cult.2011.03.003
86. de Rooij SE, Abu-Hanna A, Levi M, de Jonge E (2005) Factors that predict outcome of intensive care treatment in very elderly patients: a review. Crit Care 9(4):R307–R314. doi:10.1186/cc3536
87. British Medical Association; Resuscitation Council (UK); Royal College of Nursing (2001) Decisions relating to cardiopulmonary resuscitation: a joint statement from the British Medical Association, the Resuscitation Council (UK) and the Royal College of Nursing. J Med Ethics 27(5):310–316
88. Huerta-Alardín AL, Varon J (2007) Cardiopulmonary resuscitation in the elderly: a clinical and ethical perspective. J Geriatr Cardiol 4(2):117–119

Secondary Assessment of Life-Threatening Conditions of Older Patients

Hubert Blain, Abdelouahab Bellou, Mehmet Akif Karamercan, and Jacques Boddaert

4.1 Introduction

After an ED visit, more than one-third of older adults return to the ED at least once in the next 6 months [1], and approximately more than two-thirds of older adults discharged from the ED have at least one unaddressed health issue [2], suggesting that traditional ED models do not meet the chronic and underlying needs of many older patients [3–5].

The current adult ED model of rapid care has been designed to deal with life-threatening conditions, trauma, and acute illness in young- or middle-aged patients, most often without underlying diseases or treatment that can interfere with medical care. Adult ED is organized model to treat the patient's primary concern without spending the necessary time to assess and treat secondary underlying complex health problems that however may aggravate outcomes of critically ill older people [3, 6–9]. This chapter outlines the main reasons justifying comprehensive secondary

---

H. Blain (✉)
Department of Internal Medicine and Geriatrics, Faculty of Medicine, University Hospital of Montpelier, Montpellier University, MacVia-LR, EA 2991, Movement To Health, Euromov, Montpelier, France
e-mail: h-blain@chu-montpellier.fr

A. Bellou, MD, PhD
Department of Emergency Medicine, Beth Israel Deaconess Medical Center, Harvard Medical School, Boston, MA, USA
e-mail: abellou@bidmc.harvard.edu

M.A. Karamercan
Emergency Medicine Department, Gazi University School of Medicine, Ankara, Turkey

J. Boddaert
Unit of Peri-Operative Geriatric Care (UPOG), Geriatric Department Pitié-Salpêtrière Hospital, 47-83 Bd de l'Hôpital (APHP) DHU Fighting Aging and Stress (FAST) CNRS UMR 8256 Pierre et Marie Curie University (UPMC Paris 6), Paris, France

© Springer International Publishing Switzerland 2018
C. Nickel et al. (eds.), *Geriatric Emergency Medicine*,
https://doi.org/10.1007/978-3-319-19318-2_4

geriatric assessment (CGA) to better accommodate the specific needs of older patients with life-threatening conditions and improve their prognosis and quality of care [10–12].

4.2 Specific Characteristics and Needs of Older Critically Ill ED Patients that Justify a Comprehensive Secondary Geriatric Assessment (CGA)

In critically ill ED patients, particularly in older patients, the rapid identification and medical care delivery are crucial. However, the main reasons justifying a secondary CGA to improve outcomes of older ED patients with life-threatening conditions are detailed as follow.

4.2.1 Atypical Signs and Symptoms of Life-Threatening Conditions in Older ED People

4.2.1.1 The Domino Effect
Acute illnesses present often in a nonspecific way among older patients. The first sign of a new disease (or of the relapse of a chronic disease) is rarely a single specific symptom that helps identify the organ or the tissue in which the disease occurs, but more often it is the expression of the incipient failure of one or several site of less resistance [13]. In patients with multisystem deterioration and loss of physiological reserve to cope with insults (frail people), a small initial insult (and even more a life-threatening condition) can induce several other conditions and a disabling cascade of adverse effects, called the "domino" effect, that can aggravate outcome of the patient [14]. For example, in a patient with preadmission impaired mental status, heart failure, and balance impairment, a single urinary tract infection can induce fever and tachycardia, which can precipitate heart failure, induce delirium, and a fall with a hip fracture. The correct approach is not to focus exclusively on the life-threatening condition which has determined ED admission (hip fracture in this scenario) but also to conduct a standardized multidimensional and multidisciplinary diagnostic process "comprehensive geriatric assessment" (CGA) in order to ensure that all problems are identified and appropriately managed (delirium, heart failure, urinary tract infection). In this case, in addition to surgery, management comprises the optimization of heart failure treatment, treatment of the urinary tract infection, appropriate management of delirium, and rapid and appropriate rehabilitation and follow-up, taking into account of socio-environmental conditions and the patient's, family's, and caregivers' preferences [15].

ED physicians (EPs) must know the main sites or functions of less resistance (less reserve) to adequately compensate for acute conditions in older people: the brain, heart, gait and posture, gut, and general status (fatigue, pain). Indeed, delirium, acute gait impairment, or a fall especially, called geriatric syndromes (because they do not fit into distinct organ-based disease categories and have multifactorial causes), might be incorrectly regarded as mild whereas they can be the specific expression of life-threatening conditions or of diseases that may become life-threatening in older frail people. This should prompt an accurate reconstitution of medical history, as far as possible, and a systematic general examination to diagnose the primary cause of geriatric syndromes and assess reserves to cope with acute diseases in older ED patients [6].

4.2.1.2 Acute Brain Failure

Delirium
Delirium is characterized by an acute and fluctuating disturbance in attention and awareness, associated with one or several other cognitive deficits (memory, disorientation, language, visuospatial ability, or perception). Delirium does not occur in the context of reduced level of arousal, such as stupor or coma [Diagnostic and Statistical Manual of Mental Disorders (DSM) 5th edition, 2013] and is the direct consequences of acute underlying conditions that must be looked for. Numerous conditions can induce a delirium, including drugs introduced in ED (see Chap. 13).

Independently of advanced age, pre-existing dementia (diagnosed or not), premorbid functional impairment, hearing impairment, a past history of cerebrovascular disease, and epilepsy are the most consistently observed vulnerability factors for delirium in ED patients [16, 17].

In ED, missing delirium is frequent [18], and CGA in ED patients should therefore systematically look for signs and symptoms of delirium and, if identified, its primary causes, which may be life-threatening [19]. Delirium, independently of its causes, is associated with higher 30-day mortality and readmission in ED patients, due in part of the delay of diagnosis and treatment of underlying conditions but also due to inappropriate management of delirious older patients [20].

Other Possible Mental Specific Symptoms of Life-Threatening Conditions
Faintness or syncope and general malaise are also possible atypical signs of life-threatening conditions including acute coronary syndromes [21, 22], pulmonary embolism [23, 24], or abdominal aortic aneurysm [25]. Sleep disorders, such as insomnia, nocturia, nocturnal agitation, and depression, can be symptoms of life-threatening conditions, such as heart failure [26].

4.2.1.3 Functional Decline
Another atypical presentation of severe conditions in older ED patients is the sudden decline of functional abilities, such as acute gait imbalance and falls (due to infection, especially), fatigue and weakness (due to heart failure or hypo-/hyperthyroidism, especially) in people with pre-existing low muscle (sarcopenia), or postural reserve [27]. This explains why the main indexes of frailty comprise assessment of muscle strength, walking speed, and usual physical activities; those are considered as functional reserve assessments [28]. A life-threatening condition, including sepsis and acute coronary syndrome especially, has therefore to be eliminated in older patients attending ED with a sudden functional loss.

4.2.1.4 Digestive Symptoms

Independently of serious abdominal conditions, many non-abdominal life-threatening conditions may present atypically with anorexia, nausea, vomiting, and body weight loss, in frail older people. These conditions include stroke [29], acute coronary syndromes (inferior infarction especially) [21, 30], metabolic disorders (hyponatremia), and serious drug adverse effects (i.e., opioids, digoxin toxicity). Dyspepsia (usually epigastric discomfort with bloating, nausea, or early satiety) is often the only symptom of peptic ulcers. Signs of malnutrition, such as weight loss, are vulnerability factors, associated with a certain inability to cope with acute conditions [28].

4.2.1.5 Referred Pain and Symptoms

Many non-abdominal life-threatening conditions may present atypically with abdominal pain [31]. Acute coronary syndrome (ACS) is the most important diagnosis to be considered since one-third of women above the age of 65 who have an acute myocardial infarction only present with abdominal pain [21, 30]. This atypical presentation is most common in diabetics and in patients with inferior infarctions [32]. Pneumonia, pulmonary embolism, pleural effusion, pneumothorax, diabetic ketoacidosis, hypercalcemia, herpes zoster (in a case of well-localized abdominal pain), and genitourinary issues (cystitis, pyelonephritis, prostatitis) are other common causes of abdominal pain in older people [25].

Chest or back pain is the most commonly reported chief complaint of acute aortic dissection and intramural hematoma [33].

Fecal impaction is often revealed by shortness of breath [21, 22] and atypical symptoms linked to complications (infectious, systemic inflammatory response syndrome, cardiopulmonary complications) [34]. A cough can be the unique symptom of cardiac failure or pulmonary embolism [23, 24].

4.2.1.6 Atypical Presentations Due to Subnormal Response to Acute Conditions in Older People

A cough may be mild in pneumonia, without copious, purulent sputum, especially in dehydrated patients. Older patients with sepsis (diverticulitis, appendicitis, etc.) are often afebrile, and many have a normal white blood cell count [35].

In contrast, abdominal pain and tenderness may be absent in abdominal acutely life-threatening conditions, such as acute mesenteric ischemia (mortality estimates above 50%), and patients presenting often initially with vomiting and diarrhea and with complaints of intermittent abdominal pain when eating [25].

Systematic geriatric clinical and biological assessment is necessary for older ED patients, even in the lack of vital signs, to avoid misdiagnosis of life-threatening conditions and conditions that are associated with poor prognosis and intensive care unit admission in older patients with vulnerability factors [36, 37].

4.2.2 Assessment of Preadmission Functional and Health Status in Older ED Patients

Older patients have often preadmission morbidities, functional deficits, complaints, and treatments that complicate diagnosis and treatment of acute life-threatening conditions. Careful examination is therefore required to compare accurate changes in health status between the preadmission and admission.

4.2.2.1 Examples of Clinical and Biological Results in the Normal Range that Must Be Considered as Abnormal Signs and Symptoms

Clinical Pitfalls
In patients with a usual high blood pressure, a normal blood pressure must be considered as a relative hypotension that can be the first sign of an acute bleeding or a life-threatening sepsis [25]. An impaired mental status can be wrongly interpreted as a usual mental status in demented patients, whereas it can be due to delirium (worsening of mental status), stressing the importance of the question considering any difference with the daily usual mental status from a proxy family member. Similarly, pain due to serious conditions can be wrongly considered as a normal state in older patients with chronic pain and under-recognized in demented patients [38]. Acute stroke can be easily misdiagnosed in older people with poststroke locomotor disorders [29].

Biological Pitfalls
In a patient with signs of extracellular dehydration, increased hemoglobin is expected, and normal hemoglobin indicates anemia. Similarly, hemoglobin concentration may be normal in the first few hours after a major bleed because hemoglobin concentrations only fall after hemodilution occurs. Decisions regarding blood transfusion in actively bleeding patients rely on estimated blood loss and tissue hypoxia more than hemoglobin level.

A normal level of serum creatinine in a very aged older person can indicate kidney failure and result in overdosing of renal excreted and/or metabolized drugs or in using contraindicated iodine. To avoid renal failure misdiagnosis, determination of serum creatinine should be systematically accompanied by an estimate of the glomerular filtration rate in older ED patients, as calculated by CKD-EPI, MDRD, Cockcroft, and Gault, or BIS1 equations [39], even though these formulas are validated only in stable conditions [40].

Electrocardiogram
As indicated previously, electrocardiogram should be systematically performed in older ED patients to diagnose coronary, rhythm, metabolic (kaliemia), and drug

(digoxin) disorders. However, myocardial infarction may be challenging in the presence of left bundle branch block, requiring specific diagnosis criteria [41]. Measurement of serum troponin levels has the potential to refine the risk stratification in this case [42] (see Chap. 17). Older people presenting to the ED are also commonly found to have measurable troponin levels using high-sensitivity cardiac troponin T assays. In one study conducted in ED, it was impossible with high-sensitivity assays to assign a working diagnosis of AMI using only a serum troponin concentration, especially among older patients [43].

4.2.2.2 Examples of Expected Clinical and Biological Findings, Not in the Normal Range

For example, pupil diameter can be wrongly interpreted as abnormal in older patients with prior cataract surgery or who use ophthalmic eye drops or systemic drugs (i.e., opioids) [44]. Neck stiffness can wrongly be considered as meningism in patients with Parkinson's disease. Comparison with baseline status may be particularly difficult in older patients with preadmission cognitive impairment or dementia, in whom direct questioning can be unspecific or non-informative. In this case, obtaining a detailed history from a proxy family member, a caregiver, or a nursing home staff is critical to understand the exact situation.

4.2.2.3 Medication History

Older patients consume one-third of all prescription drugs and purchase 40% of over-the-counter medications [45, 46]. Adverse drug events account up to 16% of emergency visits of older patients [47]. Inappropriate prescribing accounts for at least 17 million ED visits and 8.7 million hospital admissions annually in the United States [48, 49]. Two-thirds of emergency hospitalizations occur due to four medication classes: warfarin, oral antiplatelet agents, insulin, and oral hypoglycemic agents [50].

Alcohol consumption and recent dosage changes and removal or additions to the patient's medication regimen should be looked for since significant ingestion or withdrawal from drugs as well as increased dosages and history of taking over the counter can induce serious adverse effects, such as bleeding or acute delirium [19]. Alternative medications also have to be looked for since choking and pill-induced dysphagia can be due to dietary supplements among older adults [51]. Nevertheless, only 40–60% of adverse drug events (ADE) are recognized in the ED. For example, hyponatremia secondary to thiazide diuretics that induces malaise/lethargy, dizziness, and vomiting is often not diagnosed in EDs [52]. Detecting and avoiding ADEs could be aided by using lists of potentially inappropriate drugs for older patients [53], such as Beers criteria [54] or STOPP/START [55, 56]. Medication reconciliation during admission to an ED involving a pharmacist and drawing up a history of complete medication could contribute toward reducing the risk of drug-related adverse effects and improve follow-up of patients' medication-based therapy [57]. When appropriate, the name of the medication, dose of concern, recommendations for safer medications, and modifications to doses should be concerned and documented in the ED.

4.2.3 Assessment of Homeostatic Reserves in Older ED People

Contrary to robust and young people, outcomes of acute conditions in older frail ED patients depend not only on the acute condition but also on homeostatic reserves to cope with the acute condition and treatment required by the condition. Determining whether the older patient is frail, i.e., his (her) medical, psychological, and functional ability to cope with the acute condition is weak, is crucial to adapt care of older ED people with life-threatening conditions. Indeed, patients who are vulnerable or frail will require a relatively benign insult to developing functional and mental decline and multiorgan failures [16]. For example, in the case of pneumonia, older patient's functional status is a much better predictor of mortality than bacterial virulence [58].

Patients with vulnerability factors are those who have already functional disabilities, those with comorbidities (and polypharmacy), or those who are at risk of disability.

4.2.3.1 Assessment of Functional Disability

Functional ability refers to an individual's capacity to complete everyday tasks necessary to live independently, commonly divided into basic activities of daily living (BADL) (including grooming, feeding, and toileting) [59], especially useful in already disabled older people (nursing home residents or who need assistance at home) and instrumental activities of daily living (IADL) (more cognitively complex activities such as operating a motor vehicle, managing finances, and cooking) [60] useful to assess in older patients at the early stage of disability.

Change in mobility and balance from preadmission to admission can be assessed by assessing loss of independence in getting out of the bed and walking or using the Barthel Index (independence in feeding, walking on level surface/moving from wheelchair to bed, personal toilet, getting on/off toilet, bathing, ascend/descend stairs, dressing, controlling bowels and bladder) [61].

Patients who need assistance are at high risk for poor outcome after ED admission [62].

4.2.3.2 Assessment of Morbid Conditions and Their Functional Consequences

The Rockwood Frailty Index includes variables of symptoms, signs, laboratory values, morbid conditions, and items of functional disability (e.g., problems getting dressed, problems with bathing, and impaired mobility), considering that single deficit may be not directly correlated with a negative outcome but contribute to increase the vulnerability of the patient [63–65]. A more simple version of this index is the Clinical Frailty Scale, which can be completed in 40 s and should prompt a more holistic assessment if frailty is identified [66].

4.2.3.3 Other Indicators of Poor Homeostatic Reserves in Older ED Patients

Preadmission sarcopenia [67, 68], unintentional weight loss, muscle weakness, exhaustion, slow walking speed, low level of physical activity [28], history of dementia or delirium [69, 70], anemia [71, 72], protein-energy undernutrition [73], polypharmacy [74], frequent infections, falls, taking three pills or more [62], hospitalization in the past 6 months or visual impairment [62], fluctuating disability, and living in a nursing home as well as living home alone [75] can also be used as vulnerability factors to identify ED patient at poor outcomes for whom preventative strategies and resource allocation should be tailored [76].

4.3 Secondary Assessment for Older ED Patients with Life-Threatening Conditions

As indicated previously, the correct approach to care older ED patients with life-threatening conditions is to identify, without delaying management and treatment, all problems and failures that can aggravate outcomes through an appropriate secondary assessment, considering that:

- Minor functional, mental, or health symptoms can be atypical signs of life-threatening conditions or of conditions that can become life-threatening in older patients with low homeostatic reserves, reserves that have therefore to be assessed.
- All medical and biological findings have to be interpreted as "expected" or "unexpected" signs based on baseline preadmission mental, functional, psychological, and health status and medical and surgical history.
- Adverse drug effects are frequent causes of life-threatening conditions in older people, justifying an extensive review of prescription and of over-the-counter and alternative drugs.
- Assessment of pain, identification of psychosocial, and spiritual problems are part of the optimized palliative care necessary to improve the quality of life of older patients and their families facing life-threatening conditions.
- Emergency physicians are under huge time constraints. Secondary geriatric assessment cannot be exhaustive, and tools must be adapted to the specific case of critically ill older patients. The secondary assessment goal is therefore to identify problems or failures that can aggravate short- or medium-term outcome of the patient. A more comprehensive (tertiary) geriatric assessment will be performed in a second step (including the assessment risk of malnutrition that has no interest in the early care of critically ill older patients) when the life of the patient will not anymore be threatened. This tertiary CGA, which will use tools in order to develop a coordinated and integrated plan for treatment, rehabilitation, and long-term follow-up, is not presented in the present document [15, 77, 78].

After the primary assessment based on the airway, breathing, circulation (ABC) approach (see Chap. 3), the secondary geriatric assessment of patients with life-threatening conditions should include:

4.3.1 Assessment of Preadmission Functional, Mental, Psychological, and Health Status, Medical and Surgical History, and Vulnerability Factors (cf Sects. 4.2.2 and 4.2.3)

Findings in ED patients must be interpreted as expected or unexpected findings based on comprehensive preadmission assessment. Prior diagnoses of venous thromboembolism or recent surgery or trauma are, for example, important information to collect to rule out pulmonary embolism [79]. Advanced directives, health-care power of attorney, and living will have to be looked for. History can be obtained with the patient or inpatient with acute brain dysfunction or communication difficulties, with a family member, caregivers, or a nursing home staff if the patient resides in one.

4.3.2 Vital Signs and General Appearance

- All findings at the presentation examination must be classified as expected or unexpected in comparison with baseline status (no change, worsening).
- Blood pressure must be interpreted based on usual blood pressure, considering that antihypertensive drugs have perhaps been withdrawn due to the life-threatening condition. As indicated previously, a normal blood pressure can be the first sign of shock in a patient with a usual high blood pressure.
- Temperature must be interpreted with caution in older critically ill patients because fever is frequently absent in older people in diseases known to cause fever in adults [80]. Acetaminophen and anti-inflammatory drugs can modify the response of older patients. Hypothermia is a risk factor for mortality in older ED patients with sepsis [81]. C-reactive protein, absolute neutrophil count, and procalcitonin (for ruling out bacteremia) may be useful in the diagnosis process [82].
- Body weight: a medical history of acute or subacute weight loss may be indicative of dehydration or undernutrition, and acute and subacute weight gain may be indicative of heart or kidney failure [83, 84].
- Pain: Pain severity can be assessed overall, and in 15 parts of the body, using a 0–10 numeric rating scale [85, 86] or using the Pain Assessment in Advanced Dementia (PAINAD) in patients with advanced dementia [38, 87–89] (see Chap. 22).

The patient should be completely exposed, and the skin should be examined for medication patches (e.g., fentanyl or scopolamine). Initial skin observation includes color (pale, cyanotic, etc.), signs of tissue ischemia, bruises, infection, pressure ulcers, and signs of skin frailty (thin, friable skin). Indeed, materials such as medical tape and adhesive devices may result in frail people in skin injury, improperly positioned drainage catheters, and loss of intravenous access. In older patients with mobility impairment, pressure ulcer risk should be assessed by using a validated tool, such as the Braden Scale [90, 91].

4.3.3 Head to Toe Examination

As indicated in the chapter "Primary assessment and stabilization of life-threatening conditions of older patients," the Richmond Agitation-Sedation Scale (RASS) should be used to determine consciousness in any older ED patients. The Richmond Agitation-Sedation Scale (RASS) ranges from −5 (unresponsive to pain and voice) to +4 (extreme combativeness) [92], with stupor (RASS −4) (deep sleep in a patient who can be aroused only with vigorous and continuous stimulation) and coma (RASS −5) (state of unresponsiveness in which the patient cannot be aroused with any stimuli) [92]. In the case of stupor or coma, a validated coma scale such as the GCS should be used, considering that the more the level of consciousness is disturbed, the more the underlying life-threatening acute medical illness is concerning [19].

As written above, delirium is often missed in older ED patients and should be screened using RASS [93]. If RASS is of −3 and above, a brief delirium assessment, such as mRASS, or for higher sensitivity the CAM-ICU should be used [93–96]. Establishing comparison with baseline mental status of patients with caregivers is critical, delirium being characterized by an acute worsening of pre-existing mental status [95] (see Chap. 13). Some simple tests such as the Mini Clock Drawing Test [98, 99], the Six-Item Screener (SIS) [three questions on temporal orientation (day, month, and year) and three-item recall: A score of 4 or less indicates a positive screen for cognitive impairment] [100, 101], or the Mini-Cog, which consists of three-item recall and a clock drawing [102, 103], can adequately detect dementia in older ED patients who are not delirious [104, 105].

Depression tends to amplify both symptoms of illnesses, including pain and discomfort. Besides, increased severity of medical illness could also lead to increased symptoms of depression [106]. Conversely, symptoms, such as short breathiness, pain, or fatigue, due to life-threatening conditions, such as heart failure, pulmonary embolism or acute coronary syndrome, can be wrongly interpreted as due to depression [107]. Short questionnaires such as the three-question screening test developed by Arroll et al. can be used to screen older people at risk of depression. In patients with at least two out of three questions answered positive, a complementary psychiatric examination should be proposed [108].

Head examination should look for cyanosis, conjunctival pallor suggesting anemia [109], and any signs of recent trauma. Modified pupil size can be due to surgery history or drugs (i.e., opioid toxicity) [110, 44]. Focal, lateralizing neurological symptoms are suggestive of a central nervous system insult (e.g., cerebrovascular accident, intraparenchymal hemorrhage, or mass effect). The presence of repetitive movement of the eyelids, eyes, or extremities may be suggestive of a seizure.

The sensory exam is also important since poor vision and hearing are risk factors of delirium and poor vision is a risk factor for ED admission for falls [111] and adverse health outcome after ED admission [62]. Patients with poor hearing are disadvantaged in their ability to understand speech, thus limiting their participation in decision-making. After provision of usual aids, vision and hearing can be assessed with a validated test such as the Snellen eye chart [112] for vision and a brief hearing loss screener [113], for hearing, respectively. The mouth has to be inspected after removal of dentures, especially to check the absence of the foreign body in case of respiratory failure.

Neck examination should look for thyromegaly, which can be associated with hypo-/hyperthyroidism, and meningismus. The impairment of airway protective reflexes, i.e., swallowing and cough reflexes, is thought to be one of the major causes of aspiration pneumonia in older people.

Pulmonary and heart examination: Cardiac and pulmonary diseases often acutely affect one another in older patients. Pulses and blood pressure are checked in both arms. Pulse is taken for 30 s, and any irregularity is noted. A rate of >25 breaths/min or tachycardia may be the first sign of a lower respiratory tract infection, heart failure, or another disorder. Because signs and symptoms of acute pulmonary and heart diseases are often atypical, blood biomarkers are increasingly used to assist in rapid decision-making in the ED [114].

Abdomen examination should look for any acute surgical emergencies such as acute appendicitis, diverticulitis, cholecystitis, abdominal aortic aneurysms, or urinary retention.

Severe low back pain, with marked sacral tenderness, may indicate spontaneous osteoporotic fractures. Back pain can be referral pain of underlying life-threatening abdominal conditions (i.e., abdominal aortic aneurysm).

Rectal examination should look for fecal impaction, especially in patients with chronic constipation and use drugs that induce constipation (anticholinergic drugs, opioids especially) [115, 116], and for signs of prostatitis. Fecal occult blood testing might also be done.

Lower limbs: The exam looks for signs of hip and leg fracture in fallers, arterial insufficiency (signs of ischemia including abnormal nail bed capillary refill and decreased pulses), phlebitis (unilateral leg swelling) [79], and heart failure (proximal and distal edema, while more peripheral edema is a sign of venous insufficiency), ulcers (arterial ulcers present distally with claudication and ischemia, while venous ulcers present painlessly and are usually located near the medial malleoli), and signs of extracellular dehydration (skin turgor), which is not a reliable sign in older patients.

Patient's comorbidity can be assessed with the Modified Cumulative Illness Rating Scale (CIRS). The CIRS evaluates 14 biological systems, ranging from 0 (absence of a disorder) to 4 (acute organ insufficiency requiring emergency therapy). The total CIRS ranges from 0 to 56, with a higher score indicating a higher level of comorbidity [117].

4.3.4 Further Testing

4.3.4.1 Electrocardiogram

The high risk to older patients attending ED with atypical signs and symptoms of life-threatening conditions such as infection, impaired perfusion, terminal vascular events, medication reaction(s), toxicological events, and ischemia should prompt the utilization of electrocardiogram (ECG) and laboratory screening for cardiovascular injury and metabolic disturbance(s) to be routine. A 12-lead electrocardiogram should be systematically performed in all older ED patients and may be completed by right and posterior derivations in case of coronary syndrome suspicion. Myocardial infarction is a challenged diagnosis in the presence of left bundle branch block. Measurement of serum troponin levels has the potential to help for the risk stratification in this case [42]. Prolongation of the heart rate-corrected QT interval (QTc) should also be systematically looked for, since it is an independent risk factor for predicting future acute coronary syndrome (ACS) occurrence or mortality in patients with at least one cardiac risk factor presenting with chest pain to the ED [118].

4.3.4.2 Laboratory Testing

Systematically Ordered

Stick blood glucose should be obtained immediately to rule out hypoglycemia, especially in the case of a neurological symptom.

Serum electrolytes should also be routinely obtained to rule out electrolyte abnormalities such as hypernatremia, hyponatremia, hypokalemia, hyperkalemia, hypercalcemia, or hypocalcemia.

Blood urea nitrogen and serum creatinine (to estimate glomerular filtration rate) must be systematically ordered because renal failure can precipitate delirium or functional decline, may contra-indicate enhanced CT, can be the marker of a urinary retention, sepsis, and abdominal emergencies, such as acute mesenteric ischemia [119], and is a significant risk factor for drug adverse effects in older ED patients [120], a [23, 24].

Levels of C-Reactive Protein should be measured systematically, since a quarter of pneumonia and urinary tract infections lack the typical symptoms (presenting with delirium or functional decline, without fever, especially) ([121–125]).

Transaminases and gamma-glutamyl transferase (GGT) should be systematically ordered because biliary disorders may result in nonspecific mental and physical deterioration without jaundice, fever, or abdominal pain [126]. Elevated serum aspartate and alanine aminotransferase (AST and ALT) are also signs of hypoxic liver injury in case of acute heart failure necessitating prompt strategies to improve hemodynamic profile [127, 128], are elevated in case of rhabdomyolysis in the absence of significant liver injury or hypothyroidism [129, 130], and may be a sign of drug adverse effects [131].

4.3.4.3 Context-Dependent Testings

Creatine kinase may be measured after a fall or in case of elevated aminotransferase.

Thyroid-stimulating hormone and free T4 can also be considered in the presence of signs of hyperthyroidism or hypothyroidism, which are often atypical in older ED patients [83].

High-sensitivity troponin: Because signs and symptoms of acute coronary syndrome are often atypical in older ED patients, high-sensitivity troponin, such as ECG, is routinely used in older ED patients.

B-type natriuretic peptide (BNP) is not valuable when heart failure is obvious at the clinical examination but should be used in case of dyspnea of unknown cause, to mainly rule out heart failure, when <100 pg/ml [132]. BNP is elevated in both decompensated right- and left-sided HF. NT-proBNP generally shows similar diagnostic implications to BNP.

D-dimer can be used to rule out pulmonary embolism when <500 ng/ml [133]. However, D-dimer levels increase with age. Therefore, D-Dimer cutoff value to rule out pulmonary embolism should be adjusted for age (age × 10 μg/l above age 50 years) [134–136].

Urinalysis: Because urinary tract infections are frequent and common causes of ED visits, a urinalysis should be performed in patients with atypical symptoms, such as delirium and functional decline without an obvious source (see Chap. 16).

Procalcitonin, which is not useful in patients with typical signs of bacterial infection, may be valuable in case of fever or respiratory complaints without source and for prognosis (in pneumonia) [137, 138] and for meningitis diagnosis [139]. Procalcitonin levels in early stages of sepsis are significantly lower among survivors as compared with nonsurvivors of sepsis [140, 141].

Arterial or venous blood gas should be considered in patients with respiratory complaints or issues.

Serum drug levels should also be ordered if the patient is on medications that can be measured in the serum (i.e., digoxin).

A lumbar puncture can be considered if no other etiologies for delirium, stupor, or coma are found [142].

4.3.5 Special Considerations During the Secondary Assessment

4.3.5.1 Trauma in Older Patients
Rates of ED-treated unintentional injuries, driven mainly by falls among older adults, increase in the United States and Europe [143]. Adults older than 65 years currently account for almost a quarter of all traumas [144–146].

Head injury constitutes one of the most common and severe injuries sustained in older fallers who attend the ED [71] and a predictor of subsequent ED visits [147]. Head and neck CT scan should be done more systematically [148–151].

Hip fracture is the perfect example of an acute condition in which baseline homeostatic reserves play a significantly higher role in outcome than the condition itself. Indeed, handgrip strength, functional and health status, depression, and cognitive impairment are the main predictors of short-term outcome in hip-fractured patients attending the ED [152–154]. Management of people with older hip fractures should therefore not focus only on the primary concern (hip fracture surgery) but identify all problems that can interfere with the primary concern. The British Orthopedic Association and the British Geriatrics Society have produced the Blue Book, which summarizes current evidence and best practice consensus in the care and secondary prevention of fragility fractures (http://www.bgs.org.uk/pdf_cms/pubs/Blue%20Book%20on%20fragility%20fracture%20care.pdf).

All patients who attend the ED with a hip fracture should be admitted to an acute orthopedic ward within 4 h of presentation and have surgery within 48 h of admission wherever possible, and management with geriatrician should be organized. All patients presenting with fragility fracture should also be assessed to determine their need for bone protection and should be offered a fall multidisciplinary assessment and intervention to prevent future falls and fractures [155].

The American Geriatrics Society and British Geriatrics Society have published in 2011 guidelines for older ED adult fallers that recommend multifactorial fall risk evaluations for modifiable factors such as orthostatic hypotension, vision, hearing, balance and gait, instrumental and non-instrumental activities of daily living, cognition, depression, neurological, and musculoskeletal function, alcohol use, certain comorbidities and health problems, review of lighting in the environment and other environmental hazards, fall history, exercise, behavior modification, feet, footwear, assistive devices, and medications [156]. Gradual withdrawal of psychotropic medication especially reduces rate of falls in older fallers [157].

The implementation of specific measures in ED older fallers has shown a beneficial impact on the fall recurrence rate [158].

4.3.5.2 Abdominal Symptoms in Older ED Patients

Acute abdominal pain accounts for 13% of ED visits in older patients [159]. Diagnosis of acute abdominal pain in older persons is a challenge, given the unreliability of clinical and biological predictors of disease, overlapping presentations and coexisting disease in this population [160]. Acute bowel infarction may be indicated by acute confusion. Abdominal pain and tenderness may be absent in severe abdominal conditions. Appendicitis pain tends to begin in the right lower quadrant rather than periumbilical. Eventually, pain may be diffuse in the abdomen rather than localized to the right lower quadrant. However, tenderness in this quadrant is a significant early sign. Because of common atypical presentation, the use of enhanced CT scanning allows making diagnosis of abdominal emergencies in a timely fashion [161, 162].

4.3.5.3 Care for Older People with Cognitive Impairment in Emergency Departments (SQIs)

Indicators of quality of care have been defined to assess care for older people with cognitive impairment (SQIs) in EDs. Indeed, clinical assessment is often made difficult by a low reliability of the medical history. Family and usual caregivers must be involved for getting the most accurate information. Indicators of quality of care of older people with cognitive impairment include therefore the presence in the ED of a policy outlining the management of older people with cognitive impairment and their caregivers and prevention, assessment, and management of behavioral symptoms, delirium, and pain [163].

4.4 Strategies to Improve Quality of Care and Outcomes

4.4.1 Liaison Services

The first strategy tested in order to improve the prognosis of older ED patients is called referral or liaison service. This strategy consists of the screening by a care provider (usually a nurse or a social worker) of older patients potentially at risk for poor outcomes after the ED visit, followed by recommendations or referral for follow-up with the regular or other physicians [164–168].

Different assessment geriatric tools have been developed to screen ED patients at risk of repeat visits or poor outcome [164–166, 169–176]. These tools comprise quite similar items, including a high number of medications (indicator of multiple chronic conditions and risk factor of adverse effect; see Sect 4.4.2.), previous ED use, hospital or community services, issues of self-care, history of falls, caregiving responsibilities and living alone, age, and cognitive impairment [172]. Referral or liaison service strategy may reduce with a small to moderate success the number of return visits to the ED, admissions to nursing homes, and death in older people [164–167].

The assessment can be a comprehensive geriatric assessment, implemented by a care coordination team comprising a geriatrician, a nurse, and a social worker, in order to provide an individualized care plan including counseling, education, treatment changes, and referrals to community services and interdisciplinary teams. This plan can be associated with a follow-up at home [169, 170]. This strategy is effective in reducing ED revisits rates and hospitalizations [169, 170]. This strategy seems more effective when the comprehensive geriatric assessment and the care plan are implemented by a team comprising a geriatrician [171].

Taken together, and despite inconsistencies across validity of the screening tools, interventions, and reported outcomes [177], the above studies suggest that interventions based on risk prediction tool to screen frail older people [178, 179] followed by individualized, integrated care, including advice by a geriatrician, may be effective in improving outcomes in older adults after ED discharge [77, 78, 180, 181]. The difficulty is the practical and broad implementation of this integrated care model, due to its complex nature [182].

4.4.2 The Geriatric Emergency Health-Care Centers

In 1992, the Society for Academic Emergency Medicine has recognized the special needs of older patients in ED and has made recommendations for increasing expertise in geriatrics among emergency medical specialists and for investigating the point of setting up emergency health-care centers analogous to trauma centers or pediatric centers [183]. Just as pediatric population, geriatric patients are a unique population and require specialized environment, protocols, medications, and equipment to provide the best evidence-based care. The goal of a geriatric ED should be to create, operate, and sustain safe and effective emergency services that meet the complex and uncertain needs of older patients and those who care for them. In 2014, the American College of Emergency Physicians, American Geriatrics Society, Emergency Nurses Association, and Society Academic Emergency Medicine have published new "Geriatric Emergency Departments Guidelines" to characterize the essential attribute of a "Geriatric ED" [184]. The geriatric ED guidelines consisted of 40 specific recommendations in 6 general categories: staffing (recommendations for the medical director and nurse manager and accessibility to specialist ancillary services), transitions of care (discharge processes, appropriate collaboration with home health services, and home safety assessments), nurse and physician education, care indicators (including falls prevalence and prevention), equipment/supplies (including reclining chairs and pressure-redistributing foam mattresses to reduce the incidence of pressure ulcers), and different tools to facilitate screening for older adults at increased risk for post-ED discharge functional decline, recidivism, or institutionalization, as well as validated and ED-feasible screening instruments for geriatric syndromes like delirium, polypharmacy, falls, and dementia. Guidelines are freely available on each organization's website (i.e., http://www.saem.org/docs/default-source/education/geri_ed_guidelines_final.pdf?sfvrsn=4). The authors insisted on the fact that the general principles defined in the guidelines had to be tailored for each ED based on patient needs and available resources and that effective implementation of these recommendations would require time to attain. Indeed, and, for example, for older patients who have ED fall visit, the current evaluation is discordant with general and ED-specific [156] Geriatric Emergency Department Guidelines [181].

Conclusion

People aged 65 years and older have a high rate of ED use for life-threatening conditions, poorer outcome, and a higher risk of a revisit. In order to improve prognosis of older ED patients and prevent revisits, it is now recommended to incorporate geriatric assessment into the ED to make care recommendations, particularly for those with complex issues, poor homeostatic reserves (disability, cognitive impairment, comorbidities, and signs of frailty), in whom expression of life-threatening conditions are often atypical. Without delaying management of immediate life-threatening conditions, comprehensive functional, mental, health, medication, psychosocial, and spiritual geriatric assessment in ED patients allow to reduce misdiagnosis of serious conditions with atypical presentation; identify all problems and failures that can aggravate outcome; adapt care to characteristics of patients, especially for demented or delirious patients and to desires of patients; and offer optimized palliative care necessary to improve the quality of life of older patients and their families facing life-threatening conditions. Even if the attribute of geriatric EDs is now well characterized [184], efforts must be pursued to promote the practical and broad implementation of integrated care models for older ED people, with a tailored organization for each ED based on patient needs and available resources.

References

1. McCusker J, Cardin S, Bellavance F, Belzile E (2000) Return to the emergency department among elders: patterns and predictors. Acad Emerg Med 7:249–259
2. Rosted E, Wagner L, Hendriksen C, Poulsen I (2012) Geriatric nursing assessment and intervention in an emergency department: a pilot study. Int J Older People Nursing 7:141–151
3. Adams JG, Gerson LW (2003) A new model for emergency care of geriatric patients. Acad Emerg Med 10:271–274
4. Gruneir A, Silver MJ, Rochon PA (2011) Emergency department use by older adults: a literature review on trends, appropriateness, and consequences of unmet health care needs. Med Care Res Rev 68:131–155
5. Schumacher JG (2005) Emergency medicine and older adults: continuing challenges and opportunities. Am J Emerg Med 23:556–560
6. Aminzadeh F, Dalziel WB (2002) Older adults in the emergency department: a systematic review of patterns of use, adverse outcomes, and effectiveness of interventions. Ann Emerg Med 39:238–247
7. Foo CL, Siu VW, Tan TL, Ding YY, Seow E (2012) Geriatric assessment and intervention in an emergency department observation unit reduced re-attendance and hospitalisation rates. Australas J Ageing 31:40–46
8. Hwang U, Morrison RS (2007) The geriatric emergency department. J Am Geriatr Soc 55:1873–1876
9. Lowenstein SR, Crescenzi CA, Kern DC, Steel K (1986) Care of the elderly in the emergency department. Ann Emerg Med 15:528–535
10. Basic D, Conforti DA (2005) A prospective, randomised controlled trial of an aged care nurse intervention within the emergency department. Aust Health Rev 29:51–59
11. McCoy HV, Kipp CW, Ahern M (1992) Reducing older patients' reliance on the emergency department. Soc Work Health Care 17:23–37
12. McCusker J, Dendukuri N, Tousignant P, Verdon J, Poulin de Courval L, Belzile E (2003) Rapid two-stage emergency department intervention for seniors: impact on continuity of care. Acad Emerg Med 10:233–243
13. Besdine RW (1983) The educational utility of comprehensive functional assessment in the elderly. J Am Geriatr Soc 31:651–656
14. Heppenstall CP, Wilkinson TJ, Hanger HC, Keeling S (2009) Frailty: dominos or deliberation? N Z Med J 122:42–53
15. Rubenstein LZ, Stuck AE, Siu AL, Wieland D (1991) Impacts of geriatric evaluation and management programs on defined outcomes: overview of the evidence. J Am Geriatr Soc 39:8S–16S
16. Han JH, Zimmerman EE, Cutler N et al (2009) Delirium in older emergency department patients: recognition, risk factors, and psychomotor subtypes. Acad Emerg Med 16:193–200
17. Kennedy M, Enander RA, Wolfe RE, Marcantonio ER, Shapiro NI (2012) Identification of delirium in elderly emergency department patients. Acad Emerg Med 19:S147
18. Han JH, Eden S, Shintani A, Morandi A, Schnelle J, Dittus RS, Storrow AB, Ely EW (2011) Delirium in older emergency department patients is an independent predictor of hospital length of stay. Acad Emerg Med 18:451–457
19. Han JH, Wilber ST (2013) Altered mental status in older patients in the emergency department. Clin Geriatr Med 29:101–136
20. Kennedy M, Enander RA, Tadiri SP, Wolfe RE, Shapiro NI, Marcantonio ER (2014) Delirium risk prediction, healthcare use and mortality of elderly adults in the emergency department. J Am Geriatr Soc 62:462–469
21. Gillis NK, Arslanian-Engoren C, Struble LM (2014) Acute coronary syndromes in older adults: a review of literature. J Emerg Nurs 40:270–275
22. Grosmaitre P, Le Vavasseur O, Yachouh E, Courtial Y, Jacob X, Meyran S, Lantelme P (2013) Significance of atypical symptoms for the diagnosis and management of myocardial infarction in elderly patients admitted to emergency departments. Arch Cardiovasc Dis 106:586–592

23. Hendriksen JM, Geersing GJ, Lucassen WA, Erkens PM, Stoffers HE, van Weert HC, Büller HR, Hoes AW, Moons KG (2015) Diagnostic prediction models for suspected pulmonary embolism: systematic review and independent external validation in primary care. BMJ 351:h4438
24. Righini M, Le Gal G, Bounameaux H (2015) Venous thromboembolism diagnosis: unresolved issues. Thromb Haemost 113:1184–1192
25. Spangler R, Van Pham T, Khoujah D, Martinez JP (2014) Abdominal emergencies in the geriatric patient. Int J Emerg Med 7:43
26. Asplund R (2005) Nocturia in relation to sleep, health, and medical treatment in the elderly. BJU Int 96(Suppl 1):15–21
27. Rockwood K, Rockwood MR, Andrew MK, Mitnitski A (2008) Reliability of the hierarchical assessment of balance and mobility in frail older adults. J Am Geriatr Soc 56:1213–1217
28. Fried LP, Tangen CM, Walston J, Newman AB, Hirsch C, Gottdiener J et al (2001) Frailty in older adults: evidence for a phenotype. J Gerontol A Biol Sci Med Sci 56:M146–M156
29. Arch AE, Weisman DC, Coca S, Nystrom KV, Wira CR, Schindler JL (2016) Missed ischemic stroke diagnosis in the emergency department by emergency medicine and neurology services. Stroke 47:668–673
30. Coventry LL, Bremner AP, Jacobs IG, Finn J (2013) Myocardial infarction: sex differences in symptoms reported to emergency dispatch. Prehosp Emerg Care 17:193–202
31. Leuthauser A, McVane B (2016) Abdominal pain in the geriatric patient. Emerg Med Clin North Am 34:363–375
32. Canto JG, Shlipak MG, Rogers WJ, Malmgren J, Frederick P, Lambrew CT, Ornato JP, Kiefe CI (2000) Prevalence, clinical characteristics and mortality among patients with myocardial infarction presenting without chest pain. JAMA 283:3223–3229
33. Mussa FF, Horton JD, Moridzadeh R, Nicholson J, Trimarchi S, Eagle KA (2016) Acute aortic dissection and intramural hematoma: a systematic review. JAMA 316:754V763
34. Halawi HM, Maasri KA, Mourad FH, Barada KA (2012) Faecal impaction: in-hospital complications and their predictors in a retrospective study on 130 patients. Color Dis 14:231–236
35. Dickinson M, Leo MM (2014) Geriatric emergency medicine: principles and practice. In: Kahn JH, Maguaran BG Jr, Olshaker JS (eds) Gastrointestinal emergencies in the elderly. Cambridge University Press, New York, pp 207–218
36. Ellis G, Marshall T, Ritchie C (2014) Comprehensive geriatric assessment in the emergency department. Clin Interv Aging 9:2033–2043
37. Fan JS, Kao WF, Yen DH, Wang LM, Huang CI, Lee CH (2007) Risk factors and prognostic predictors of unexpected intensive care unit admission within 3 days after ED discharge. Am J Emerg Med 25:1009–1014
38. Somes J, Donatelli NS (2013) Pain assessment in the cognitively impaired or demented older adult. J Emerg Nurs 39:164–167
39. Musso CG, Alvarez-Gregori J, Jauregui J, Núñez JF (2015) Are currently GFR estimating equations and standard Kt/V value adequate for advanced chronic kidney disease (CKD) frail elderly patients? Int Urol Nephrol 47:1231–1232
40. Rosner MH (2013) Acute kidney injury in the elderly. Clin Geriatr Med 29:565–578
41. Meyers HP, Limkakeng AT Jr, Jaffa EJ, Patel A, Theiling BJ, Rezaie SR, Stewart T, Zhuang C, Pera VK, Smith SW (2015) Validation of the modified Sgarbossa criteria for acute coronary occlusion in the setting of left bundle branch block: a retrospective case-control study. Am Heart J 170:1255–1264
42. Ayer A, Terkelsen CJ (2014) Difficult ECGs in STEMI: lessons learned from serial sampling of pre- and in-hospital ECGs. J Electrocardiol 47:448–458
43. Menacer S, Claessens YE, Meune C et al (2013) Reference range values of troponin measured by sensitive assays in elderly patients without any cardiac signs/symptoms. Clin Chim Acta 417:45–47
44. Slattery A, Liebelt E, Gaines LA. Common ocular effects reported to a poison control center after systemic absorption of drugs in therapeutic and toxic doses. Curr Opin Ophthalmol. 2014;25(6):519–23.

45. Hanlon JT, Fillenbaum GG, Ruby CM, Gray S, Bohannon A (2001) Epidemiology of over-the-counter drug use in community dwelling elderly: United States perspective. Drugs Aging 18:123–131
46. Hustey FM, Mion LC, Connor JT, Emerman CL, Campbell J, Palmer RM (2007) A brief risk stratification tool to predict functional decline in older adults discharged from emergency departments. J Am Geriatrics Soc 55:1269–1274
47. Zed PJ, Abu-Laban RB, Balen RM, Loewen PS, Hohl CM, Brubacher JR, Wilbur K, Wiens MO, Samoy LJ, Lacaria K, Purssell RA (2008) Incidence, severity and preventability of medication-related visits to the emergency department: a prospective study. CMAJ 178:1563–1569
48. Bates DW, Spell N, Cullen DJ, Burdick E, Laird N, Petersen LA et al (1997) The costs of adverse drug events in hospitalized patients. Adverse drug events prevention study group. JAMA 277:307
49. Johnson JA, Bootman JL (1995) Drug-related morbidity and mortality. A cost-of-illness model. Arch Int Med 155:1949–1956
50. Budnitz DS, Lovegrove MC, Shehab N, Richards CL (2011) Emergency hospitalizations for adverse drug events in older Americans. N Engl J Med 365:2002–2012
51. Geller AI, Shehab N, Weidle NJ, Lovegrove MC, Wolpert BJ, Timbo BB, Mozersky RP, Budnitz DS (2015) Emergency department visits for adverse events related to dietary supplements. N Engl J Med 373:1531–1540
52. Sardar GK, Eilbert WP (2015) Severe hyponatremia associated with thiazide diuretic use. J Emerg Med 48(3):305–309
53. Brown JD, Hutchison LC, Li C, Painter JT, Martin BC (2016) Predictive validity of the beers and screening tool of older persons' potentially inappropriate prescriptions (STOPP) criteria to detect adverse drug events, hospitalizations, and emergency department visits in the United States. J Am Geriatr Soc 64:22–30
54. American Geriatrics Society 2012 Beers Criteria Update Expert Panel (2012) American Geriatrics Society updated beers criteria for potentially inappropriate medication use in older adults. J Am Geriatr Soc 60:616–631
55. Gallagher P, O'Mahony D (2008) STOPP (screening tool of older persons' potentially inappropriate prescriptions): application to acutely ill elderly patients and comparison with beers' criteria. Age Ageing 37:673–679
56. Hill-Taylor B, Walsh KA, Stewart S, Hayden J, Byrne S, Sketris IS (2016) Effectiveness of the STOPP/START (screening tool of older persons' potentially inappropriate prescriptions/screening tool to alert doctors to the right treatment) criteria: systematic review and meta-analysis of randomized controlled studies. J Clin Pharm Ther 41:158–169
57. Becerra-Camargo J, Martínez-Martínez F, García-Jiménez E (2015) The effect on potential adverse drug events of a pharmacist-acquired medication history in an emergency department: a multicentre, double-blind, randomised, controlled, parallel-group study. BMC Health Serv Res 15:337
58. Polverino E, Torres A, Menendez R, Cilloniz C, Valles JM, Capelastegui A et al (2013) Microbial aetiology of healthcare associated pneumonia in Spain: a prospective, multicentre, case-control study. Thorax 68:1007–1014
59. Katz S, Ford AB, Moskowitz RW, Jackson BA, Jaffe MW (1963) Studies of illness in the aged. The index of Adl: a standardized measure of biological and psychosocial function. JAMA 185:914–919
60. Lawton MP, Brody EM (1969) Assessment of older people: self-maintaining and instrumental activities of daily living. Gerontologist 9:179–186
61. Mahoney FI, Barthel DW (1965) Functional evaluation: the Barthel index. Md State Med J 14:61–65
62. McCusker J, Bellavance F, Cardin S, Trépanier S, Verdon J, Ardman O (1999) Detection of older people at increased risk of adverse health outcomes after an emergency visit: the ISAR screening tool. J Am Geriatr Soc 47:1229–1237
63. Nydegger UE, Luginbühl M, Risch M (2015) The aging human recipient of transfusion products. Transfus Apher Sci 52:290–294

64. Overdyk F, Dahan A, Roozekrans M, van der Schrier R, Aarts L, Niesters M (2014) Opioid-induced respiratory depression in the acute care setting: a compendium of case reports. Pain Manag 4:317–325
65. Rockwood K (2005) Frailty and its definition: a worthy challenge. J Am Geriatr Soc 53:1069–1070
66. Wallis SJ, Wall J, Biram RW, Romero-Ortuno R (2015) Association of the clinical frailty scale with hospital outcomes. QJM 108:943–949
67. Calvani R, Marini F, Cesari M, Tosato M, Anker SD, von Haehling S, Miller RR, Bernabei R, Landi F, Marzetti E, SPRINTT consortium (2015) Biomarkers for physical frailty and sarcopenia: state of the science and future developments. J Cachexia Sarcopenia Muscle 6:278–286
68. Du Y, Karvellas CJ, Baracos V, Williams DC, Khadaroo RG, Acute Care and Emergency Surgery (ACES) Group (2014) Sarcopenia is a predictor of outcomes in very elderly patients undergoing emergency surgery. Surgery 156:521–527
69. Avila-Funes JA, Amieva H, Barberger-Gateau P, Le Goff M, Raoux N, Ritchie K et al (2009) Cognitive impairment improves the predictive validity of the phenotype of frailty for adverse health outcomes: the three-city study. J Am Geriatr Soc 57:453–461
70. Eeles EM, White SV, O'Mahony SM, Bayer AJ, Hubbard RE (2012) The impact of frailty and delirium on mortality in older inpatients. Age Ageing 41:412–416
71. Cartagena LJ, Kang A, Munnangi S, Jordan A, Nweze IC, Sasthakonar V, Boutin A, George Angus LD (2016) Risk factors associated with in-hospital mortality in elderly patients admitted to a regional trauma center after sustaining a fall. Aging Clin Exp Res 29(3):427–433. doi:10.1007/s40520-016-0579-5
72. Röhrig G (2016) Anemia in the frail, elderly patient. Clin Interv Aging 11:319–326
73. Guyonnet S, Secher M, Vellas B (2015) Nutrition, frailty, cognitive frailty and prevention of disabilities with aging. Nestle Nutr Inst Workshop Ser 82:143–152
74. Gómez C, Vega-Quiroga S, Bermejo-Pareja F, Medrano MJ, Louis ED, Benito-León J (2015) Polypharmacy in the elderly: a marker of increased risk of mortality in a population-based prospective study (NEDICES). Gerontology 61:301–309
75. Dramé M, Lang PO, Jolly D, Narbey D, Mahmoudi R, Lanièce I, Somme D, Gauvain JB, Heitz D, Voisin T, de Wazières B, Gonthier R, Ankri J, Saint-Jean O, Jeandel C, Couturier P, Blanchard F, Novella JL (2012) Nursing home admission in elderly subjects with dementia: predictive factors and future challenges. J Am Med Dir Assoc 13:83
76. Clegg A, Young J, Iliffe S, Rikkert MO, Rockwood K (2013) Frailty in elderly people. Lancet 381:752–762
77. Ellis G, Whitehead MA, Robinson D, O'Neill D, Langhorne P (2011) Comprehensive geriatric assessment for older adults admitted to hospital: metaanalysis of randomised controlled trials. BMJ 343:d6553
78. Ellis G, Whitehead MA, O'Neill D, Langhorne P, Robinson D (2011) Comprehensive geriatric assessment for older adults admitted to hospital. Cochrane Database Syst Rev 7:CD006211
79. Kline JA, Courtney DM, Kabrhel C, Moore CL, Smithline HA, Plewa MC, Richman PB, O'Neil BJ, Nordenholz K (2008) Prospective multicenter evaluation of the pulmonary embolism rule-out criteria. J Thromb Haemost 6:772–780
80. Limpawattana P, Phungoen P, Mitsungnern T, Laosuangkoon W, Tansangworn N (2016) Atypical presentations of older adults at the emergency department and associated factors. Arch Gerontol Geriatr 62:97–102
81. Hofman SE, Lucke JA, Heim N, de Gelder J, Fogteloo AJ, Heringhaus C, de Groot B, de Craen AJ, Blauw GJ, Mooijaart SP (2016) Prediction of 90-day mortality in older patients after discharge from an emergency department: a retrospective follow-up study. BMC Emerg Med 16:26
82. Kim SY, Jeong TD, Lee W, Chun S, Min WK (2015) Procalcitonin in the assessment of bacteraemia in emergency department patients: results of a large retrospective study. Ann Clin Biochem 52:654–659
83. Guo F, Xu T, Wang H (2009) Early recognition of myxedematous respiratory failure in the elderly. Am J Emerg Med 27:212–215

84. Lesperance ME, Bell SE, Ervin NE (2005) Heart failure and weight gain monitoring. Lippincotts Case Manage 10:287–293
85. Miro J, Huguet A, Nieto R, Paredes S, Baos J (2005) Evaluation of reliability, validity, and preference for a pain intensity scale for use with the elderly. J Pain 6:727–735
86. Platts-Mills TF, Flannigan SA, Bortsov AV, Smith S, Domeier RM, Swor RA, Hendry PL, Peak DA, Rathlev NK, Jones JS, Lee DC, Keefe FJ, Sloane PD, SA ML (2016) Persistent pain among older adults discharged home from the emergency department after motor vehicle crash: a prospective cohort study. Ann Emerg Med 67:166–176.e1
87. Mosele M, Inelmen EM, Toffanello ED, Girardi A, Coin A, Sergi G, Manzato E (2012) Psychometric properties of the pain assessment in advanced dementia scale compared to self assessment of pain in elderly patients. Dement Geriatr Cogn Disord 34:38–43
88. Platts-Mills TF, Esserman DA, Brown DL, Bortsov AV, Sloane PD, McLean SA (2014) Older US emergency department patients are less likely to receive pain medication than younger patients: results from a national survey. Ann Emerg Med 60:199–206
89. van der Steen JT, Sampson EL, Van den Block L, Lord K, Vankova H, Pautex S, Vandervoort A, Radbruch L, Shvartzman P, Sacchi V, de Vet HC, Van Den Noortgate NJ, EU-COST Action TD1005 Collaborators (2015) Tools to assess pain or lack of comfort in dementia: a content analysis. J Pain Symptom Manag 50:65975.e3
90. Cooper L, Vellodi C, Stansby G, Avital L (2015) The prevention and management of pressure ulcers: summary of updated NICE guidance. J Wound Care 24:179–181
91. Cohen RR, Lagoo-Deenadayalan SA, Heflin MT, Sloane R, Eisen I, Thacker JM, Whitson HE (2012) Exploring predictors of complication in older surgical patients: a deficit accumulation index and the Braden Scale. J Am Geriatr Soc 60(9):1609–1615
92. Ely EW, Truman B, Shintani A et al (2003) Monitoring sedation status over time in ICU patients: reliability and validity of the richmond agitation-sedation scale (RASS). JAMA 289:2983–2991
93. Han JH, Wilson A, Graves AJ, Shintani A, Schnelle JF, Dittus RS, Powers JS, Vernon J, Storrow AB, Ely EW (2014) Validation of the confusion assessment method for the intensive care unit in older emergency department patients. Acad Emerg Med 21:180–187
94. Han JH, Vasilevskis EE, Schnelle JF, Shintani A, Dittus RS, Wilson A, Ely EW (2015) The diagnostic performance of the richmond agitation sedation scale for detecting delirium in older emergency department patients. Acad Emerg Med 22:878–882
95. Morandi A, Han JH, Meagher D, Vasilevskis E, Cerejeira J, Hasemann W, MacLullich AM, Annoni G, Trabucchi M, Bellelli G (2016) Detecting delirium superimposed on dementia: evaluation of the diagnostic performance of the richmond agitation and sedation scale. J Am Med Dir Assoc 17(9):828–833
96. Van de Meeberg EK, Festen S, Kwant M, Georg RR, Izaks GJ, Ter Maaten JC (2016) Improved detection of delirium, implementation and validation of the CAM-ICU in elderly emergency department patients. Eur J Emerg Med. doi:10.1097/MEJ.0000000000000380
97. Hustey FM, Meldon SW, Smith MD, Lex CK (2003) The effect of mental status screening on the care of elderly emergency department patients. Ann Emerg Med 41:678–684
98. Davis KK, Allen JK (2013) Identifying cognitive impairment in heart failure: a review of screening measures. Heart Lung 42:92–97
99. Kirby M, Denihan A, Bruce I, Coakley D, Lawlor BA (2001) The clock drawing test in primary care: sensitivity in dementia detection and specificity against normal and depressed elderly. Int J Geriatr Psychiatry 16:935–940
100. Callahan CM, Unverzagt FW, Hui SL, Perkins AJ, Hendrie HC (2002) Six-item screener to identify cognitive impairment among potential subjects for clinical research. Med Care 40:771–781
101. Wilber ST, Lofgren SD, Mager TG, Blanda M, Gerson LW (2005) An evaluation of two screening tools for cognitive impairment in older emergency department patients. Acad Emerg Med 12:612–616
102. Borson S, Scanlan J, Brush M, Vitaliano P, Dokmak A (2000) The mini-cog: a cognitive "vital signs" measure for dementia screening in multi-lingual elderly. Int J Geriatr Psychiatry 15:1021–1027

103. Scanlan J, Borson S (2001) The mini-cog: receiver operating characteristics with expert and naive raters. Int J Geriatr Psychiatry 16:216–222
104. Lin JS, O'Connor E, Rossom RC, Perdue LA, Eckstrom E (2013) Screening for cognitive impairment in older adults: a systematic review for the U.S. preventive services task force. Ann Intern Med 159:601–612
105. McCabe JJ, Kennelly SP (2015) Acute care of older patients in the emergency department: strategies to improve patient outcomes. Open Access Emerg Med 7:45–54
106. Choi NG, Marti CN, Bruce ML, Kunik ME (2012) Relationship between depressive symptom severity and emergency department use among low-income, depressed homebound older adults aged 50 years and older. BMC Psychiatry 12:233
107. Lutwak N, Dill C (2012) A depressed post-menopausal woman. J Emerg Med 43:815–819
108. Arroll B, Goodyear-Smith F, Kerse N, Fishman T, Gunn J (2005) Effect of the addition of a "help" question to two screening questions on specificity for diagnosis of depression in general practice: diagnostic validity study. BMJ 331:884
109. Sheth TN, Choudhry NK, Bowes M, Detsky AS (1997) The relation of conjunctival pallor to the presence of anemia. J Gen Intern Med 12:102–106
110. Porath-Waller AJ, Beirness DJ (2010) Simplifying the process for identifying drug combinations by drug recognition experts. Traffic Inj Prev 11(5):453–459. doi:10.1080/15389588.2010.489199
111. Scheffer AC, van Hensbroek PB, van Dijk N, Luitse JS, Goslings JC, Luigies RH, de Rooij SE (2013) Risk factors associated with visiting or not visiting the accident & emergency department after a fall. BMC Health Serv Res 13:286
112. Chou R, Dana T, Bougatsos C (2009) Screening older adults for impaired visual acuity: a review of the evidence for the U.S. preventive services task force. Ann Int Med 151:44–58
113. Demers K (2013) Hearing screening in older adults: a brief hearing loss screener. In: Try this: best practices in nursing care to older adults. Hartford Institute for Geriatric Nursing, College of Nursing, New York University, New York:issue 12
114. Suzuki T, Lyon A, Saggar R, Heaney LM, Aizawa K, Cittadini A, Mauro C, Citro R, Limongelli G, Ferrara F, Vriz O, Morley-Smith A, Calabrò P, Bossone E (2016) Editor's Choice-Biomarkers of acute cardiovascular and pulmonary diseases. Eur Heart J Acute Cardiovasc Care 5(5):416–433
115. Collamati A, Martone AM, Poscia A, Brandi V, Celi M, Marzetti E, Cherubini A, Landi F (2016) Anticholinergic drugs and negative outcomes in the older population: from biological plausibility to clinical evidence. Aging Clin Exp Res 28:25–35
116. Roulet L, Ballereau F, Hardouin JB, Chiffoleau A, Potel G, Asseray N (2014) Adverse drug event nonrecognition in emergency departments: an exploratory study on factors related to patients and drugs. J Emerg Med 46:857–864
117. Salvi F, Miller MD, Grilli A, Giorgi R, Towers AL, Morichi V, Spazzafumo L, Mancinelli L, Espinosa E, Rappelli A, Dessì-Fulgheri P (2008) A manual of guidelines to score the modified cumulative illness rating scale and its validation in acute hospitalized elderly patients. J Am Geriatr Soc 56:1926–1931
118. de Venecia TA, Lu MY, Nwakile CC, Figueredo VM (2015) Utility of the QT interval in predicting outcomes in patients presenting to the emergency department with chest pain. Coron Artery Dis 26:422–424
119. Huang HH, Chang YC, Yen DH, Kao WF, Chen JD, Wang LM, Huang CI, Lee CH (2005) Clinical factors and outcomes in patients with acute mesenteric ischemia in the emergency department. J Chin Med Assoc 68:299–306
120. Chen YC, Fan JS, Chen MH, Hsu TF, Huang HH, Cheng KW, Yen DH, Huang CI, Chen LK, Yang CC (2014) Risk factors associated with adverse drug events among older adults in emergency department. Eur J Int Med 25:49–55
121. Bafadhel M, Clark TW, Reid C, Medina MJ, Batham S, Barer MR, Nicholson KG, Brightling CE (2011) Procalcitonin and C-reactive protein in hospitalized adult patients with community-acquired pneumonia or exacerbation of asthma or COPD. Chest 139:1410–1418
122. Albazzaz MK, Pal C, Berman P, Shale DJ. Inflammatory markers of lower respiratory tract infection in elderly people. Age Ageing. 1994;23(4):299–302.

123. Haran JP, Beaudoin FL, Suner S, Lu S. C-reactive protein as predictor of bacterial infection among patients with an influenza-like illness. Am J Emerg Med. 2013 Jan;31(1):137–44.
124. Hortmann M, Singler K, Geier F, Christ M (2015) Recognition of infections in elderly emergency patients. Z Gerontol Geriatr 48:601–607
125. Schuetz P, Daniels LB, Kulkarni P, Anker SD, Mueller B (2016) Procalcitonin: a new biomarker for the cardiologist. Int J Cardiol 223:390–397
126. Zarnescu NO, Costea R, Zarnescu Vasiliu EC, Neagu S (2015) Clinico-biochemical factors to early predict biliary etiology of acute pancreatitis: age, female gender, and ALT. J Med Life 8:523–526
127. Moon J, Kang W, Oh PC, Seo SY, Lee K, Han SH, Ahn T, Shin E (2014) Serum transaminase determined in the emergency room predicts outcomes in patients with acute ST-segment elevation myocardial infarction who undergo primary percutaneous coronary intervention. Int J Cardiol 177:442–447
128. Moreira-Silva S, Urbano J, Moura MC, Ferreira-Coimbra J, Bettencourt P, Pimenta J (2016) Liver cytolysis in acute heart failure: what does it mean? Clinical profile and outcomes of a prospective hospital cohort. Int J Cardiol 221:422–427
129. Weibrecht K, Dayno M, Darling C, Bird SB (2010) Liver aminotransferases are elevated with rhabdomyolysis in the absence of significant liver injury. J Med Toxicol 6(3):294–300
130. Burra P (2013) Liver abnormalities and endocrine diseases. Best Pract Res Clin Gastroenterol 27:553–563
131. Fontana RJ, Hayashi PH, Barnhart H, Kleiner DE, Reddy KR, Chalasani N, Lee WM, Stolz A, Phillips T, Serrano J, Watkins PB (2015) DILIN investigators. Persistent liver biochemistry abnormalities are more common in older patients and those with cholestatic drug induced liver injury. Am J Gastroenterol 110:1450–1459
132. McMurray JJ, Adamopoulos S, Anker SD, Auricchio A, Böhm M, Dickstein K, Falk V, Filippatos G, Fonseca C, Gomez-Sanchez MA, Jaarsma T, Køber L, Lip GY, Maggioni AP, Parkhomenko A, Pieske BM, Popescu BA, Rønnevik PK, Rutten FH, Schwitter J, Seferovic P, Stepinska J, Trindade PT, Voors AA, Zannad F, Zeiher A, Bax JJ, Baumgartner H, Ceconi C, Dean V, Deaton C, Fagard R, Funck-Brentano C, Hasdai D, Hoes A, Kirchhof P, Knuuti J, Kolh P, McDonagh T, Moulin C, Popescu BA, Reiner Z, Sechtem U, Sirnes PA, Tendera M, Torbicki A, Vahanian A, Windecker S, McDonagh T, Sechtem U, Bonet LA, Avraamides P, Ben Lamin HA, Brignole M, Coca A, Cowburn P, Dargie H, Elliott P, Flachskampf FA, Guida GF, Hardman S, Iung B, Merkely B, Mueller C, Nanas JN, Nielsen OW, Orn S, Parissis JT, Ponikowski P, ESC Committee for Practice Guidelines (2012) ESC guidelines for the diagnosis and treatment of acute and chronic heart failure 2012: the task force for the diagnosis and treatment of acute and chronic heart failure 2012 of the European Society of Cardiology. Developed in collaboration with the heart failure association (HFA) of the ESC. Eur J Heart Fail 14:803–869
133. Erbel R, Aboyans V, Boileau C, Bossone E, Bartolomeo RD, Eggebrecht H, Evangelista A, Falk V, Frank H, Gaemperli O, Grabenwöger M, Haverich A, Iung B, Manolis AJ, Meijboom F, Nienaber CA, Roffi M, Rousseau H, Sechtem U, Sirnes PA, Allmen RS, Vrints CJ, ESC Committee for Practice Guidelines (2014) 2014 ESC guidelines on the diagnosis and treatment of aortic diseases: document covering acute and chronic aortic diseases of the thoracic and abdominal aorta of the adult. The task force for the diagnosis and treatment of aortic diseases of the European society of cardiology (ESC). Eur Heart J 35:2873–2926
134. Konstantinides SV, Torbicki A, Agnelli G, Danchin N, Fitzmaurice D, Galiè N, Gibbs JS, Huisman MV, Humbert M, Kucher N, Lang I, Lankeit M, Lekakis J, Maack C, Mayer E, Meneveau N, Perrier A, Pruszczyk P, Rasmussen LH, Schindler TH, Svitil P, Vonk Noordegraaf A, Zamorano JL, Zompatori M, Task Force for the Diagnosis and Management of Acute Pulmonary Embolism of the European Society of Cardiology (ESC) (2014) 2014 ESC guidelines on the diagnosis and management of acute pulmonary embolism. Eur Heart J 35:3033–3069
135. Righini M, Van Es J, Den Exter PL, Roy PM, Verschuren F, Ghuysen A, Rutschmann OT, Sanchez O, Jaffrelot M, Trinh-Duc A, Le Gall C, Moustafa F, Principe A, Van Houten AA, Ten Wolde M, Douma RA, Hazelaar G, Erkens PM, Van Kralingen KW, Grootenboers MJ,

Durian MF, Cheung YW, Meyer G, Bounameaux H, Huisman MV, Kamphuisen PW, Le Gal G (2014) Age-adjusted D-dimer cutoff levels to rule out pulmonary embolism: the ADJUST-PE study. JAMA 311:1117–1124
136. Schouten HJ, Geersing GJ, Koek HL, Zuithoff NP, Janssen KJ, Douma RA, van Delden JJ, Moons KG, Reitsma JB (2013) Diagnostic accuracy of conventional or age adjusted D-dimer cut-off values in older patients with suspected venous thromboembolism: systematic review and meta-analysis. BMJ 346:f2492
137. van der Does Y, Rood PP, Haagsma JA, Patka P, van Gorp EC, Limper M (2016) Procalcitonin-guided therapy for the initiation of antibiotics in the ED: a systematic review. Am J Emerg Med 34:1286–1293
138. Park JH, Wee JH, Choi SP, Oh SH (2012) The value of procalcitonin level in community-acquired pneumonia in the ED. Am J Emerg Med 30:1248–1254
139. Ko BS, Ryoo SM, Ahn S, Sohn CH, Seo DW, Kim WY (2016) Usefulness of procalcitonin level as an outcome predictor of adult bacterial meningitis. Intern Emerg Med. doi:10.1007/s11739-016-1509-4
140. Arora S, Singh P, Singh PM, Trikha A (2015) Procalcitonin levels in survivors and nonsurvivors of sepsis: systematic review and meta-analysis. Shock 43:212–221
141. de Azevedo JR, Torres OJ, Beraldi RA, Ribas CA, Malafaia O (2015) Prognostic evaluation of severe sepsis and septic shock: procalcitonin clearance vs Δ sequential organ failure assessment. J Crit Care 30:219.e9–219.12
142. Metersky ML, Williams A, Rafanan AL (1997) Retrospective analysis: are fever and altered mental status indications for lumbar puncture in a hospitalized patient who has not undergone neurosurgery? Clin Infect Dis 25:285–288
143. DeGrauw X, Annest JL, Stevens JA, Xu L, Coronado V (2016) Unintentional injuries treated in hospital emergency departments among persons aged 65 years and older, United States, 2006–2011. J Saf Res 56:105–109
144. Bonne S, Schuerer DJ (2013) Trauma in the older adult: epidemiology and evolving geriatric trauma principles. Clin Geriatr Med 29:137–150
145. Keller JM, Sciadini MF, Sinclair E, O'Toole RV (2012) Geriatric trauma: demographics, injuries, and mortality. J Orthop Trauma 26:e161–e165
146. Pfortmueller CA, Kunz M, Lindner G, Zisakis A, Puig S, Exadaktylos AK (2014) Fall-related emergency department admission: fall environment and settings and related injurypatterns in 6357 patients with special emphasis on the elderly. Sci World J 2014:256519
147. Southerland LT, Stephens JA, Robinson S, Falk J, Phieffer L, Rosenthal JA, Caterino JM (2016) Head trauma from falling increases subsequent emergency department visits more than other fall-related injuries in older adults. J Am Geriatr Soc 64:870–874
148. Hoffman JR, Mower WR, Wolfson AB, Todd KH, Zucker MI (2000) Validity of a set of clinical criteria to rule out injury to the cervical spine in patients with blunt trauma. National emergency X-radiography utilization study group. N Engl J Med 343:94–99
149. Kavalci C, Aksel G, Salt O, Yilmaz MS, Demir A, Kavalci G, Akbuga Ozel B, Altinbilek E, Durdu T, Yel C, Durukan P, Isik B (2014) Comparison of the Canadian CT head rule and the new orleans criteria in patients with minorhead injury. World J Emerg Surg 9:31
150. Stiell IG, Wells GA, Vandemheen K, Clement C, Lesiuk H, Laupacis A (2001) The Canadian CT head rule for patients with minor head injury. Lancet 357:1391–1396
151. Tran J, Jeanmonod D, Agresti D, Hamden K, Jeanmonod RK (2016) Prospective validation of modified NEXUS cervical spine injury criteria in low-risk elderly fall patients. West J Emerg Med 17:252–257
152. Ariza-Vega P, Jiménez-Moleón JJ, Kristensen MT (2014) Non-weight-bearing status compromises the functional level up to 1 yr after hip fracturesurgery. Am J Phys Med Rehabil 93:641–648
153. Di Monaco M, Castiglioni C, De Toma E, Gardin L, Giordano S, Tappero R (2015) Handgrip strength is an independent predictor of functional outcome in hip-fracture women: a prospective study with 6-month follow-up. Medicine (Baltimore) 94:e542

154. He D, Xue Y, Li Z, Tang Y, Ding H, Yang Z, Zhang C, Zhou H, Zhao Y, Zong Y (2014) Effect of depression on femoral head avascular necrosis from femoral neck fracture in patients younger than 60 years. Orthopedics 37:e244–e251
155. Blain H, Masud T, Dargent-Molina P, Martin FC, Rosendahl E, van der Velde N, Bousquet J, Benetos A, Cooper C, Kanis JA, Reginster JY, Rizzoli R, Cortet B, Barbagallo M, Dreinhöfer KE, Vellas B, Maggi S, Strandberg T, EUGMS Falls and Fracture Interest Group, European Society for Clinical and Economic Aspects of Osteoporosis and Osteoarthritis (ESCEO), Osteoporosis Research and Information Group (GRIO), International osteoporosis Foundation (IOF) (2016) A comprehensive fracture prevention strategy in older adults: the European Union geriatric medicine society (EUGMS) statement. J Nutr Health Aging 20:647–652
156. American Geriatrics Society, British Geriatrics Society (2011) Panel on prevention of falls in older persons. Summary of the updated American Geriatrics Society/British Geriatrics Society clinical practice guideline for prevention of falls in older persons. J Am Geriatr Soc 59:148–157
157. Gillespie LD, Robertson MC, Gillespie WJ, Sherrington C, Gates S, Clemson LM, Lamb SE (2012) Interventions for preventing falls in older people living in the community. Cochrane Database Syst Rev 9:CD007146
158. Ageron FX, Ricard C, Perrin-Besson S, Picot F, Dumont O, Cabillic S, Haesevoet M, Dalmon P, Gaillard C, Cezard O, Belle L, Couturier P (2016) Effectiveness of a multimodal intervention program for older individuals presenting to the emergency department after a fall in the northern French alps emergency network. Acad Emerg Med 23(9):1031–1039. doi:10.1111/acem.12989
159. Lewis LM, Banet GA, Blanda M, Hustey FM, Meldon SW, Gerson LW (2005) Etiology and clinical course of abdominal pain in senior patients: a prospective, multicenter study. J Gerontol A Biol Sci Med Sci 60:1071–1076
160. Laurell H, Hansson LE, Gunnarsson U (2006) Acute abdominal pain among elderly patients. Gerontology 52:339–444
161. Millet I et al. (2017) Systematic unenhanced CT for acute abdominal symptoms in the elderly patients improves both emergency department diagnosis and prompt clinical management. Eur Radiol 27(2):868–877
162. Segev L, Keidar A, Schrier I, Rayman S, Wasserberg N, Sadot E (2015) Acute appendicitis in the elderly in the twenty-first century. J Gastrointest Surg 19:730–735
163. Schnitker LM, Martin-Khan M, Burkett E, Brand CA, Beattie ER, Jones RN, Gray LC (2015) Research collaboration for quality care of older persons: emergency care panel. Structural quality indicators to support quality of care for older people with cognitive impairment in emergency departments. Acad Emerg Med 22:273–284
164. Guttman A, Afilalo M, Guttman R et al (2004) An emergency department-based nurse discharge coordinator for elder patients: does it make a difference? Acad Emerg Med 11:1318–1327
165. Hegney D, Buikstra E, Chamberlain C et al (2006) Nurse discharge planning in the emergency department: a Toowoomba, Australia, study. J Clin Nurs 15:1033–1044
166. Miller DK, Lewis LM, Nork MJ, Morley JE (1996) Controlled trial of a geriatric case-finding and liaison service in an emergency department. J Am Geriatr Soc 44:513–520
167. Mion LC, Palmer RM, Meldon SW et al (2003) Case finding and referral model for emergency department elders: a randomized clinical trial. Ann Emerg Med 41:57–68
168. Moss JE, Flower CL, Houghton LM, Moss DL, Nielsen DA, Taylor DM (2002) A multidisciplinary care coordination team improves emergency department discharge planning practice. Med J Aust 177:435–439
169. Ballabio C, Bergamaschini L, Mauri S, Baroni E, Ferretti M, Bilotta C, Vergani C (2008) A comprehensive evaluation of elderly people discharged from an emergency department. Intern Emerg Med 3:245–249
170. Bird SR, Kurowski W, Dickman GK, Kronborg I (2007) Integrated care facilitation for older patients with complex health care needs reduces hospital demand. Aust Health Rev 31:451–461. discussion 449–450

171. Caplan GA, Williams AJ, Daly B, Abraham K (2004) A randomized, controlled trial of comprehensive geriatric assessment and multidisciplinary intervention after discharge of elderly from the emergency department – the DEED II study. J Am Geriatr Soc 52:1417–1423
172. Lee JS, Hurley MJ, Carew D, Fisher R, Kiss A, Drummond N (2007) A randomized clinical trial to assess the impact on an emergency response system on anxiety and health care use among older emergency patients after a fall. Acad Emerg Med 14:301–308
173. McCusker J, Verdon J, Tousignant P, de Courval LP, Dendukuri N, Belzile E (2001) Rapid emergency department intervention for older people reduces risk of functional decline: results of a multicenter randomized trial. J Am Geriatr Soc 49:1272–1281
174. Mion LC, Palmer RM, Anetzberger GJ, Meldon SW (2001) Establishing a case-finding and referral system for at-risk older individuals in the emergency department setting: the SIGNET model. J Am Geriatr Soc 49:1379–1386
175. Salvi F, Morichi V, Lorenzetti B, Rossi L, Spazzafumo L, Luzi R, De Tommaso G, Lattanzio F (2012) Risk stratification of older patients in the emergency department: comparison between the identification of seniors at risk and triage risk screening tool. Rejuvenation Res 15:288–294
176. Sirois MJ, Griffith L, Perry J, Daoust R, Veillette N, Lee J, Pelletier M, Wilding L, Émond M (2017) Measuring frailty can help emergency departments identify independent seniors at risk of functional decline after minor injuries. J Gerontol A Biol Sci Med Sci 72(1):68–74
177. Yao JL, Fang J, Lou QQ, Anderson RM (2015) A systematic review of the identification of seniors at risk (ISAR) tool for the prediction of adverse outcome in elderly patients seen in the emergency department. Int J Clin Exp Med 8:4778–4786
178. Beland F, Bergman H, Lebel P, Dallaire L (2006) Integrated services for frail elders (SIPA): a trial of a model for Canada. Can J Aging 25:5–42
179. Kodner DL (2006) Whole-system approaches to health and social care partnerships for the frail elderly: an exploration of north American models and lessons. Health Soc Care Community 14:384–390
180. Lowthian JA, McGinnes RA, Brand CA, Barker AL, Cameron PA (2015) Discharging older patients from the emergency department effectively: a systematic review and meta-analysis. Age Ageing 44:761–770
181. Tirrell G, Sri-on J, Lipsitz LA, Camargo CA Jr, Kabrhel C, Liu SW (2015) Evaluation of older adult patients with falls in the emergency department: discordance with national guidelines. Acad Emerg Med 22:461–467
182. Glendinning C (2003) Breaking down barriers: integrating health and care services for older people in England. Health Policy (New York) 65:139–151
183. Sanders AB (1992) Care of the elderly in emergency departments: conclusions and recommendations. Ann Emerg Med 21:830–834
184. Carpenter CR, Bromley M, Caterino JM, Chun A, Gerson LW, Greenspan J, Hwang U, John DP, Lyons WL, Platts-Mills TF, Mortensen B, Ragsdale L, Rosenberg M, Wilber S (2014) Optimal older adult emergency care: introducing multidisciplinary geriatric emergency department guidelines from the American College of Emergency Physicians, American Geriatrics Society, emergency nurses association, and Society for Academic Emergency Medicine. Acad Emerg Med 21:806–809

Clinical Assessment and Management of Older People: What's Different?

Gertrude Chikura, Simon Conroy, and Fabio Salvi

5.1 Introduction

Managing older people in any context, in particular urgent care settings, can be challenging. Unlike patient with single presenting problems, older people will usually present with a range of issues, not just medical, that require addressing in order to achieve an effective management plan. The key points to consider are the following:

- Non-specific presentations
- Multiple comorbidities and polypharmacy
- Functional decline and altered homeostasis
- Differential challenge

5.1.1 Non-Specific Presentations

Older people with frailty often present non-specifically [1, 2]. This means that the textbook clues for diagnosis may not be present. Do not interpret a lack of specificity with a lack of seriousness or urgency. Recognise the non-specific presentations (off legs, falls, immobility, delirium, etc.), and use them as a prompt to switch on your diagnostic antennae to focus upon objective pointers towards a diagnosis.

The non-specific presentation itself is a cue—it will be related to a communication barrier (think delirium, dementia, dysphasia and/or sensory impairment).

5.1.2 Multiple Comorbidities

Do not content yourself with a single-system diagnosis; there will usually be multiple active issues, which often interact and compete for prioritisation. List the active diagnoses, and stratify them in order of urgency, as this will help you prioritise those that need addressing now and those that can wait a few hours but should not be forgotten.

Multiple comorbidities often bring polypharmacy; use the urgent care episode to discern if there are active adverse drug events or opportunities for deprescribing. Older adults with polypharmacy are predisposed to drug interactions leading to preventable adverse drug events and medication-related hospitalisations. Multiple medications and age-related modifications in pharmacokinetics and pharmacodynamics participate in the higher rates of adverse drug effects. Older patients attending urgent care receive an average of 4.2 medications per day (ranging from 0 to 17 medications), with 91% receiving at least 1 and 13% receiving 8 or more presentations, and 11% of these patients receive at least 1 inappropriate medication. Clinicians should be acutely aware of the particularities of drug prescription in older adults and should be mindful when prescribing any new medications.

5.1.3 Functional Decline and Altered Homeostasis

Older people with frailty will often have pre-existing functional impairment added to which they may delay presentation with acute illness, either through inherent reticence or reduced access to support. This means that the impact of an acute event will already have started to manifest in terms of functional ability, which can be exacerbated by enforced bed rest in urgent care settings. A period of rehabilitation will often be needed—increasingly this should be done at home rather than in an institutional setting.

Older people with frailty will have altered homeostatic mechanisms, which means that their reserve is impaired, making them more vulnerable to apparently minor insults but also altering their responses, for example, altered drug handling. Remember 'start low, go slow' when introducing new drug treatments.

5.1.4 Differential Challenge

Those most in need are least able to access the services they require (inverse care law [3])—this can be due to intrinsic factors, such as cognitive or sensory impairment, or extrinsic factors, such as the lack of age-attuned services or broader socio-economic factors, such as isolation and lack of social support.

Non-specific presentations make for diagnostic uncertainty, communication barriers mandate the need to involve the patient's carers and families and almost by definition there is usually more than one active problem with interactions that make assessment and management complex.

A significant number of older people experience social isolation or lack of social networks [4]. Although there are a number of community-based services which might partially ameliorate the impact of social isolation, many of these services have been reduced or cut due to economic crisis in recent years. Some of the services still in existence face increased demand and often have long waiting lists. Another problem is families, friends or significant others who may struggle to cope with increased functional decline and as such are not able to look after their beloved one at home. Increasing support to families and reducing barriers to accessing services may in turn affect hospital admission among this patient group. Although admissions for social reasons certainly occur, clinicians should always rule out subacute or acute illness which can present as functional decline, motivating the social ED visit.

To resolve this, problem lists are helpful. These list not just medical diagnostic issues but should seek out other domains that require attention. As these patients will have multiple problems, unidimensional problem-solving results in prolonged lengths of stay or readmission—in one series, over 50% of frail older people were readmitted to an acute unit within a year post-discharge [5]. By working in a team and coordinating care through structured but rapid communication (e.g. board-round concept), the full range of assessment can be undertaken rapidly without any one individual team member having to do everything.

5.1.5 Comprehensive Geriatric Assessment

Comprehensive geriatric assessment (CGA) offers a useful structure to ensure that your assessment is holistic and therefore more likely to result in a management plan that will be successful. Mentally check off if you have sought out and identified issues in each of the domains of CGA (see below) when formulating your management plan:

Medical: Have you got a working primary diagnosis, as well as a list of comorbidities that are active or important that also require attention?
Psychological: Have you assessed for the presence of delirium, dementia or depression/anxiety? These will have a substantial impact upon ongoing management.
Functional ability: You may have made a diagnosis, but how will you get the patient 'clinically stable for transfer'? Being 'medically fit' is meaningless if the person cannot mobilise to the toilet and back safely.
Social circumstances: What support exists? What more is needed to enable a return home? Do you know how to access resources that can help?
Environment: Is the home setting conducive to ongoing care needs, or is adaptation required? Do you know how to organise a home hazards review for people who have fallen?

5.2 Identifying Older People with Frailty in Urgent Care

Frailty is a distinctive late-life health state in which apparently minor stressor events are associated with adverse health outcomes. The two established international models are the frailty phenotype [6] and the cumulative deficit model [7], both of which have been validated in large population studies. The models identify people at increased risk of a range of adverse outcomes including dependency, institutionalisation and premature mortality. However, there is limited evidence for the discriminant ability of frailty scales in the urgent care context [8].

When defining a population for intervention in clinical practice, acceptability and ease of use are important considerations as well as discriminant ability [9]. Until more accurate tools become available, simple, clinically acceptable criteria are used to identify a large proportion of frail older people (sensitivity); the risks are that some older people without frailty will be included (specificity—usually inversely related to sensitivity). An example for frailty identification criteria can include the following:

- Aged 65+ and presenting with one or more frailty syndromes (confusion, Parkinson's disease, presenting with fragility fractures and/or falls, care home residents) or people aged 85+
- Moderate or severe frailty (grades 6–9) using the Canadian Frailty Scale

The purpose of focussing on older people with frailty is that they represent a relatively small proportion of all those accessing urgent care settings, but moving through the system, increasing proportion of those at risk of harms and increasing resource use. Depending upon definitions, the setting and local service configuration, about 5–10% of all ED attendees [10] and about 30% of patients in acute medical units [8] will be identified as older people with frailty. Frailty identification can also be helpful when considering the use of disease-specific prognostic or stratification tools, which should be always interpreted in the light of the presence of frailty and multimorbidity.

Early identification of older people with frailty in urgent care facilitates and enhanced focus on pathways that can deliver evidence-based care (see Chap. 6), in an attempt to improve patient and service-level outcomes.

5.2.1 Communication with Patients, Carers and Families

Competent communication is essential. Communication involves the reciprocal process in which messages are sent and received between two or more people. Effective communication is a two-way open conversation where patients are informed of the nature of their disease and treatment and are encouraged to express their concerns and emotions [11]. Communication is essential in empowering patients and improving quality of life. Clinicians' interactions and behaviours have a significant impact on how older people participate in decision-making and sense of control of their own life. Empathetic communication such as trust, mutual understanding and self-efficacy is among other factors that are shown to correlate with positive health outcomes and positive relationships with older people [12].

Obtaining a coherent story can be difficult due to hearing, visual or cognitive impairment [13]. It is useful to interact in a well-lit environment, taking care to eliminate as much as possible sources of noise; speak with a deep voice, slowly, stepping in front of the patient so that he/she can lip-read; formulate the questions in plain language, avoiding technical terms or jargon; and ask specific questions with respect to potentially significant symptoms. In some cases, you may need to write in large letters the questions posed allowing time to read, understand and answer (it is not a timed quiz, and not always the first answer is the one that counts!). It is essential to determine as soon as possible the reliability of the information provided by the patient, assessing cognitive status—this can usually be inferred from the opening discussion, without resorting to the need for formal cognitive tests at this stage—these may upset the flow and can usually be deferred until later time. It is especially important to differentiate delirium from dementia when cognitive impairment is present. Again an experienced clinician will be able to do this from a natural conversation, supported by a key informant perspective (carer, loved one, etc.), but there are tools available to help those less experienced (see below).

5.2.2 History Taking

Collecting a complete medical history of an older adult during an ED visit can be time-consuming and difficult. The focus should be placed on 'value-added' critical information to be taken in a few minutes. Often there will be existing information on past medical history, medications and so on available in accompanying correspondence or computer records. Ascertaining this information ahead of the discussion with the patient allows time to be focussed on eliciting that information that helps move the diagnosis and management forwards, rather than repeating or duplicating. This is easier on patients as well as staff.

Often, the list of medications could help to identify unreported diseases; otherwise, this could be a good time for preliminary reconciliation of therapy (i.e. a significant disease being untreated, a taken/prescribed drug without a corresponding disease).

The reason for ED presentation is the core of medical history collection in the ED: a predefined list of presenting complaints should be used at triage (i.e. Canadian Emergency Department Information System; Manchester Triage System) [14].[1] Procedures for defining details about the main symptom differ among all possible presenting complaints: structured interviews or diagnostic/prognostic rules specific for the main symptom (dyspnoea, chest or abdominal pain, syncope) could be useful. Particular attention should be paid for older adults with non-specific complaints (weakness, dizziness, anorexia, confusion, etc.) [15]. Screening for specific geriatric problems (geriatric syndromes) could be also quickly performed at this time: falls (yes/no; how many in the last year), incontinence, nutritional problems (weight loss, anorexia, dysphagia), living situation (the presence of a reliable caregiver, institution/nursing home), mobility problems/evident disability and the presence of pressure ulcers.

---

[1] http://www.triagenet.net/en.

5.2.3 Physical Examination

As in younger patients, the priority for physical examination of an older adult in the ED is based on urgency. For resuscitation/emergency patients, the ABCD (airways, breath, circulation, defibrillation) approach and the ALS treatment algorithm are mandatory [16], unless the patient is clearly terminally ill or there is a known do not resuscitate order (DNR). In these patients, always keep in mind, check and treat reversible causes: the four Hs (hypoxia, hypovolaemia, hypothermia and hyperkalaemia/hypokalaemia/hypoglycaemia/hypocalcaemia/acidaemia and other metabolic disorders) and the 4Ts (thrombosis, coronary or pulmonary; tension pneumothorax; tamponade, cardiac; toxins).

For less-urgent patients, physical examination should focus on the organ system(s) more closely related with the presenting symptom, but it should never neglect other aspects (remember the 'weakest link' concept, e.g. in an agitated/delirious patient, check systematically for acute urinary retention, faecal impaction and/or pain). A critical cornerstone in older patients is to differentiate sequelae of old illnesses from new-onset pathological signs (e.g. crackles due to old/new-onset pleural effusion, old/new-onset hemiplegia or weakness). Another important issue is to differentiate subtle clinical signs, such as crackles due to acute pulmonary oedema or aspiration pneumonia.

The presence of a family member or carer is often necessary to ease clinical examination where there is cognitive impairment or severe disability: the caregiver can help to position the patient sitting or standing, to mimic gestures and to perform open-mouth deep breaths (patients with dementia do not understand the commands but are often still able to imitate). Another little trick to get open-mouth deep breaths in the uncooperative and not-able-to-imitate demented patient can be to close nostrils: this will stimulate open-mouth breathing. Particular attention should be paid to non-verbal communication, especially in cognitively impaired patients, who are often unable to describe symptoms or pain. For example, during the palpation of the abdomen or limb, you should watch the patient's face, observing for grimaces or changes in facial expression that suggest the presence of pain; also an increase in agitation or the appearance of aggression or clumsy attempts to get away should be considered a possible expression of pain or, more generally, a 'sign'. Furthermore, it may be useful to distract the patient by talking of pleasant memories or familiar subjects whilst visiting aching parts or making medical procedures; similarly, in demented patients, mobility of the upper limbs can be assessed by asking to perform simple orders (e.g. pick up a suspended pen with right or left hand).

5.2.4 Communication Between Professionals

A challenge common to different health settings is the effective sharing of information. This is particularly relevant in establishing a reliable past medical history and record of current and previous medications and allergies, as well as accessing prior investigations. Such information can supplement the details known by the patient and carer and facilitate better-informed decision-making and reduce avoidable error by making inappropriate recommendations of medications known to have adverse effects and reduce waste by repeating investigations. The benefits of accessing information are higher in relation to decisions such as those around resuscitation and the levels of treatment which patients accept in a life-threatening situation (e.g. non-invasive ventilation, intravenous antibiotics, etc.). Healthcare professionals are often uncertain about such decisions, particularly if original documentation is not available. In such situations, the presumption is rightly to intervene; however, this can often be due to a lack of information and uncertainty. In the highly digitalised age, moves towards coordinated electronic records spanning primary, secondary and community care services are essential. Written and standardised transfer forms with essential health information (i.e. reason for transfer and tests requested, resuscitation status, medication list and allergies, health problem list, contact information) in patients who are resident in nursing homes have been proposed to improve the flow of information between the home and the ED [17]. Rapidly access to the primary care information should always be available, particularly when the patient is alone and unable to provide a reliable history or when important questions arise concerning medical history or drug therapies.

Similarly when an individual is transferred or discharged from the emergency department, effective communication with their other health and care providers is a useful way of acting on the recommendations made and ensuring care is contemporaneous. Accurate discharge letters, phone calls and short message text or email have been proposed and tested.

Aim to be clear, concise and comprehensive, and document your findings in a succinct and legible format. The progress report should also follow the same standards as the initial assessment.

5.2.4.1 Multidisciplinary Meeting in Urgent Care Settings

A cornerstone of comprehensive geriatric assessment is an interdisciplinary communication and coordination. These have traditionally been delivered using multidisciplinary team (MDT) meetings—typically on a weekly or occasionally daily basis. Clearly this frequency is not well adapted to the ED setting, so alternative mechanisms are necessary.

In some settings, it might be possible to bring the team together for a rapid MDT discussion about patients, for example, in 'observation units'; such meetings should be at a fixed time every day and for a fixed duration so that expectations for attendance and duration are clear to all team members. On average, each patient discussion should be for no more than 1 minute, and it might be helpful to structure the discussion using the domains of comprehensive geriatric assessment—physical/medial issues, functional/mobility issues, cognition/mood, social support networks and environment (home setting). For an example, see here: https://vimeo.com/132073531.

In the main area of the ED ('majors'), coordination and communication can be more difficult, as it will be unusual to be able to have multiple staff involved in the same patient at the same time. In this scenario, standardised documentation again based on the principles of CGA can help staff more easily navigate the issues that have been addressed and identify where 'value can be added'. Even in a busy and noisy major area, it is possible to bring most clinicians together every hour or two for a quick run through the patients. In addition to addressing the domains of CGA, it is useful to consider situational awareness issues in this context.

5.2.5 Communication About Older People with Frailty

Language is important—it betrays our attitudes, and attitudes influence behaviour and action. How we speak also impacts upon patients and their loved ones—how would you like to be described as having 'acopia' or being a 'social admission' or 'bed-blocker'. Such terms are dehumanising and reflect the ignorance of the staff using such language in how to assess and manage older people with frailty—in that sense, they can be helpful as the use of the phrase 'acopia' tells you more about the clinician using the phrase (and their competence) than it does about the patient themselves. The customary diagnostic rigour, which we have been trained to apply as standard, can be mysteriously replaced in older patients by ageist, diagnostic abdication and therapeutic nihilism.

There is no perfect term that suits all, but there are a few phrases that should most certainly be avoided—to quote Falconer [18] 'Nobody wants to be elderly. No-one wants to buy an elderly car or travel in an elderly aeroplane. The word elderly as an adjective, and particularly when used as a noun, is a pejorative term. In a Europe wide survey, older people expressed a clear preference for the use of the adjective 'older' 'or 'senior' to describe their age group, rather than terms such as 'elderly', 'aged' and 'old.' This is also reflected by the Human Rights Commission of the United Nations in the International Covenant on Economic, Social and Cultural Rights, which outlined why the term 'older' should be used. What would you think about a man who says that he is fascinated by the allure of elderly women? Yet to be attracted to the older woman (or man) is a well-recognised phenomenon'.

This is not just about 'political correctness'—the term 'elderly' homogenises and ascribes a general state to older people which we know is not true. 'Frail older people' or more recently 'older people living with frailty' is the preferred term as it immediately asks the question 'what is frail'—and we can start a conversation about frailty; or it asks 'older than what' which introduces relativism rather than absolutism and encourages thinking about individuals. Although some will argue that this is political niceties, it is more about attitude/behaviour and role modelling, all of which are crucial to improvement.

Aside from the 'philosophy of care' (holistic assessment, value-driven decision-making), the effective management of older people with frailty requires specific knowledge about presentations in this group.

5.2.6 Geriatric Giants

5.2.6.1 Delirium and Dementia

Dementia and delirium are syndromes, not pathologies, and so the diagnosis is entirely dependent on the skill of health professionals [cross reference].

Cognitive impairment is present in 15–40% of older ED patients (especially if over 80 years old and/or institutionalised), but it's recognised only in 27–50% of the cases with implication in clinical data collection (undertriage, delay in diagnosis/therapy) and understanding of discharge indications (ADRs, reduced compliance, caregiver presence/reliability) [19, 20]. Routine assessment of cognition will identify moderate to severe cognitive impairment, but more subtle presentations can be missed. The four-point Abbreviated Mental Test score (4-AMT) is quick to complete and has good correlation with the ten-point scale but is easier to apply requiring only place, age, date of birth and year [21]. However, other tools do exist to be used in the ED, such as the six-item screener or the short blessed test [22] or more recently, the Ottawa 3DY Scale [23].

The evaluation of cognitive impairment in the ED context should always be accompanied by an assessment for delirium.

Delirium has acute onset, the course typically over days and weeks. Importantly, delirium is usually an acute medical condition related to infection, metabolic disturbance, intoxication, medication or a combination of these factors. Under-detection in emergency departments is associated with a sevenfold hazard for increased mortality [24, 25] and is an independent predictor of hospital length of stay [20]. Symptoms may not only be cognitive, but they may be behavioural, psychotic (hallucinations, delusions) or mood symptoms with little or absent signs of disorientation or cognitive impairment; hypoactive delirium is the most difficult to recognise. For example, symptoms of depression in a delirious individual may be indistinguishable from people suffering from depressive disorder. The key is to suspect delirium with any sudden change of mental state or behaviour in older people and to systematically search for the cause. Characteristic signs of delirium, which also help distinguish this from dementia, are:

- Clouding of consciousness
- Reduced attention and concentration
- A fluctuating pattern of symptoms

It may not be possible for an ED clinician to be able to tell whether the cognitive impairment they have detected is different from the usual state. Information from carers or third parties is essential and will often hold the key. Specific tools like CAM-ICU, mCAM-ED or combination of delirium triage screen (DTS) and bCAM are able to increase the accuracy of delirium recognition in the ED, in order to start prompt diagnostic pathways to identify underlying medical cause(s) responsible for the altered cognitive status [26–28]. Moreover, the 4-AMT (used to evaluate cognition) has recently been included in the four As test (4AT) for rapid delirium screening [29].

Both dementia and delirium impact upon the diagnostic approach and treatment, for example, through raising questions about a person's capacity to make health and welfare decisions or practical issues such as concordance with therapies.

5.2.6.2 Sepsis

Sepsis is a huge challenge in older people with frailty, being both over- and under-diagnosed. Key is a familiarity with non-specific presentations (i.e. acute functional decline, delirium/confusion, general weakness), a careful focus on objective signs that constellate towards the most probable diagnosis, and treatment, to include

Table 5.1 Considerations when implementing the Sepsis Six in older people

Deliver high-flow oxygen	Remember CO_2 retention
Take blood cultures	Be careful delirium-related agitation does not result in injury (to patient or staff)
Administer empiric intravenous antibiotics	Balanced against the risk of *Clostridium difficile*, antibiotic resistance, missed non-infective diagnoses (the patient was given antibiotics, so it must be sepsis… and missing the subdural)
Measure serum lactate and send full blood count	Validation studies based in 60-year-olds [31]; unclear if prognostic significance holds up in older people with frailty and multiple comorbidities[a]
Start intravenous fluid resuscitation	Important as premorbid dehydration is common, and volume depletion is exacerbated by acute illness; but beware of fluid overload—careful boluses titrated against clinical response are mandatory
Commence accurate urine output measurement	But do not rush to insert urinary catheters: catheter-associated sepsis is common [32, 33] as is subsequent incontinence due to deconditioning of the detrusor muscle; reducing unnecessary catheterisations improves patient safety [34]. Can the response to hydration not be assessed using blood pressure, pulse and JVP?

[a]Experience-based vs. evidence-based assertion–study required

volume replacement in nearly all cases unless fluid overload is evident (remember sacral oedema may be the only sign). Bundles such as 'Sepsis Six' can be helpful as guides [30] but have generally not been validated or designed for older people with frailty. Consider the Sepsis Six criteria applied to a typical older person with frailty, presenting with delirium on a background of COPD, heart failure and detrusor instability—Table 5.1.

On the other hand, many abnormalities in older people are incidental, best exemplified by the ubiquitous 'dipstick-positive UTI' (aka 'acute trimethoprim deficiency'[2]). The conundrum here is that asymptomatic bacteriuria, which commonly causes positive urine dips, is prevalent (up to 50% of care home residents will have this abnormality); the treatment of positive urinary dips confers no benefit. Very simply, a clinical diagnosis of urinary tract infection requires the presence of one or more of dysuria, frequency, suprapubic tenderness (or acute urinary retention), urgency, polyuria and haematuria in the absence of any other good explanation for the apparent sepsis [35]. When suspecting lower urinary tract infections in people unable to express themselves, urine dipstick testing should only be considered in patients with unexplained systemic sepsis (which may manifest as delirium). A urine dip should not be used to diagnose a urinary tract infection in coherent patients without lower urinary tract symptoms; it can be misleading [36].

Prognostic scores (APACHE II, MEDS, etc.) and biomarkers (i.e. C-reactive protein, procalcitonin, etc.) can be useful in the diagnosis of sepsis although they require further studies in older ED patients. Moreover, in older patients with atypical presentations, the diagnosis of sepsis can become more evident over time; therefore, disposition planning improves after observation [37].

---

[2] Phrase coined by Dr. Chris Roseveare, Southampton; @CRoseveare.

5.2.6.3 Falls and Syncope

Falls are the commonest single reason for older people to present to urgent care. Falls are not an inevitable part of ageing but are often due to underlying disease or impairment that may be amendable to treatment or modification.

Key in urgent care settings is to carefully differentiate between syncopal and non-syncopal falls; this is not always easy because of ante- and retrograde amnesia, which is common. All too often, direct witness accounts are not available, meaning that the clinicians have to base their assessment on the balance of probabilities.

An understanding of cerebral perfusion pressure in older people is important, minor perturbations of which can result in (pre-) syncope. Whilst national drivers promulgate a focus upon tight BP control, there is ongoing debate about the ideal BP, which is linked to perfusion pressure in older people [38]. Whilst detailed discussion about BP control is beyond the scope of this section, it is worth noting that blood pressures less than 120 systolic in older people, especially where variation with lower troughs is evident, should prompt a careful examination of whether or not syncope is likely [39]. It is useful to ask 'do you remember hitting the floor?' and not to accept vague assertions such as 'I must have tripped', as plausible explanations for the fall. The pattern of injury can also provide clues—facial bruising in particular is highly suspicious of syncope. The presence of syncope should prompt a review of medication and a search for underlying causes, at the very least a 12-lead ECG and routine bloods; other tests may be indicated[3].

5.2.6.4 Injuries

Older people presenting with poly-trauma need to be managed according to advanced trauma and life support (ATLS) principles with special consideration of the fact that they do not respond well to prolonged immobilisation. Advanced imaging including early CT scanning is important for quicker and definitive diagnosis, and as an adjunct to clinical assessment.

There is an association between increasing age and poor outcome following trauma, although any individual factor or combinations fail to predict an unacceptable outcome. Hence, it is usually advisable to embark on aggressive therapy irrespective of age or injury, except in the initially moribund individual. Older people who do not respond to this initial resuscitation have adverse outcomes. Responders have a good prognosis, including a complete return to their premorbid state [40].

5.2.6.5 Pain

The use of traditional pain scales can be difficult because of communication barriers, such as cognitive impairment; alternative assessment processes that rely on non-verbal cues may be more useful in some older people. Pain management in people with dementia may be challenging not only because of comorbidities but also because of polypharmacy. The importance of assessing changes in the individual's normal behaviour patterns as an indicator of increasing stress levels or

---
[3] http://www.nice.org.uk/CG021.

potential pain cannot be underestimated. The modified Abbey Pain Scale [41] emphasises involving the person's carers/family.

5.2.6.6 Medication

Particular attention must be devoted to determine the details of a patient's medication regimen prior to presentation. Community resources such as general practitioners and community pharmacists are valuable, as are patient medication lists and electronic 'smart cards' have been explored. One simple parameter that improves prescribing accuracy in the ED is the availability of patients' own medications brought to the ED by ambulance paramedics [42]. Whilst there has been a substantial focus on 'deprescribing' in older people, driven by guidance such as the STOPP/START criteria, urgent care presentations do present an additional opportunity to review medication appropriateness and even to introduce important drugs for the patients that were not currently prescribed. Consideration should be given as to where a patient is in their life—a consideration of trajectory [43], informed, when possible, by a description of physical and cognitive function over the last year. Some patients will be clearly entering a more palliative phase of life (consider the 'surprise question'—would you be surprised if your patient were to die in the next 6–12 months?), in which case, is it really helpful to continue anti-platelets or anti-coagulants (side effects such as bruising, bleeding and low-grade anaemia are common, and their impact is often underestimated in older people with frailty)? Does someone who is bed bound really require high-dose antianginals if they are no longer exerting themselves? Each deprescribing scenario should consider the patient values or best interest formulations, the rationale for continuing the treatment (how will it help?) and the opportunity costs of continuing prescribing (e.g. remembering that time spent administering medication is time not spent on comfort care). This can be a challenging task, but informed by guidance, practice and clinical supervision could and arguably should be a routine part of urgent care assessments. Any changes and the rationale for the changes should be clearly communicated to primary care and carers.

5.2.7 Risk Assessments

Hospitalisation of an older person can be a sentinel event that heralds an intensive period of health and social care service use [5, 44, 45]. But as older people are a heterogeneous group, risk assessment tools have been developed to try and segment the population. The use of screening instruments may allow point-of-care identification of older patients who are at increased risk for readmission or other adverse outcomes, opening opportunities for emergency clinicians to alter ED or post-ED trajectories for these vulnerable patients using observation units, mobile acute care for the older teams and other healthcare resources. The identification of seniors at risk (ISAR) is a self-report questionnaire that was originally developed and validated in Canada: it concisely investigates functional status, previous hospital admission, complaints of cognitive and visual impairment and polypharmacy. An ISAR score ≥ 2 (in a range from 0 to 6) suggests an increased risk for functional decline, repeated ED visits, hospital admissions, institutionalisation and death within 6 months after an ED visit [46]. The triage risk screening tool (TRST), developed in the USA to be used by nurses [47], includes the possible presence of cognitive impairment or a score ≥2 in the remaining risk factors (loneliness or absence of a caregiver, difficulties with walking or transfer or history of recent falls, previous hospital admission or ED visit and polypharmacy) or professional evaluation and suggests an increased risk for functional decline, subsequent ED use, hospitalisation and nursing home admission 30 and 120 days after an ED visit [19, 48–50].

The Silver Code (SC) is a prognostic tool based solely on administrative data and was developed and validated in Italy [51]. A score is assigned to age, sex, marital status, admission to a day hospital, admission to regular ward with corresponding discharge diagnosis and polypharmacy 3–6 months prior to the index ED visit. One-year mortality increases linearly with the SC score, and the tool was found to be able to predict 6-month ED return and hospital admission [51].

Although most scales perform better than chance in predicting a range of poor outcomes, none of them performed adequately, and most perform either poorly or very poorly [50, 52]. New insights in this field are expected by the ongoing evaluation/validation of the interRAI ED screener, a novel tool of the interRAI family of instruments that is based on the Assessment Urgency Algorithm (a risk scale derived from the interRAI ED Contact Assessment) that was found to be a good predictor of hospital admissions, prolonged hospital stays and the need for referral to geriatric services.

5.2.8 Assessing for Older Abuse

Whenever an older and potentially vulnerable patient is admitted to the emergency department, staff should be alert to the possibility of abuse. Abuse is defined as 'a single or repeated act or lack of appropriate action, occurring within any relationship where there is an expectation of trust, which causes harm or distress to an older person'. A 2007 UK study estimated a prevalence rate of abuse as 1 in 40 people over the age of 65. Signs of abuse include patterns of injuries which are likely to be nonaccidental, differing versions of events between patients and another individual and the vulnerable patient seeming to appear scared or withdrawn when certain individuals are present.

Clinicians working in these areas will come across cases of abuse and have a responsibility to take immediate and appropriate action, just as with child or domestic abuse.

5.2.9 Functional Assessments

Particularly important in the older adult is the rapid deterioration of functional status: a family member or the caregiver could report that the patient 'yesterday was walking' whilst today 'cannot get out (of bed)' or 'does not stand up' or 'has fallen' or 'has become incontinent' or even 'does not eat, has no appetite' or 'cannot swallow'. These 'symptoms' should never be underestimated and are often not strictly related to neurological problems: indeed, they often underlie an acute illness that is not yet presenting with its conventional symptoms, such as heart failure, infectious diseases (e.g. pneumonia; urinary tract infections: urinary frequency becomes 'incontinence' in older people, too slow to get to the bathroom, but we should not forget the possibility of acute urinary retention), bowel obstruction or faecal impaction.

5.3 Summary

In this chapter, we have tried to highlight the key issues that make the clinical assessment and management of older people with frailty. The take-home message can be encapsulated in these points:

- Non-specific presentations are common and potentially dangerous.
- Multiple comorbidities and polypharmacy.
- Functional decline and altered homeostasis.
- Differential challenge.

Interdisciplinary communication and coordination built upon the principles of comprehensive geriatric assessment are key, and we have highlighted how this might be achieved in the ED setting. We have also considered some specific clinical scenarios and pointed out how current protocol-driven approaches need to be adapted to the needs of older people with frailty.

Finally, building upon the arguments detailed above, we advocate for a social movement around geriatric emergency medicine, which has the power to deliver a paradigm shift in the care of older people in the ED, with benefits for patients, staff and the system.

References

1. Limpawattana P, Phungoen P, Mitsungnern T (2016) Atypical presentations of older adults at the emergency department and associated factors. Arch Gerontol Geriatr 62:97–102
2. Jarrett PG, Rockwood K, Carver D et al (1995) Illness presentation in elderly patients. Arch Intern Med 155(10):1060–1064
3. Tudor Hart J (1971) The inverse care law. Lancet 297(7696):405–412
4. Samaras N, Chevalley T, Samaras D et al (2010) Older patients in the emergency department: a review. Ann Emerg Med 56(3):261–269
5. Woodard J, Gladman J, Conroy S (2010) Frail older people at the interface. Age Ageing 39(S1):i36
6. Fried L, Tangen C, Walston J et al (2001) Frailty in older adults: evidence for a phenotype. J Gerontol Med Sci 56A(3):M146–M156
7. Rockwood K, Song X, MacKnight C et al (2005) A global clinical measure of fitness and frailty in elderly people. Can Med Assoc J 173(5):489–495

8. Conroy S, Dowsing T (2013) The ability of frailty to predict outcomes in older people attending an acute medical unit. Acute Med 12(2):74–76
9. Adams ST, Leveson SH (2012) Clinical prediction rules
10. Ferguson C, Woodard J, Banerjee J et al (2010) Operationalising frailty definitions in the emergency department – a mapping exercise. Age Ageing 39(S1):i7
11. Caswell G, Pollock K, Harwood R et al (2015) Communication between family carers and health professionals about end-of-life care for older people in the acute hospital setting: a qualitative study. BMC Palliat Care 14:35
12. Bridges J, Flatley M, Meyer J (2010) Older people's and relatives' experiences in acute care settings: systematic review and synthesis of qualitative studies. Int J Nurs Stud 47(1):89–107
13. Williamson R, Lauricella K, Browning A et al (2014) Patient factors associated with incidents of aggression in a general inpatient setting. J Clin Nurs 23(7–8):1144–1152
14. Grafstein E, Bullard M, Warren D et al (2008) The CTAS National Working Group Revision of the Canadian emergency department information system (CEDIS) presenting complaint list version 1.1. Can J Emerg Med 10:151–161
15. Nemec M, Koller M, Nickel C (2010) Patients presenting to the emergency department with non-specific complaints: the basel non-specific complaints (BANC) study. Acad Emerg Med 17(3):284–292
16. Soar J, Nolan J, Böttiger B (2015) European resuscitation council guidelines for resuscitation 2015: section 3. Adult advanced life support. Resuscitation 95:100–147
17. Terrell KM, Hustey FM, Hwang U et al (2009) Quality indicators for geriatric emergency care. Acad Emerg Med 16(5):441–449
18. Falconer M, O'Neill D (2007) Personal views: out with "the old," elderly, and aged. BMJ 334:316
19. Hustey FM, Meldon SW (2002) The prevalence and documentation of impaired mental status in elderly emergency department patients. Ann Emerg Med 39(3):248–253
20. Han JH et al (2011) Delirium in older emergency department patients: recognition, risk factors, and psychomotor subtypes. Acad Emerg Med 18:451–457
21. Swain DG et al (2000) Cognitive assessment in elderly patients admitted to hospital. Relationship between shortened version of AMT and the AMT and MMSE. Clin Rehabil 13(6):608–610
22. Carpenter CR, Bassett ER, Fischer GM et al (2011) Four sensitive screening tools to detect cognitive dysfunction in geriatric emergency department patients: brief Alzheimer's screen, short blessed test, Ottawa 3DY, and the caregiver-completed AD8. Acad Emerg Med 18(4):374–384
23. Wilding L, Eagles D, Molnar F et al (2016) Prospective validation of the Ottawa 3DY scale by geriatric emergency management nurses to identify impaired cognition in older emergency department patients. Ann Emerg Med 67(2):157–163
24. Han J, Wilson A, Wesley E (2010) Delirium in the older emergency department patient: a quiet epidemic. Emerg Med Clin N Am 28:611–631
25. Young J, Inouye S (2007) Delirium in older people. BMJ 334:842–846
26. Han JH, Wilson A, Graves AJ et al (2014) Validation of the confusion assessment method for the intensive care unit in older emergency department patients. Acad Emerg Med 21(2):180–187
27. Grossmann F, Hasemann W, Graber A et al (2014) Screening, detection and management of delirium in the emergency department – a pilot study on the feasibility of a new algorithm for use in older emergency department patients: the modified confusion assessment method for the emergency department (mCAM-ED). Scand J Trauma Resusc Emerg Med 22(1):19
28. Han JH, Wilson A, Vasilevskis EE et al (2013) Diagnosing delirium in older emergency department patients: validity and reliability of the delirium triage screen and the brief confusion assessment method. Ann Emerg Med 62(5):457–465
29. Bellelli G, Morandi A, Davis D (2014) Validation of the 4AT, a new instrument for rapid delirium screening: a study in 234 hospitalised older people. Age Ageing 43:496–502
30. Dellinger RP, Levy MM, Carlet JM et al (2008) Surviving sepsis campaign: international guidelines for management of severe sepsis and septic shock: 2008. Crit Care Med 36(1):296–327

31. Shapiro NI, Fisher C, Donnino M et al (2010) The feasibility and accuracy of point-of-care lactate measurement in emergency department patients with suspected infection. J Emerg Med 39(1):89–94
32. Jain P, Parada J, David A et al (1995) Overuse of the indwelling urinary tract catheter in hospitalized medical patient. Arch Intern Med 155(13):1425–1429
33. Hazelett S, Tsai M, Gareri M et al (2006) The association between indwelling urinary catheter use in the elderly and urinary tract infection in acute care. BMC Geriatr 6:15
34. Elpern E, Killeen K, Ketchem A et al (2009) Reducing use of indwelling urinary catheters and associated urinary tract infections. Am J Crit Care 18:535–541
35. Scottish Intercollegiate Guidelines Network (2006) Management of suspected bacterial urinary tract infection in adults
36. Banerjee J, Conroy S (2012) The silver book: quality care for older people with urgent & emergency care needs. Secondary the silver book: quality care for older people with urgent & emergency care needs. http://www.bgs.org.uk/index.php/bgscampaigns-715/silverbook
37. Misch F, Messmer AS, Nickel CH et al (2014) Impact of observation on disposition of elderly patients presenting to emergency departments with non-specific complaints. PLoS One 9(5):e98097
38. van der Wardt V (2015) Should guidance for the use of antihypertensive medication in older people with frailty be different? Age Ageing 44(6):912–913
39. Ogliari G, Westendorp RGJ, Muller M et al (2015) Blood pressure and 10-year mortality risk in the Milan geriatrics 75+ cohort study: role of functional and cognitive status. Age Ageing 44(6):932–937
40. The Eastern Association for the Surgery of Trauma (2001) The EAST practice management guidelines workshop: practice management guidelines for geriatric trauma
41. Abbey J, Piller N, De Bellis A et al (2004) The Abbey pain scale: a 1-minute numerical indicator for people with end-stage dementia. Int J Palliat Nurs 10(1):6–13
42. Chan EW, Taylor SE, Marriott J et al (2010) An intervention to encourage ambulance paramedics to bring patients' own medications to the ED: impact on medications brought in and prescribing errors. Emerg Med Australas 22(2):151–158
43. Gill TM, Gahbauer EA, Han L et al (2010) Trajectories of disability in the last year of life. N Engl J Med 362(13):1173–1180
44. Krumholz HM (2013) Post-hospital syndrome – an acquired, transient condition of generalized risk. N Engl J Med 368(2):100–102
45. Sager MA, Franke T, Inouye SK et al (1996) Functional outcomes of acute medical illness and hospitalization in older persons. Arch Intern Med 156(6):645–652
46. McCusker J, Bellavance F, Cardin S et al (2000) Prediction of hospital utilization among elderly patients during the 6 months after an emergency department visit. Ann Emerg Med 36(5):438–445
47. Mion LC, Palmer RM, Meldon SW et al (2003) Case finding and referral model for emergency department elders: a randomized clinical trial. [see comment]. Ann Emerg Med 41(1):57–68
48. Meldon SWML, Palmer RM et al (2003) A brief risk-stratification tool to predict repeat emergency department visits and hospitalizations in older patients discharged from the emergency department. Acad Emerg Med 10:224–232
49. Lee JS, Schwindt G, Langevin M et al (2008) Validation of the triage risk stratification tool to identify older persons at risk for hospital admission and returning to the emergency department. J Am Geriatr Soc 56(11):2112–2117
50. Carpenter CR, Shelton E, Fowler S et al (2015) Risk factors and screening instruments to predict adverse outcomes for undifferentiated older emergency department patients: a systematic review and meta-analysis. Acad Emerg Med 22(1):1–21
51. Di Bari M, Salvi F, Roberts AT et al (2012) Prognostic stratification of elderly patients in the emergency department: a comparison between the "identification of seniors at risk" and the "silver code". J Gerontol Ser A Biol Sci Med Sci 67(5):544–550
52. Graf CE, Giannelli SV, Herrmann FR et al (2012) Can we improve the detection of old patients at higher risk for readmission after an emergency department visit? J Am Geriatr Soc 60(7):1372–1373

Comprehensive Geriatric Assessment in the Emergency Department

6

Els Devriendt and Simon Conroy

6.1 Frail Older People in the Emergency Department

Many older people who are admitted to hospital come via the emergency department (ED) which is a key interface in the health and social care system where older people with crises can be assessed. So it is important that EDs are appropriately supported in the management of older people.

The clinical assessment of frail older people is challenging because they often present non-specifically (e.g. with falls, immobility, delirium) which can make the immediate diagnosis obscure. History taking may be challenging because of sensory impairment, under-reporting of problems, dementia or delirium. Often additional information and collateral history are needed which may not be readily accessible in the emergency setting; time pressures or lack of geriatric knowledge may prevent staff from focussing on anything other than immediate problem.

Older people are especially sensitive to the harms associated with long waits in the ED (e.g. pressure sores)—and these long waits in ED can have adverse consequences on the downstream outcomes. For example, longer waits in ED are associated with increased in-patient mortality [1].

Whilst whole system approaches are required to modify urgent care use, in particular systems that align primary, prehospital and secondary care pathways ('vertical integration') [2], the ED remains a key focus for intervention that can improve patient outcomes.

E. Devriendt (✉)
Department of Public Health and Primary Care, Academic Centre for Nursing and Midwifery, KU Leuven, Kapucijnenvoer 35/4, 3000 Leuven, Belgium

Department of Geriatric Medicine, University Hospitals Leuven,
Herestraat 49, 3000 Leuven, Belgium
e-mail: els.devriendt@uzleuven.be

S. Conroy
Department of Health Sciences, University of Leicester,
Leicester, United Kingdom

6.2 Evidence-Based Solutions for the Care of Older People: Comprehensive Geriatric Assessment

The typical profile of frail older patients accessing EDs mandates a different approach from general adult patients. To meet the complex needs of frail older patients, the process of 'comprehensive geriatric assessment' (CGA) has been developed. CGA is defined as 'a multidimensional, interdisciplinary diagnostic process to determine the medical, psychological and functional capabilities of a frail older person in order to develop a coordinated and integrated plan for the treatment and long-term follow-up' [3]. Why this is important will be addressed in this section.

Multidimensional—this highlights the importance of taking a holistic overview. In this cohort of patients, it is not sufficient to focus simply on one domain or the main problem of the patient. For example, an approach to chest pain that simply states that the troponin is negative and that a coronary angiogram is not required but fails to test for and identify the cognitive impairment that led to the individual not taking analgesia for arthritis (the true cause of the pain) is doomed to fail. Equally, a purely functional approach to falls that seeks to provide only rehabilitation and not identify the underlying reasons for a fall (of which there are many, including serious disorders such as aortic stenosis) will not succeed. It is the integrated assessment of all of the domains of CGA that allows an accurate problem list to be generated.

Interdisciplinary diagnostic process—in a mature CGA service, the hierarchy should be flattened such that all staff should feel empowered to constructively challenge within and without of their particular area of expertise. For example, the option to admit for rehabilitation by a therapist concerned about falls at home might be challenged by pointing out that admission often increases the risk of falls and that home-based rehabilitation may offer substantial benefits [4]. Equally therapists will bring useful information to the diagnostic process—for example, the patient who is 'fit to return home' that develops new dyspnoea on mobilisation might prompt a re-evaluation of respiratory function and identify potentially new diagnoses such as pulmonary embolus. That this assessment is a *process* and not a discrete event is also the key; the process should continue in an iterative manner over the course of the acute stay, and the diagnostic elements should be sensitive to deviations from the anticipated pathway. For example, if the initial treatment plan for an individual with a fall and hip pain but no fracture was to 'increase analgesia, reduce antihypertensives and aim to return home once able to walk 5 m unaided using a frame', yet after 14 h, pain remains a problem, the diagnosis may need to be revisited and further imaging may be considered.

Frail older people—targeting patients who will benefit most from CGA is important. CGA requires time and staffing resource, both of which may be in short supply in a hospital, e.g. busy ED environment. The use of accurate and easy-to-use case-finding or screening tools should be a critical first step. A wide range of screening tools are available, but none are perfect and none have an area under the curve of greater than 0.7—so the current tools *alone* are insufficient to identify the population of interest, although they can be used to reliably screen out those that do not require CGA as their specificity (and hence negative predictive value tends to be good) [5–7]. The most common targeting criteria are a combination of age, physical disease, geriatric syndromes, impairment of functional ability and social problems [8].

Coordinated and integrated plan for treatment—reinforces that the team caring for an individual needs to know and respect each other's roles and know and understand what each is doing and how the medical treatment will impact upon the rehabilitation goals and vice versa. For example, whilst therapists would not need to know the detailed intricacies of the management of acute heart failure, it is important that they know that intravenous diuretics might be required for the first few days that will result in polyuria and then be able to incorporate continence needs into the rehabilitation plan. Equally, doctors will need to appreciate that just because a patient has grade 5 power on the MRC grading system, that does not necessarily translate into useful functional ability.

Follow-up—as many older people will have multiple long-term conditions, they will usually require some form of ongoing care and support. How this is delivered will vary from country to country, but there is little point in providing excellent acute care if conditions are only going to be allowed to decline because of a lack of ongoing support. For example, a 2-week admission during which Parkinson's disease medications are carefully titrated and optimised in conjunction with the multi-disciplinary rehabilitation process can easily be reversed if there is no ongoing titration of L-Dopa once the patient returns home.

So whilst integrating standard medical diagnostic evaluation, CGA emphasises problem-solving, team working and a patient-centred approach.

6.2.1 The History of Comprehensive Geriatric Assessment

CGA has evolved over time; three generations of CGA instruments are used in clinical practice. First-generation CGA instruments use an assortment of individually validated instruments that each focus on one clinical domain (e.g. mini-mental state examination [9] evaluating cognition or the index of activities of daily living [10] evaluating physical function [11]). The 'impression' of clinicians is usually the trigger to initialise the assessment of a specific domain [12].

Second-generation CGA instruments encompass all geriatric domains, are setting specific [13] and have been validated in each specific setting (e.g. Minimum Data Set (MDS) 2.0 [11, 14]). Whilst the first and the second generation of instruments conducts a systematic and standardised assessment of the patient, the items of the different instruments are not uniform, a characteristic required to transfer information across different settings (e.g. home care, long-time care and acute care).

Third-generation instruments, such as the interRAI Suite, allow data transfer between healthcare settings and within the healthcare setting between different wards (e.g. ED and ACE unit), based on a common set of standardised items [13, 15]. Electronic standardised clinical data systems can support the transfer of this data which can improve the coordination and quality of care.

6.3 The Evidence Base for Comprehensive Geriatric Assessment

CGA improves outcomes for older people in various settings. Meta-analyses have shown reduced mortality or deterioration (odds ratio 0.76), improved cognition (odds ratio 1.11), improved quality of life, reduced length of stay and reduced rates of long-term care use (odds ratio 0.78) and are associated with reduced costs [16–18].

In the urgent hospital care context in, there are three main models or settings where CGA has been tested:

1. Acute care for the older (ACE) units: these are post-ED receiving wards (sometime referred to as acute medical units or acute frailty units). ACE units typically assess frail older people over the first 1–3 days of their stay.
2. Geriatric evaluation and management (GEM) units: these units deliver CGA to frail older people who require a longer in-patient stay within a specific geographical area (ward).
3. Interdisciplinary geriatric consultation services (IGCS): liaison services or teams that care for frail older people wherever they might be found in the hospital, rather than in a specific ward-based area.

There is reasonable evidence that CGA works better in ACE or GEM units compared to IGCS [19, 20]. Core principles underpinning the development of ACE and GEM units include [21, 22]:

- A dedicated environment: environments designed to prevent cognitive and physical functional decline through early mobilisation, orientation, way finding, familiarity and socialisation. Examples might include the installation of clocks, calendars, elevated toilet seats, easy-to-use door levers, corridor handrails, communal areas, designated spaces for personal items, carpeted flooring, visually contrasting floor and wall coverings, enhanced lighting and reducing trip hazards.

- Patient-centred care: assessment, identification and intervention of risks (mobility, hydration and nutrition, cognition, self-care and skin integrity) for each individual. Intervention might include standing or mobilising as soon and as often as possible; providing nutritious snacks, high-protein meals, and 'four glasses of water a day—prescribed and administered like a drug'; providing orientation cues ensuring eyeglasses and hearing aids are worn; encouraging families to visit; administering regular analgesia when indicated and strategies to promote sleep; encouraging self-washing, dressing, feeding etc.; and providing care to prevent sores.
- Preservation of ADLs through multidisciplinary assessment and working: improving mobility to decrease the risk of falling and improving self-care ability by providing adaptive or assistive devices and exercise.
- Early discharge planning: involving social workers and families or caregivers in care planning, liaising with community care providers and devising a care plan outlining patient functional goals and home care needs with a target for the length of stay.
- Reducing iatrogenesis: this includes accurate diagnosis, medication reviews and avoiding unnecessary harms such as overtreatment and under-treatment, unnecessary procedures especially urinary catheters and venous access/venepuncture, and prevention of harms such as venous thromboembolism.

6.4 The Evidence Base for Comprehensive Geriatric Assessment in the Emergency Department

The delivery of such complex interventions such as CGA is challenging within a busy, time-constrained ED. It is difficult to recreate the ACE or GEM unit model of care in the ED context. Several studies have examined the role of a team identifying older people in the ED and delivering coordinated care in the community setting upon discharge immediately after ED visit [23–29], and a meta-analysis of these studies provides some evidence of improved outcomes [30]. On the other hand, a few studies looked at a more embedded CGA service in the ED which leans towards the unit model [31–33]. Table 6.1 gives an overview of the existing evidence.

The current evidence base is limited by methodological issues and overall poor quality of the studies (e.g. lack of power), and heterogeneity in intervention and outcomes makes the comparison of the existing literature difficult. Positive elements include interventions with targeting of a population at risk, discrete beds for geriatric patient on the ED, specialised trained caregivers, a multidisciplinary approach and home-based follow-up to improve adherence to the given recommendations.

Table 6.1 A summary of controlled evaluation of interventions for frail older people attending emergency departments

Trial	Population	Intervention	Team	Readmission	Hospitalisation	Functional decline	Admission to LTC	Mortality
			CGA in the ED					
Miller [29] Non-randomised controlled trial	65+	Geriatric case finding and liaison service: CGA → team discussion → further work-up in the ED—evaluations during hospitalisation—referral → information transfer → telephone follow-up	Geriatric nurse Consultation with ED staff	3 m ↔	N/A	N/A	↕	↕
Mc Cusker [26, 34] RCT	65+, ISAR ≥2, expected to be discharged	CGA → problem identification → team discussion → referral → limited follow-up after the ED visit	Nurses Consultation with ED staff and geriatric staff	30d ↑	N/A	4 m ↓	N/A	N/A
Mion [27] RCT	65+, living at home, expected to be discharge home	CGA → identification of unmet needs → team discussion → discharge plan → information transfer → referral → short-term telephone follow-up	Advanced practice nurse specialised in geriatrics Consultation with ED staff	30d ↔ 120d ↔	N/A	N/A	30d ↓ 120d ↔	30d ↔ 120d ↔
Caplan [28] RCT	75+, discharged from the ED	CGA on the ED or at home → discussion with GP + weekly interdisciplinary team meeting → care plan—initiation of urgent interventions → referrals → follow-up for 4 weeks	Nurse Consultation with geriatric team	30d ↓ 18 m ↓	N/A	6 m ↓	↕	↕

					During HOS ↔	N/A	N/A
Basic [35] RCT	Older people AND Functional impairment OR psychological disability OR social disability OR active multisystem disease OR readmission	CGA → problem identification → referral when discharged—suggestions and recommendations in the file when admitted	Geriatric nurse	N/A	↔		
Foo [36] Pre-post evaluation	65+, living at home	CGA → problem list → team discussion → intervention if necessary → referral or admission	ED nurse trained in geriatric care Consultation with ED physician or geriatric nurse clinician	3 m ↓ 6 m ↓ 9 m ↓ 12 m ↓	N/A	N/A	↔
Arendts [37, 38] Non-randomised trial	65+ and criteria based on clinical presentation	Early allied health intervention: Comprehensive functional assessment → initiation of services based on identified needs	Allied health personnel Other specialists when required	28d ↓ 1y ↑	→	N/A	28d ↔ 1y ↔
Wright [23] Pre-post cohort study	70+ with complex medical and social needs	CGA → prompt intervention → referral → follow-up at home	Multidisciplinary geriatric team	N/A	→	N/A	N/A

(continued)

Table 6.1 (continued)

Trial	Population	Intervention	Team	Readmission	Hospitalisation	Functional decline	Admission to LTC	Mortality
Foo [39] Quasi RCT	65+, TRST ≥2, living at home, planned for discharge	Focused geriatric screening (15-item screening form) → intervention if necessary → referral	GEM nurse	3 m, 6 m, 9 m, 12 m ↔	N/A	3 m ↓ 6 m ↓ 9 m ↓ 12 m ↓	N/A	↔
Embedded CGA—service in the ED
Ellis [31] Pre-post evaluation	65+ AND Functional impairment OR cognitive impairment OR falls or other GER syndromes OR care home pat	ACE unit: rapid and thorough CGA → admission avoidance or specialty admission Specific policy, geriatric infrastructure	Geriatrician and experienced older people nurse	7d ↔ 30d ↔	↔	N/A	12m ↔	12m ↔
Keyes [32] (Retrospective) pre-post evaluation	65+	Senior ED: CGA → problem identification → case management Staff training and education, geriatric infrastructure	Nurses, social workers, pharmacist and physician	30d ↔	↓	N/A	N/A	N/A
Conroy [33] Pre-post cohort study	Frail older people	Emergency frailty unit: Embedded CGA service—vertically integrated care pathways Staff education	Geriatrician + ED staff	7d ↔ 30d ↔ 90d ↓	↓	N/A	N/A	N/A

6.5 Practical Examples of Comprehensive Geriatric Assessment

Before CGA

Vera, an 80-year-old lady, attended the ED following a fall. A primary survey revealed no major injuries, and there was no evidence of any head trauma. The assessing doctor felt that the fall was 'mechanical' and that there was no suggestion of any syncope. Near-patient tests revealed slightly low sodium. The doctor assessing Vera felt that she was safe to go home and arranged for her daughter to collect her and asked that they see the GP in a week to get the sodium levels looked into.

Vera was taken home by her daughter feeling reassured but had a second fall 2 days later; on this occasion she injured her hip; she was again taken to the ED where an X-ray revealed a hip fracture that required surgery. The surgery was successful, but post-operatively Vera developed delirium thought to be related to infection; antibiotics were given which caused some diarrhoea, but all eventually settled. After a period of convalescence in a community hospital, Vera returned home after 6 weeks, although her confidence remained low.

After CGA

…same doctor assessment….

The admitting nurse had completed a frailty screening tool which indicated that Vera had some cognitive impairment and polypharmacy and needed help with activities of daily living indicating that she was at high risk of readmission (ISAR score 3). Whilst the doctor was awaiting the blood test results, the nurse arranged for a review by the frailty team. The frailty nurse undertook a holistic assessment, which revealed that Vera had significant cognitive impairment (MMSE 24/30). The frailty nurse phoned Vera's daughter who confirmed what appeared to be a history of undiagnosed dementia and also mentioned how stressed she had been over recent weeks, as she was the main carer for her mum. There had been several falls, and Vera's confusion had been worsening over the last few days. The frailty nurse asked the duty geriatrician to review Vera; this led to diuretics being stopped as a likely cause of the low sodium. A referral to the falls service was made; in addition, the intermediate care team were asked to see Vera at home and support her for a few weeks. The geriatricians discussed Vera's case with her GP, who was happy to monitor the sodium levels and fluid status—he also agreed to refer to the memory clinic. Vera left the department and made a gradual but uneventful recovery at home without readmission.

6.6 How to Conduct Comprehensive Geriatric Assessment in the Emergency Department

The ED provides an early opportunity to initiate CGA in a targeted population of frail older patients. Within the ED, it is possible and useful to initiate CGA and to identify domains at risk within the older patient and identify management strategies; these might be delivered in the acute hospital or in the community according to individual needs. A suggested approach to delivering CGA in the ED is outlined here.

6.6.1 Problem Detection

6.6.1.1 Problem Detection: Identification of the High-Risk Population

Older people are a heterogeneous group. Current triage at the front door of the hospital prioritises using physiological parameters. Conventional triage often fails to detect and identify the complexity seen in frail older people; frailty itself is a marker of poor outcomes following an acute care episode [40]. The identification of high-risk patients using the frailty paradigm during the ED visit is important to identify the need for additional assessment.

Frailty has an important role in the identification of patients at risk for adverse events following discharge from ED. Many tools have been developed, but they have significant limitations when operationalised in the ED. Examples include the identification of seniors at risk (ISAR) and the triage risk-stratification tool (TRST) [41–45]. The tools are relatively easy to use but have limitations in their predictive accuracy, as mentioned above. Those instruments can give some direction but cannot be used as a stand-alone test and should be combined with clinical judgement.

6.6.1.2 Problem Detection: Domains of Assessment

As the most important tasks of the ED are focused on diagnosis and appropriate discharge management, e.g. *discharge home with referral for ambulatory follow-up or admission to an acute geriatric unit for the high-risk patients*, the assessment of functional problems, cognitive impairment, polypharmacy, falls and existing help must be seen as essential information in the ED. During the ED admission, it is important to detect those problems and manage them as where possible within the complex ED environment.

6.6.1.2.1 Functionality
Loss of *function* can lead to a loss of self-care and lead to a risk of loss of independence and institutionalisation. Functional decline is nearly always related to an underlying disease process and should be interpreted accordingly [46]. It is important to compare the premorbid function with function at the time of the ED visit. After the diagnosis and treatment of underlying diseases, interventions including rehabilitation and optimisation of home care can be initiated in the ED. Different, easy-to-complete scales (such as Katz [10] and/or Barthel [47]) can be used to map the functional evolution of the patient.

6.6.1.2.2 Cognition
The identification *of cognitive impairment*, whether dementia or delirium, is essential in the ED. The detection of previously unknown subclinical cognitive impairment is very useful in the ED. A positive screen requires further evaluation, first differentiating delirium (see Chap. 13) from dementia (see Chap. 13). Several short instruments can be used, e.g. 4-AT and Mini-Cog [48, 49]. In addition to identifying the immediate clinical scenario, diagnosing cognitive impairment may well have an impact on clinical decision-making and prognosis.

Delirium is associated with poor outcomes and may be related to the underlying disorders. It is associated with a longer length of stay, in-patient harm, reduced quality of life and death [50]. Early detection of symptoms and a search for the underlying cause must be started as soon as possible in the first few hours after ED admission.

6.6.1.2.3 Depression
Depression is the most common mental health problem in old age, and aetiological factors such as social isolation and chronic physical illness mean that an ageing population will be a more depressed one too. The Geriatric Depression Scale-5 [51] is a quick useful tool to screen for depression. Older people who self-harm have high levels of suicidal intent [52, 53] and often have ongoing suicidal ideation after presentation. The adverse effects on cognitive function of common drugs used in self-harm, such as tricyclic antidepressants, may make detection of the act more difficult. Additionally, older people with delirium or dementia may present with unintentional self-harm which, if undetected, could have adverse consequences.

6.6.1.2.4 Polypharmacy
The intake of several medications may affect the care for older people at the ED. Adverse drug events account for approximately 6.5% of all hospital admissions

[54], but more in older people, leading to increased hospital stay and significant morbidity and mortality [55, 56]. Making a list of all medications taken (medicines reconciliation) and identification of polypharmacy can be an important first step during the ED admission period. Restricted time on the ED limits an in-depth medication review but is an excellent opportunity to gather information for subsequent intervention in or out of hospital. There are examples of pharmacists based in the ED who can support this process and liaise with community pharmacists, adding value to the patient journey.

6.6.1.2.5 Falls
Falls is one of the most common reasons for admission in older people visiting the ED. The main priority in the ED is to recognise and manage any injury related to fall, to identify the underlying pathology and to list the causes of the fall. As the cause of a fall is often related to multiple factors, the presence of a fall should be an indicator for multidimensional assessment. A referral to a specialised falls service is important for a further multifactorial intervention. A robust process for identifying any possible predisposition to injury (e.g. fracture risk) is sensible in older people attending the ED with falls,

6.6.1.2.6 Early Discharge Planning
It is important to get an overview of the existing help at home and home circumstances in order to decide on a safe discharge destination after ED visit. The first port of call is of course the patient. But informal and formal carers may also provide important information on the home situation, including the ambulance service. It is also important to consider the possible caregiver burden.

6.6.1.3 Problem Detection: Comprehensive Geriatric Assessment Instruments
A variety of CGA instruments have been developed to capture the complexity of the patient. Given the time constraints and complexity of the emergency setting, it is important to work with validated and short instruments that are able to detect problems requiring prompt action or areas which need further investigation after the ED visit. Both instruments of the second and third generation are useful and make a standardised way of detecting problems possible. There are instruments covering a range of domains of the patient, e.g. interRAI instruments (www.interRAI.org) and instruments focusing on one domain, e.g. cognitive functioning: 4-AT test [49].

6.6.1.4 Problem Detection: Importance
Conducting a limited CGA during the ED visit can result in the identification of additional underlying problems, which are not automatically detected by usual clinical investigations [57]. CGA can make a subjective clinical opinion more objective. Organising and prioritising the multiple concerns will help prioritise the severity of the situation and the most appropriate settings where the issues can be addressed.

6.6.2 Care Plan

The next step following the problem identification is to get to work with the information gathered from the CGA. Initiating CGA in the ED leads to a proactive approach and can provide a time course against each action that will inform the evolution of the condition of the patient.

CGA usually gives a lot of information that needs prioritisation by developing a stratified problem list—which will be informed by the multiple domains described above. The care plan should be an individual plan for each patient and is preferably discussed with all healthcare workers, the patient himself and informal caregivers involved in the care for the patient.

As the ED plays an important role in the screening and identification of problems, an important part of the further planning will be referral to other services in- and outside the hospital, e.g. depending on the identified problems such as referral to memory clinic, falls clinic, CGA unit and primary care provider.

CGA can give diagnostic insights on problems that are presented with functional decline, and early initiation of CGA can avoid further decline [57].

Having an overall picture of the older patient in the ED through geriatric assessment can enhance the decision-making process with regard to orientation of the patient (admission or discharge) and may impact indirectly patient flow in the ED. An admission to the hospital can be avoided and replaced by a safe discharge or alternatives to admission (day hospital) [57] or hospital at home services [4, 58].

Objective CGA information may have an impact on treatment decisions. For example, describing the initial presenting problem (such as chest pain) in the context of global decline related to dementia with features of end-of-life care might dissuade the clinician from an active course (e.g. anti-platelets, anticoagulants) more towards a palliative approach.

6.6.3 Follow-Up

Studies suggest that follow-up after ED discharge is important to implement the recommendations or make a further evaluation of problems detected. Follow-up after discharge can be organised by the hospital or by primary care providers. Follow-up implies that information transfer should be optimal and fast (see Chap. 23). The coordination of referrals and coordination of implementation of recommendations will improve the chance of success.

6.7 Summary: Comprehensive Geriatric Assessment in the Emergency Department

Frail older people are important users of EDs. Multidimensional assessment and interdisciplinary management—often referred to as CGA—can improve outcomes for frail older people in the ED. Important domains of assessment over and above the standard diagnostic approach include cognition, function, mood, medications and home support. The multidimensional assessment should trigger an interdisciplinary intervention, in hospital or at home depending upon the individual's needs.

Whilst the evidence base for CGA in general is robust, in the ED specifically, the evidence is still evolving. Future research will need to refine risk-stratification tools, determine optimal methods of service configuration and develop interventions that can be transferred between settings.

References

1. Carter EJ, Pouch SM, Larson EL (2013) The relationship between emergency department crowding and patient outcomes: a systematic review. J Nurs Scholarsh 46(2):106–115
2. Ernst & Young (2012) National Evaluation of the Department of Health's integrated care pilots. RAND Europe, Cambridge, UK
3. Rubenstein LZ, Rubenstein LV (1991) Multidimensional assessment of elderly patients. Adv Intern Med 36:81–108
4. Shepperd S, Doll H, Broad J, Gladman J, Iliffe S, Langhorne P, et al (2009) Early discharge hospital at home. Cochrane Database Syst Rev Issue 1
5. Carpenter CR, Shelton E, Fowler S, Suffoletto B, Platts-Mills T, Rothman RE et al (2015) Risk factors and screening instruments to predict adverse outcomes for undifferentiated older emergency department patients: a systematic review and meta-analysis. Acad Emerg Med 22(1):1–21
6. Salvi F, Belluigi A, Cherubini A (2013) Predictive validity of different modified versions of the identification of seniors at risk. J Am Geriatr Soc 61(3):462–464
7. Di Bari M, Salvi F, Roberts AT, Balzi D, Lorenzetti B, Morichi V et al (2012) Prognostic stratification of elderly patients in the emergency department: a comparison between the "identification of seniors at risk" and the "silver code". J Gerontol A Biol Sci Med Sci 67(5):544–550
8. Ellis G, Langhorne P (2004) Comprehensive geriatric assessment for older hospital patients. Br Med Bull 71:45–59
9. Folstein MF, Folstein SE, McHugh PR (1975) "Mini-mental state". A practical method for grading the cognitive state of patients for the clinician. J Psychiatr Res 12(3):189–198
10. Katz S, Ford AB, Moskowitz RW, Jackson BA, Jaffe MW (1963) Studies of illness in the aged. The index of Adl: a standardized measure of biological and psychosocial function. JAMA 185:914–919
11. Wellens NI, Deschodt M, Flamaing J, Moons P, Boonen S, Boman X et al (2011) First-generation versus third-generation comprehensive geriatric assessment instruments in the acute hospital setting: a comparison of the minimum geriatric screening tools (MGST) and the interRAI acute care (interRAI AC). J Nutr Health Aging 15(8):638–644
12. Rubenstein LZ, Stuck AE, Siu AL, Wieland D (1991) Impacts of geriatric evaluation and management programs on defined outcomes: overview of the evidence. J Am Geriatr Soc 39(9 Pt 2):8S–16S. discussion 17S-18S
13. Bernabei R, Landi F, Onder G, Liperoti R, Gambassi G (2008) Second and third generation assessment instruments: the birth of standardization in geriatric care. J Gerontol A Biol Sci Med Sci 63(3):308–313
14. Carpenter GI, Teare GF, Steel K, Berg K, Murphy K, Bjornson J et al (2001) A new assessment for elders admitted to acute care: reliability of the MDS-AC. Aging 13(4):316–330
15. Gray LC, Berg K, Fries BE, Henrard JC, Hirdes JP, Steel K et al (2009) Sharing clinical information across care settings: the birth of an integrated assessment system. BMC Health Serv Res 9:71
16. Beswick AD, Rees K, Dieppe P, Ayis S, Gooberman-Hill R, Horwood J et al (2008) Complex interventions to improve physical function and maintain independent living in elderly people: a systematic review and meta-analysis.[see comment]. Lancet 371(9614):725–735

17. Ellis G, Whitehead M, O'Neill D, Robinson D, Langhorne P (2011) Comprehensive geriatric assessment for older adults admitted to hospital. Cochrane Library: Cochrane collaboration
18. Ellis G, Whitehead MA, Robinson D, O'Neill D, Langhorne P (2011) Comprehensive geriatric assessment for older adults admitted to hospital: meta-analysis of randomised controlled trials. BMJ 343:d6553
19. Deschodt M, Flamaing J, Haentjens P, Boonen S, Milisen K (2013) Impact of geriatric consultation teams on clinical outcome in acute hospitals: a systematic review and meta-analysis. BMC Med 11(1):48
20. Van Craen K, Braes T, Wellens N, Denhaerynck K, Flamaing J, Moons P et al (2010) The effectiveness of inpatient geriatric evaluation and management units: a systematic review and meta-analysis. J Am Geriatr Soc 58(1):83–92
21. Fox MT, Sidani S, Persaud M, Tregunno D, Maimets I, Brooks D et al (2013) Acute care for elders components of acute geriatric unit care: systematic descriptive review. J Am Geriatr Soc 61(6):939–946
22. Fox MT, Persaud M, Maimets I, O'Brien K, Brooks D, Tregunno D et al (2012) Effectiveness of acute geriatric unit care using acute care for elders components: a systematic review and meta-analysis. J Am Geriatr Soc 60(12):2237–2245
23. Wright PN, Tan G, Iliffe S, Lee D (2014) The impact of a new emergency admission avoidance system for older people on length of stay and same-day discharges. Age Ageing 43(1):116–121
24. Davison J, Bond J, Dawson P, Steen IN, Kenny RA (2005) Patients with recurrent falls attending Accident & Emergency benefit from multifactorial intervention--a randomised controlled trial.[see comment]. Age Ageing 34(2):162–168
25. Close J, Ellis M, Hooper R, Glucksman E, Jackson S, Swift C (1999) Prevention of falls in the elderly trial (PROFET): a randomised controlled trial. Lancet 353:93–97
26. McCusker J, Dendukuri N, Tousignant P, Verdon J, Poulin de Courval L, Belzile E (2003) Rapid two-stage emergency department intervention for seniors: impact on continuity of care. Acad Emerg Med 10(3):233–243
27. Mion LC, Palmer RM, Meldon SW, Bass DM, Singer ME, Payne SM et al (2003) Case finding and referral model for emergency department elders: a randomized clinical trial. Ann Emerg Med 41(1):57–68
28. Caplan GA, Williams AJ, Daly B, Abraham K (2004) A randomized, controlled trial of comprehensive geriatric assessment and multidisciplinary intervention after discharge of elderly from the emergency department--the DEED II study. J Am Geriatr Soc 52(9):1417–1423
29. Miller DK, Lewis LM, Nork MJ, Morley JE (1996) Controlled trial of a geriatric case-finding and liaison service in an emergency department. J Am Geriatr Soc 44(5):513–520
30. Conroy SP, Stevens T, Parker SG, Gladman JRF (2011) A systematic review of comprehensive geriatric assessment to improve outcomes for frail older people being rapidly discharged from acute hospital: 'interface geriatrics'. Age Ageing 40(4):436–443
31. Ellis G, Jamieson CA, Alcorn M, Devlin V (2012) An acute Care for Elders (ACE) unit in the emergency department. Eur Geriatr Med 3(4):261–263
32. Keyes DC, Singal B, Kropf CW, Fisk A (2014) Impact of a new senior emergency department on emergency department recidivism, rate of hospital admission, and hospital length of stay Ann Emerg Med 63(5):517–524
33. Conroy SP, Ansari K, Williams M, Laithwaite E, Teasdale B, Dawson J et al (2014) A controlled evaluation of comprehensive geriatric assessment in the emergency department: the 'Emergency frailty Unit'. Age Ageing 43(1):109–114
34. McCusker J, Verdon J, Tousignant P, de Courval LP, Dendukuri N, Belzile E (2001) Rapid emergency department intervention for older people reduces risk of functional decline: results of a multicenter randomized trial. J Am Geriatr Soc 49(10):1272–1281
35. Basic D, Conforti DA (2005) A prospective, randomised controlled trial of an aged care nurse intervention within the emergency department. Aust Health Rev 29(1):51–59
36. Foo CL, Siu VW, Tan TL, Ding YY, Seow E (2012) Geriatric assessment and intervention in an emergency department observation unit reduced re-attendance and hospitalisation rates. Australas J Ageing 31(1):40–46

37. Arendts G, Fitzhardinge S, Pronk K, Donaldson M, Hutton M, Nagree Y (2012) The impact of early emergency department allied health intervention on admission rates in older people: a non-randomized clinical study. BMC Geriatr 12:8
38. Arendts G, Fitzhardinge S, Pronk K, Hutton M (2013) Outcomes in older patients requiring comprehensive allied health care prior to discharge from the emergency department. Emerg Med Australas 25(2):127–131
39. Foo CL, Siu VW, Ang H, Phuah MW, Ooi CK (2014) Risk stratification and rapid geriatric screening in an emergency department - a quasi-randomised controlled trial. BMC Geriatr 14:98
40. Eeles EMP, White SV, O'Mahony SM, Bayer AJ, Hubbard RE (2012) The impact of frailty and delirium on mortality in older inpatients. Age Ageing 41(3):412–416
41. Dendukuri N, McCusker J, Belzile E (2004) The identification of seniors at risk screening tool: further evidence of concurrent and predictive validity. J Am Geriatr Soc 52(2):290–296
42. Deschodt M, Wellens NIH, Braes T, De Vuyst A, Boonen S, Flamaing J et al (2011) Prediction of functional decline in older hospitalized patients: a comparative multicenter study of three screening tools. Aging Clin Exp Res 23(5-6):421–426
43. Braes T, Moons P, Lipkens P, Sterckx W, Sabbe M, Flamaing J et al (2010) Screening for risk of unplanned readmission in older patients admitted to hospital: predictive accuracy of three instruments. Aging Clin Exp Res 22(4):345–351
44. Lee JS, Schwindt G, Langevin M, Moghabghab R, Alibhai SMH, Kiss A et al (2008) Validation of the triage risk stratification tool to identify older persons at risk for hospital admission and returning to the emergency department. J Am Geriatr Soc 56(11):2112–2117
45. Graf CE, Giannelli SV, Herrmann FR, Sarasin FP, Michel J-P, Zekry D et al (2012) Can we improve the detection of old patients at higher risk for readmission after an emergency department visit? J Am Geriatr Soc 60(7):1372–1373
46. Schumacher JG (2005) Emergency medicine and older adults: continuing challenges and opportunities. Am J Emerg Med 23(4):556–560
47. Wade DT, Collin C (1988) The Barthel ADL index: a standard measure of physical disability? Int Disabil Stud 10:64–67
48. Borson S, Scanlan JM, Chen P, Ganguli M (2003) The mini-cog as a screen for dementia: validation in a population-based sample. J Am Geriatr Soc 51(10):1451–1454
49. Bellelli G, Morandi A, Davis DH, Mazzola P, Turco R, Gentile S et al (2014) Validation of the 4AT, a new instrument for rapid delirium screening: a study in 234 hospitalised older people. Age Ageing 43(4):496–502
50. Bradshaw LE, Goldberg SE, Lewis SA, Whittamore K, Gladman JRF, Jones RG et al (2013) Six-month outcomes following an emergency hospital admission for older adults with co-morbid mental health problems indicate complexity of care needs. Age Ageing 42(5):582–588
51. Rinaldi P, Mecocci P, Benedetti C, Ercolani S, Bregnocchi M, Menculini G et al (2003) Validation of the five-item geriatric depression scale in elderly subjects in three different settings. J Am Geriatr Soc 51(5):694–698
52. Dennis MS, Wakefield P, Molloy C, Andrews H, Friedman T, Dennis MS et al (2007) A study of self-harm in older people: mental disorder, social factors and motives. Aging Ment Health 11(5):520–525
53. Hawton K, Harriss L, Hawton K, Harriss L (2006) Deliberate self-harm in people aged 60 years and over: characteristics and outcome of a 20-year cohort. Int J Geriatr Psychiatry 21(6):572–581
54. Pirmohamed M, James S, Meakin S, Green C, Scott AK, Walley TJ et al (2004) Adverse drug reactions as cause of admission to hospital: prospective analysis of 18 820 patients. BMJ 329(7456):15–19
55. Beijer H, de Blaey C (2002) Hospitalisations caused by adverse drug reactions (ADR): a meta-analysis of observational studies. Pharm World Sci 24:46–54
56. Mannesse CK, Derkx FH, de Ridder MA, Man In't Veld AJ, van der Cammen TJ (2000) Contribution of adverse drug reactions to hospital admission of older patients. Age Ageing 29(1):35–39

57. Ellis G, Marshall T, Ritchie C (2014) Comprehensive geriatric assessment in the emergency department. Clin Interv Aging 9:2033–2043
58. Shepperd S, Doll H, Angus R, Clarke M, Iliffe S, Kalra L, et al (2008) Admission avoidance hospital at home. Cochrane Database Syst Rev Issue 4

Part II
Management of Common Conditions

Pitfalls in the Management of Older Patients in the Emergency Department

Fredrik Sjöstrand and Christian Nickel

7.1 Vital Signs

The four signs, heart rate, blood pressure, body temperature and respiratory rate create the core components of an examination for both doctors and nurse, although these objective assessments cannot tell what disease is causing the change in vital signs (specificity). Furthermore, vital signs are often evaluated after a single-point examination although research suggests that changes from an individual reference point are more informative [1]. We therefore suggest inquiring about baseline values of vital signs.

The diversity of physiological age-related changes in older patients makes single-point measurements of vital signs a true pitfall in the ED as normal ranges for adults do not apply. The risk of misinterpreting vital signs increases even more for those older patients with comorbidities.

As an example, someone who suffers from hypertension but at the point of admission to the ED has "normal" blood pressure may actually present a warning sign of a serious disease process. Another aspect is the adverse effect of drugs. A beta-blocker, for example, might prevent tachycardia as a warning sign.

F. Sjöstrand (✉)
Section of Emergency Medicine, Department of Clinical Research & Education,
Karolinska Institutet, Stockholm, Sweden
e-mail: fredrik.sjostrand@ki.se

C. Nickel
Emergency Department, University Hospital Basel,
Petersgraben 2, CH-4032 Basel, Switzerland
e-mail: christian.nickel@usb.ch

7.1.1 Heart Rate (HR)

Using heart rate (HR) in the clinical assessment and prognostication of older patients can be challenging although it is indeed of great value. The challenges concern age-related matters and adverse chronotropic effect of common drugs.

The *maximal* HR typically falls with increasing age due to the diminished response of the sympathetic nervous system [2]. The *resting* HR, however, is often increased with age. The pulse pressure may also be influenced by age-related conditions such as hypertension, atherosclerosis and arrhythmias.

Using HR as a *single* vital sign is of less value to the ED staff when it comes to older people, but it increases significantly if also having access to a baseline value from the patient's habitual HR. Repeated or continuous measurements of HR give the clinical staff better information on trends that is of extra value, e.g. when administering various drugs to the patient in the ED.

There are specific clinical situations where HR is of extra prognostic value. One example is patients, admitted for a myocardial infarction, that have an increased risk for ischemic stroke if presenting with a high HR [3, 4]. Another example is patients with vascular disease that have an increased mortality risk if having an elevated resting HR [5].

7.1.2 Blood Pressure

The blood pressure increases with age. However, older patients are also at greater risk for hypotension as their abilities to respond appropriately and rapidly to stressors are reduced. Moreover, the ageing process causes a decline in autonomic sensitivity [1], which often leads to orthostatic hypotension (OH). OH is a problem for as many as 30% of older outpatients and up to 50% of nursing home residents [6], and it represents a risk factor for falls in these individuals [7]. There are clinical trials that have shown that antihypertensive drugs improve the outcomes for older people by reducing cardiovascular events [8]. However, it is unknown whether the populations recruited to these studies are representative. Butt et al. presented clear differences in characteristics between older people seen in routine clinical practice and those participating in antihypertensive drug trials [9]. Older patients seen in routine practice have higher prevalence of diabetes, dementia and cardiovascular and renal diseases that increases risks of adverse effects of antihypertensive treatment, e.g. orthostatic hypotension. In conclusion, there is a lack of well-balanced studies, which might be one important reason why there is no consistent international guideline on treatment of hypertensive in older people [9].

A true pitfall for the ED doctor is the management of medication in hypertensive older people. It is recommended that the list of medication be reviewed for drugs that aggravate OH.

7.1.3 Body Temperature

The level of a normal body temperature does not change much with ageing, but the control of the body temperature is significantly impaired in older ages.

A decrease in the amount of fat below the skin makes it harder to stay warm. However, there is also a risk for overheating (heat stroke) as the ability to sweat is reduced.

Unless the patient was exposed to high temperatures, fever (>37.8 °C oral, 38.1 °C rectal temperature) in older ED patients is often a marker of a serious illness; especially, bacterial infections should be suspected [10].

On the other hand, a normal body temperature is not a sign of a less serious condition. Examples are acute cholecystitis and appendicitis in which the prevalence of fever is only 50% [11].

Older patients with fever should be considered for urgent assessment, particularly when presenting clinical features such as oral temperature > 39 °C combined with respiratory rate > 30, heart rate > 120 and leucocytosis (>11.0 × 10^9/L) [10].

7.1.4 Respiratory Rate

Respiratory rate (RR) is often described as one of the most reliable indicators of severe illness; however, measurement and documentation of the RR are often neglected in the clinical day-to-day work [12]. This is particularly problematic when neglected in older patients, as RR might be the only sign of an acute illness in this vulnerable group.

With increasing age, there are larger residual volumes and decreased vital capacity [13]. A high RR is often compensation for an unmet increase in oxygen consumption requirement.

An example of this may be complaints from older patients experiencing a slow onset of difficulties climbing stairs. They are able to walk on a level surface, but when walking on stairs (that increase the oxygen requirements), the body compensates by increasing RR to a significantly higher level than in younger ages.

Moreover, age-related changes include decreased response to various receptors. As an example, studies show that older patients have a 50% reduction in response to hypoxia and hypercapnia [14].

7.2 Atypical Presentations

Due to age-related processes in the organs and the impact of multiple diseases, it is important for the clinicians to identify the patient having an increased risk for atypical expressions or nonspecific presentations. When detecting such patients, it is justified to increase the receptiveness for subtle symptoms and to broaden the scope of examinations.

The risk groups for atypical presentation of illnesses are the oldest old patients (≥85 years of age) and those with a large number of medications and diseases [15]. Furthermore, cognitive impairment increases the risk of atypical presentations (Chap. 5).

7.2.1 Fever and Common Infections

The prevalence of infection as the main complaint is only 3% in older ED patients in the ED. One possible reason for this low prevalence may be atypical presentations [16] such as when older patients with bacteraemia do not present with fever, irregular leucocytosis or tachycardia [17], leading to under-recognition.

Lee et al. [17] compared community-acquired bloodstream infections among the "oldest old, older and adult patients" in their study: "Older" patients developed organ failure more easily and were more likely to have urinary tract infections, lower respiratory tractions and primary bacteraemia. The oldest old patients were similar in their propensity to develop organ failure, but were more likely to have a longer length of hospital stay, higher mortality rate, more disturbances in consciousness and septic shock. The 90-day mortality was higher in older patients with bacteraemia [17].

Fever in older patients is a strong indicator for bacterial infection, a high mortality and need of quick management. Marco et al. [10] reported 10% mortality in a population of older patients presenting to the ED with fever (oral temperature > 37.8 °C, rectal 38.1 °C). But occasionally fever can be representative of more rare conditions, such as neuroleptic malignant syndrome related to antipsychotics—hence the need for careful assessment.

Unfortunately, there are no well-established guidelines for identification of infections in older patients. Recently, a Geriatric Fever Score (0–3) was developed [18] to help ED physicians to stratify febrile patients into a low (4%) or a high (30%) mortality risk group by evaluating three risk factors that each give one point per positive factor: thrombocytopenia (platelets < $150 \times 10^3/mm^3$), leucocytosis (>12,000 cells/mm^3) and Glasgow Coma Scale ≤8. Patients in the low-risk group (score 0–1) are recommended to either be admitted to a general hospital ward or receive treatment in the ED and to be discharged back home after this. The patients in the high-risk group (score 2–3) should be deemed critically ill and considered for ICU admission. But given the heterogeneous nature of older people, management by scores alone should be avoided—although scores can be helpful in identifying people who need a much more careful evaluation. More recently, attention has turned towards assessing frailty in urgent care [19] and using this a frailty measure to manage patients carefully and holistically (e.g. through comprehensive geriatric assessment [20]).

7.2.2 Pneumonia

Age-related changes lead to diminished cough reflex due to decrements in the expansion of the chest wall and decreased elasticity of the alveoli. Maximum voluntary ventilation and total lung capacity decrease with old age, whereas the

7 Pitfalls in the Management of Older Patients in the Emergency Department

functional residual capacity increases which may cause collapse of small airways and air trapping [13, 14] (Chap. 18).

The high mortality associated with pneumonia in older people may, partly, be explained by atypical presentations, which leads to difficulties in finding the correct diagnosis. When comparing with autopsy results, pneumonia is one of the most frequently missed diagnoses [21, 22].

Altered mental state such as confusion, high respiratory rate and an acute decline in functional status may be the only symptoms of pneumonia.

In summary, older patients with community-acquired pneumonia report less respiratory (cough, dyspnoea) and non-respiratory (fever, chills, sweats, headache, myalgia) symptoms [23]. Even laboratory tests such as total white blood cell count may be normal.

Studies have shown that increased respiratory rate is the most reliable sign of an acute pulmonary condition, and it is an independent risk marker for in-hospital mortality [24].

7.2.3 Urinary Tract Infection and Asymptomatic Bacteriuria

UTI is the second most common infection diagnosed in the acute hospital setting and accounts for almost 5% of all emergency department visits by adults aged 65 years and older in the United States each year [25].

Although several consensus guidelines have developed UTI definitions for surveillance purposes, a universally accepted definition of symptomatic UTI in older adults does not exist [26]. As there are many ways urinary tract infections (UTI) can be presented, there are several common and important definitions for the ED staff to work with (Table 7.1).

Distinguishing UTI from ASB is problematic, as older adults may not present with typical signs and symptoms suggestive of UTI. Although challenging, it is particularly important, as antibiotics are necessary for the treatment of symptomatic UTI, but not for ASB. Moreover, there is a high risk to develop multidrug-resistant bacteria due to overprescription of antibiotics to older people with suspected UTI.

The pitfall with UTI is to diagnose, but not to overdiagnose the condition.

Table 7.1 Terminology and definitions.

Genitourinary symptoms	Dysuria, suprapubic pain or tenderness, frequency or urgency
Pyuria	>10 white blood cells (WBC)/mm^3 per high-power field (HPF)
Bacteriuria	Urinary pathogen of ≥105 colony-forming units (cfu) per mL
Laboratory-confirmed UTI	Pyuria and bacteriuria
Asymptomatic bacteriuria	Bacteriuria in the absence of genitourinary symptoms
Symptomatic UTI	Bacteriuria in the presence of genitourinary symptoms
Uncomplicated UTI	Genitourinary symptoms, pyuria and bacteriuria in a structurally normal urinary tract
Complicated UTI	Genitourinary symptoms, pyuria and bacteriuria in a structurally abnormal urinary tract

7.2.4 Pulmonary Embolism

The annual incidence of pulmonary embolus (PE) increases with age and corresponds to 3.5 per 1000 in the age group 60–74, but it almost triples to 9.0 per 1000 in the age group ≥75 [27]. The diagnosis is typically harder to identify due to increased incidence also for other cardiopulmonary conditions that may mimic the classical symptoms of PE. Compared to younger patients with PE, classical symptoms such as pleuritic chest pain and haemoptysis are less common, whereas hypoxia and syncope are more common [28]. These challenges may lead to delays in correct diagnosis and relevant treatment.

Moreover, for older patients, syncope seems to be a particularly important symptom as a study presented the incidence of syncope in 3% of younger patients but 24% in older individuals [28].

7.2.5 Thyroid Disease

Signs of primary endocrine disorder seem difficult to identify in older people. As an example, typical clinical characteristics of hypothyroidism such as lethargy, changes in cognition and constipation are often erroneously attributed to old age than signs of a primary endocrine disorder [29].

It is also difficult to identify hyperthyroidism in the old population, as classical signs such as tremor, irritability and nervousness are frequently absent. However, fatigue, anorexia, lethargy, angina, palpitations, heart failure and atrial fibrillation may occur. Age-related resistance to thyroid hormones is thought to cause these unconventional presentations in hyperthyroidism, and as many as 20% lack an enlarged gland and many lack ophthalmologic findings [30].

7.2.6 Common Electrolyte Problems

Hyponatraemia is the most common electrolyte imbalance in hospitalised older patients [31–33] and is associated with an increased risk for 30-day hospital readmission, hospital length of stay (and costs), increase in ICU admissions (and costs) and risk of falls [34].

Hyperkalaemia [35]: If hyperkalaemia is discovered, the accuracy of the measurement must be verified. A repeat serum potassium concentration is often normal, mostly because of haemolysis, distribution or excretion of recently ingested potassium, diurnal variation or laboratory error. There is a high risk of inappropriate treatment if relying on one single test result; hence, always get a second test.

ACE inhibitors are known to frequently cause hyperkalaemia as an adverse effect. Hyperkalaemia may cause ECG changes: when serum potassium reaches 5.5–6.5 mmol/L, a peaked T-wave and prolonged PR segment may be seen on the ECG. However, it is important to know that ECG is insensitive in assessing the severity of hyperkalaemia, and profound hyperkalaemia may go without ECG changes at all.

7.2.7 Back Pain

Back pain in older patients is associated with a much higher risk of a severe cause than those younger than 65 years of age [36]. Due to this risk increase, a systematic evaluation and a broader diagnostic awareness are warranted in the older patient [37]. A fairly large portion of patients presenting with non-traumatic acute back pain in the ED was reported to suffer from conditions such as ureterolithiasis, pyelonephritis, aortic disease, pancreatitis and psoas abscess [38]. Underlying orthopaedic conditions are not confined to degenerative column and disc disease but also osteoporotic fracture and purulent spondylitis.

7.2.8 Abdominal Pain

The high morbidity and mortality in older patients with abdominal pain reflect the importance of increased awareness for clinical, radiologic and prognostic actions.

Abdominal pain is the main complaint in 3–13% of ED visits in older patients. Compared to younger patients, mortality rates are six to eight times higher and surgery rates are doubled [39]. As with many other conditions in older patients, it is difficult for ED staff to identify the underlying disease. For abdominal pain, discrepancies between ED and final diagnosis concern more often gallbladder disease, appendicitis, cancer and diverticulitis.

Abdominal computed tomography (CT) is well studied and has proved its efficacy for the elucidation of causes of abdominal pain aetiology. It may also modify admission decisions, prescriptions of antibiotics and need of surgery [39]. It often modifies the primary suspected diagnosis [40].

Even though appendicitis is known to be a disease of the younger age groups, the incidence is rising due to increase in life expectancy. Perforation rates in older patients are as high as 40%. This condition carries a high risk for postoperative complications and death [41]. Moreover, appendicitis is a condition that is difficult to identify as so many have atypical presentations (75%) that, in turn, result in general delays in admission and treatment [11].

It is recommended to have a high level of suspicion and being more liberal using CT in order to avoid an unfavourable outcome (see also Chap. 15) [41].

7.3 Falls

Falls are the leading cause to morbidity and mortality in older patients [42–44].

In ED patients aged 65 years or older, about 15–30% had a recent fall as a cause of the visit, and the prevalence of an old patient having had a fall within the last 90 days has been reported to be 37% [45]. The prevalence increases with age.

Up to 10% of all falls result in a serious injury requiring hospitalisation. About 4–6% of all falls result in fractures and 1–2% cause hip fractures [44, 46, 47]. Early mobilisation is recommended in injuries following falls, such as contusion of muscles and sprains. However, hip fracture is one important exception.

Falls cause, independently of other conditions, restricted mobility and a need of assistance as these patients suffer declines in activities of daily living (ADL), e.g. dressing, bathing, shopping or housekeeping. Moreover, a fall is an independent risk factor for nursing home placement [48]. Although there is a clear relation between falling and the number of medications, the risks associated with individual classes of drugs have been more variable. However, serotonin reuptake inhibitors, tricyclic antidepressants, neuroleptic drugs, benzodiazepines, anticonvulsants and some classes of antiarrhythmic medications have been coupled to an increased risk of falling [49].

No screening tool is able to assess the risk of falling among older people either in the community or in nursing homes, and no tool has been used or certified all over Europe. However, the following tools are examples that have been used in a number of tests and clinical sites. Several assessment tools for frail older patients contain some questions around falls due to both the high risk of lethal events and the high frequency of events. One example of assessment tool for fall risks is "STRATIFY" (St Thomas Risk Assessment Tool in Falling Older Inpatients) [50, 51], which is validated for hospitalised patients although not specifically for the ED setting. A tool specifically developed for the ED is KINDER 1 and includes the following risk factors: (1) fall reason for ED visit, (2) age > 70, (3) altered mental status (including alcohol intoxication or substance use), (4) impaired mobility and (5) nurse judgement (evaluating incontinence, orthostatic hypotension and medications). A recent study showed promising results in reducing the number of falls in the ED when including KINDER 1 in Kotter's framework for a change process; however, the tool has not yet been validated [52].

A multifactorial fall-risk assessment coupled with adequate interventions to community-dwelling people over 75 years who present to the ED due to an injurious fall may prove to be helpful [53], so older people with falls or at risk of falls who attend the ED should be referred on.

In summary, the ED doctor in charge should at least check for orthostatic blood pressure before discharge, check list of medications for those associated with falls and ask about previous falls within 90 days. If the latter is positive, it is recommended to perform a fall assessment including status of vision, hearing, muscle strength, home safety and a review of the medications—usually by referral on disposition (see also Chap. 9).

7.4 Delirium and Dementia

One fourth to one third of older ED patients have an altered mental status as a result of delirium (7–10%) and dementia (15–26%) [54, 55] (Chap. 13). Due to the high prevalence of delirium, it is recommended to screen all older ED patients for cognitive dysfunction [56] and to minimise the risk of adverse outcomes as increased risks for hospital admission [55] and mortality [57]. However, 50% of the patients with delirium suffer also from dementia, and differentiating between them is not easy. Studies have shown the sensitivity for an ED physician to detect delirium in an old patient to be 24–35% [55, 58, 59]. About one third of the patients with delirium (37%) are discharged to home [55], and these patients have nearly twice the short-term mortality rate than their non-delirious counterparts. It is recommended to admit these patients to a hospital ward, unless the cause of the delirium is known and easily reversible, and there is adequate home supervision and support for the patient (see also Chap. 14).

7.5 Coronary Artery Disease

As older people frequently have atypical presentations of myocardial infarction and as older people have much worse outcome, clinicians in the ED must have a high level of suspicion for an acute cardiac event. Symptoms such as falls [46], nausea, vomiting, syncope and shortness of breath [60, 61] should alert the ED staff to consider a cardiac problem unless there are other obvious reasons for symptoms to occur.

Only 40% of patients older than 85 years and with non-ST-elevation myocardial infarction (non-STEMI) and 57% with STEMI have chest pain as their main complaint compared with 77% non-STEMI and 90% STEMI patients younger than 65 years [61]. Moreover, ECG is non-diagnostic in 43% of patients older than 85 years and with non-STEMI compared with only 23% of patients younger than 65 years [60].

Additionally, left bundle branch block on ECG is present in 34% of patients older than 85 years and with STEMI compared with only 5% of those younger than 65 years, making diagnosis harder. Because ECG abnormalities are relatively common at an advanced age, it is particularly important to obtain old ECG results whenever possible so that findings in the ED can be compared with previous changes and interpreted accordingly (Table 7.2).

Atypical presentation, difficulties in diagnostics and uncertainties in evaluating benefits and risks of a potential treatment are tough challenges for many clinicians. These issues may decrease the likelihood for a doctor prescribing treatment to an older patient. Compared to a group of 60-year-old patients with acute myocardial infarction, the matched group of 80-year-old patients receive less medication. Twenty percent of the eligible older patients were not administered with aspirin, and 40% did not get β blockers [62].

Recent evidence suggests that invasive strategy is superior conservative strategy in reducing adverse outcomes in 80-year-old (or older) patients with NSTEMI although the efficacy of the invasive strategy decreased with increasing age [63, 64].

Table 7.2 Comparison of coronary artery disease symptoms and ECG signs between age groups.

	Pain		ECG non-diagnostic	LBBB
[60, 61]	Non-STEMI	STEMI	Non-STEMI	STEMI
≤65	77%	90%	23%	5%
≥85	40%	57%	43%	34%

7.6 Adverse Drug Effect (ADE)

In a general population being admitted to the ED, only a small proportion (1–4%) have a problem related to adverse drug reactions (ADEs). In older patients the prevalence increases to 11% [65]. The risk for ADE increases by age and number of medications. In one study [65], 13% of all older patients had eight or more medications (range 0–17), and 11% had at least one inappropriate medication [66], according to the Beers Criteria, the criteria which define certain medications to be inappropriate for use in older patients [67, 68].

Almost 40% of older adults require supervision to manage their daily medications [54] (which is a part of the instrumental activity of daily living assessment, IADL). Hence, when home care situation gets unstable, the risk that the patient will suffer from an ADE increases.

It is crucial for the ED clinician to be aware of this common pitfall and to take an active part in trying to avoid future ADE problems by prescribing wisely and selecting appropriate medications. Research indicate that one third of all the ADE-related ED visits refer to intake of one of these three medications: warfarin, insulin and digoxin [69]. Tools such as STOPP-START can help guide clinical practice [70].

7.7 Abuse and Neglect

The American Medical Association defines older abuse or neglect as "actions or the omission of actions that result in harm or threatened harm to the health or welfare of the older". It includes battery, psychological abuse, abandonment, exploitation and neglect and may be intentional or unintentional.

The most important risk factors are a relationship of dependency, social isolation and psychopathology of the abuser [71].

Most studies indicate that women are at higher risk than men. Among older adults, a younger age is associated with a greater risk of abuse and neglect [72]. It is possible that a reason for this is that the "young old" more often live with a spouse or with adult children, the two groups that are the most likely abusers.

Statistics from the United States show that about one out of ten older patients living at home with an informal caregiver would suffer from neglect or abuse [73]. The lack of specific protocols and time constraints makes it difficult to detect older abuse in the ED, which result in less referral to the appropriate authorities. One study showed that approximately half the suspected cases evaluated in the ED were not reported [73].

The ED utilisation and admission data in this population suggest that older abuse victims have high health-care utilisation [52]. An effective strategy to address family violence in outpatient settings could improve the situation and perhaps reduce health-care costs at the same time.

This is indeed an area that needs further research and until reliable protocols are produced, clinicians have to raise questions whenever their experience and clinical judgement may have detected a suspicious case.

7.8 "Social Admissions" and the Search for Hidden Diseases

This refers to patients in the ED who are *thought* to suffer from poor home care services, and due to this, inadequate care is the primary cause of their ED visit. These patients are at *an increased* risk of mortality, hospital admission and ED revisits [45, 74].

In the emergency department, about three fourths of these patients have at least one "geriatric syndrome". They are dependent on others to cope with ADL declines and cognitive impairments. Even a minor acute illness might cause an altered mental status [54]. Hence, for the ED physician in charge, it is important to learn what the patient's baseline status was and, furthermore, search for causes that changed the situation.

Key in the management of acute geriatric patients is collaboration across disciplines. Fast-track management for conditions, such as stroke and hip fracture, have been shown to have potential [47, 75]. A similar fast-track management for frail older people as the primary cause of ED admittance has been suggested, but to date, data supporting this are lacking. Collaborations with ambulance services are another possibility [76]; alternatively, skilled EMS personnel may directly admit frail patients to a non-acute service after telephone consultation with a geriatrician [77].

7.9 Discharge Planning

Besides the search of a hidden disease, another key action is discharge planning, which focuses on what care the patient requires after having come home from the ED. A simple screening tool that selects those in need of extra services would be good to have, but so far, the screening instruments that have been published have had rather poor results regarding validity and reliability [78].

Hence, a couple of extra minutes need to be spent in understanding the cause of the acute change in health status from various baseline functions and what is required to get the patient back to its baseline function level. It is key to test the patient's ability to perform simple mobility tasks prior to discharge, as the accuracy of self-reported ability to perform a simple mobility task appear to be inadequate, particularly in those patients who reported some need for assistance. Direct observation of the patient's mobility by a member of the emergency care team should therefore be considered prior to discharge [79].

Besides management of medications (adverse effects of drugs) and treatment of current condition, an evaluation of substance dependency and physical abuse and neglect must also be included in a discharge evaluation.

The transfer of older patients to and from the ED has many challenges as these patients have multiple providers and comorbidities. Moreover, cognitive impairments limit their ability to participate in their care. Consequently, poor preparation of transitions is often related to morbidity and mortality risk due to medication errors, adverse drug events, lack of timely coordination of follow-up care and unnecessary rehospitalisation [80]. Standardised communication may be helpful in reducing errors related to diagnostic uncertainty and care planning see also Chap. 23.

References

1. Chester JG, Rudolph JL (2011) Vital signs in older patients: age-related changes. J Am Med Dir Assoc 12(5):337–343
2. Lakatta EG (2000) Cardiovascular aging in health. Clin Geriatr Med 16(3):419–444
3. Cronin L et al (2001) Stroke in relation to cardiac procedures in patients with non-ST-elevation acute coronary syndrome: a study involving >18 000 patients. Circulation 104(3):269–274
4. Mahaffey KW et al (1998) Risk factors for in-hospital nonhemorrhagic stroke in patients with acute myocardial infarction treated with thrombolysis: results from GUSTO-I. Circulation 97(8):757–764
5. Bemelmans RHH et al (2013) The risk of resting heart rate on vascular events and mortality in vascular patients. Int J Cardiol 168(2):1410–1415
6. Lipsitz LA (1989) Orthostatic hypotension in the elderly. N Engl J Med 321(14):952–957
7. Shaw BH et al (2015) Cardiovascular responses to orthostasis and their association with falls in older adults. BMC Geriatr 15:174
8. Thijs L et al (2004) Prevalence, pathophysiology and treatment of isolated systolic hypertension in the elderly. Expert Rev Cardiovasc Ther 2(5):761
9. Butt DA, Harvey PJ (2015) Benefits and risks of antihypertensive medications in the elderly. J Intern Med 278(6):599–626
10. Marco CA et al (1995) Fever in geriatric emergency patients: clinical features associated with serious illness. Ann Emerg Med 26(1):18–24
11. Storm-Dickerson TL, Horattas MC (2003) What have we learned over the past 20 years about appendicitis in the elderly? Am J Surg 185(3):198–201
12. Ramsay M (2015) Breathing is good. J Clin Monit Comput 29(2):221–222
13. Sharma G, Goodwin J (2006) Effect of aging on respiratory system physiology and immunology. Clin Interv Aging 1(3):253–260
14. Peterson DD et al (1981) Effects of aging on ventilatory and occlusion pressure responses to hypoxia and hypercapnia. Am Rev Respir Dis 124(4):387–391
15. Samaras N et al (2010) Older patients in the emergency department: a review. Ann Emerg Med 56(3):261–269
16. Vanpee D et al (2001) Epidemiological profile of geriatric patients admitted to the emergency department of a university hospital localized in a rural area. Eur J Emerg Med 8(4):301–304
17. Lee C-C et al (2007) Comparison of clinical manifestations and outcome of community-acquired bloodstream infections among the oldest old, elderly, and adult patients. Medicine 86(3):138–144
18. Chung MH et al (2014) Geriatric fever score: a new decision rule for geriatric care. PLoS One 9(10):e110927
19. Wallis SJ et al (2015) Association of the clinical frailty scale with hospital outcomes. QJM 108(12):943–949
20. Ellis G et al (2011) Comprehensive geriatric assessment for older adults admitted to hospital: meta-analysis of randomised controlled trials. BMJ 343:d6553
21. Ferguson RP et al (2004) Consecutive autopsies on an internal medicine service. South Med J 97(4):335–337
22. O'Connor AE et al (2002) A comparison of the antemortem clinical diagnosis and autopsy findings for patients who die in the emergency department. Acad Emerg Med 9(9):957–959
23. Metlay JP et al (1997) INfluence of age on symptoms at presentation in patients with community-acquired pneumonia. Arch Intern Med 157(13):1453–1459
24. Strauß R et al (2014) The prognostic significance of respiratory rate in patients with pneumonia: a retrospective analysis of data from 705 928 hospitalized patients in Germany from 2010–2012. Dtsch Arztebl Int 111(29-30):503–508
25. Caterino JM et al (2009) National trends in emergency department antibiotic prescribing for elders with urinary tract infection, 1996–2005. Acad Emerg Med 16(6):500–507
26. Rowe TA, Juthani-Mehta M (2014) Diagnosis and management of urinary tract infection in older adults. Infect Dis Clin N Am 28(1):75–89

27. Oger E (2000) Incidence of venous thromboembolism: a community-based study in western France. Thromb Haemost 83(5):657–660
28. Timmons S et al (2003) Pulmonary embolism: differences in presentation between older and younger patients. Age Ageing 32(6):601–605
29. Gambert SR, Escher JE (1988) Atypical presentation of endocrine disorders in the elderly. Geriatrics 43(7):69–71. 76-8
30. Nordyke RA et al (1988) Graves' disease: influence of age on clinical findings. Arch Intern Med 148(3):626–631
31. Douglas I (2006) Hyponatremia: why it matters, how it presents, how we can manage it. Cleve Clin J Med 73(Suppl 3):S4–12
32. Ghali JK (2008) Mechanisms, risks, and new treatment options for hyponatremia. Cardiology 111(3):147–157
33. Palmer BF (2010) Diagnostic approach and management of inpatient hyponatremia. J Hosp Med 5(Suppl 3):S1–S7
34. Deitelzweig S et al (2013) Health care utilization, costs, and readmission rates associated with hyponatremia. Hosp Pract 41(1):89–95
35. Sterns RH, Grieff M, Bernstein PL (2016) Treatment of hyperkalemia: something old, something new. Kidney Int 89(3):546–554
36. Waterman BR, Belmont PJ Jr, Schoenfeld AJ (2012) Low back pain in the United States: incidence and risk factors for presentation in the emergency setting. Spine J 12(1):63–70
37. Kahn Joseph H, Magauran BG, Olshaker Jonathan S (2014) In: Magauran BG, Kahn Joseph H, Olshaker Jonathan S (eds) Geriatric emergency medicine - principles and practice. Cambridge University Press, New York, p 379
38. Nagayama M, Yanagawa Y, Aihara K, Watanabe S, Takemoto M, Nakazato T, Tanaka H (2014) Analysis of non-traumatic truncal back pain in patients who visited an emergency room. Acute Med Surg 1(2):94–100
39. Lewis LM et al (2005) Etiology and clinical course of abdominal pain in senior patients: a prospective, multicenter study. J Gerontol A Biol Sci Med Sci 60(8):1071–1076
40. Esses D et al (2004) Ability of CT to alter decision making in elderly patients with acute abdominal pain. Am J Emerg Med 22(4):270–272
41. Omari AH et al (2014) Acute appendicitis in the elderly: risk factors for perforation. World J Emerg Surg 9(1):1–6
42. Gelbard R et al (2014) Falls in the elderly: a modern look at an old problem. Am J Surg 208(2):249–253
43. Laybourne AH, Biggs S, Martin FC (2008) Falls exercise interventions and reduced falls rate: always in the patient's interest? Age Ageing 37(1):10–13
44. Baraff LJ (1998) Emergency department management of falls in the elderly. West J Med 168(3):183–184
45. Costa AP (2013) Older adults seeking emergency care: an examination of unplanned emergency department use, patient profiles, and adverse patient outcomes post discharge. In: The School of Public Health and Health Systems. University of Waterloo, Waterloo
46. Sanders AB (1999) Changing clinical practice in geriatric emergency medicine. Acad Emerg Med 6(12):1189–1193
47. Ollivere B et al (2012) Optimising fast track care for proximal femoral fracture patients using modified early warning score. Ann R Coll Surg Engl 94(4):267–271
48. Tinetti ME, Williams CS (1997) Falls, injuries due to falls, and the risk of admission to a nursing home. N Engl J Med 337:1279–1284
49. Tinetti ME (2003) Clinical practice. Preventing falls in elderly persons. N Engl J Med 348:42–49
50. Oliver D et al (1997) Development and evaluation of evidence based risk assessment tool (STRATIFY) to predict which elderly inpatients will fall: case-control and cohort studies. BMJ 315(7115):1049–1053
51. Dionyssiotis Y (2012) Analyzing the problem of falls among older people. Int J Gen Med 5:805–813

52. Townsend AB, Valle-Ortiz M, Sansweet T (2016) A successful ED fall risk program using the KINDER 1 fall risk assessment tool. J Emerg Nurs 42(6):492–497. Available online May 06 2016
53. Pohl P et al (2014) Community-dwelling older people with an injurious fall are likely to sustain new injurious falls within 5 years - a prospective long-term follow-up study. BMC Geriatr 14(1):1–7
54. Gray L, Peel N, Costa A, Burkett E, Dey AB, Jonsson P, Lakhan P, Ljunggren G, Sjostrand F, Swoboda W, Wellens N, Hirdes J (2013) Profiles of older patients in the emergency department: findings from the interRAI multinational emergency department study. Ann Emerg Med 62(5):467–474
55. Hustey FM, Meldon SW (2002) The prevalence and documentation of impaired mental status in elderly emergency department patients. Ann Emerg Med 39(3):248–253
56. Wilber ST et al (2005) An evaluation of two screening tools for cognitive impairment in older emergency department patients. Acad Emerg Med 12(7):612–616
57. Kakuma R et al (2003) Delirium in older emergency department patients discharged home: effect on survival. J Am Geriatr Soc 51(4):443–450
58. Elie M et al (2000) Prevalence and detection of delirium in elderly emergency department patients. CMAJ 163(8):977–981
59. Han JH et al (2009) Delirium in older emergency department patients: recognition, risk factors, and psychomotor subtypes. Acad Emerg Med 16(3):193–200
60. Alexander KP et al (2007) Acute coronary care in the elderly, part II: ST-segment-elevation myocardial infarction: a scientific statement for healthcare professionals from the American Heart Association Council on clinical cardiology: in collaboration with the Society of Geriatric Cardiology. Circulation 115(19):2570–2589
61. Alexander KP et al (2007) Acute coronary care in the elderly, part I: Non-ST-segment-elevation acute coronary syndromes: a scientific statement for healthcare professionals from the American Heart Association Council on Clinical Cardiology: in collaboration with the Society of Geriatric Cardiology. Circulation 115(19):2549–2569
62. Magid DJ et al (2005) Older emergency department patients with acute myocardial infarction receive lower quality of care than younger patients. Ann Emerg Med 46(1):14–21
63. Psaltis PJ, Nicholls SJ (2016) Management of acute coronary syndrome in the very elderly. Lancet 387(10023):1029–1030
64. Tegn N et al (2016) Invasive versus conservative strategy in patients aged 80 years or older with non-ST-elevation myocardial infarction or unstable angina pectoris (after eighty study): an open-label randomised controlled trial. Lancet 387(10023):1057–1065
65. Hohl CM et al (2001) Polypharmacy, adverse drug-related events, and potential adverse drug interactions in elderly patients presenting to an emergency department. Ann Emerg Med 38(6):666–671
66. Chin MH et al (1999) Appropriateness of medication selection for older persons in an urban academic emergency department. Acad Emerg Med 6(12):1232–1241
67. Beers MH (1997) Explicit criteria for determining potentially inappropriate medication use by the elderly. An update. Arch Intern Med 157(14):1531–1536
68. American Geriatrics Society Beers Criteria Update Expert Panel (2015) American Geriatrics Society 2015 updated beers criteria for potentially inappropriate medication use in older adults. J Am Geriatr Soc 63(11):2227–2246
69. Budnitz DS et al (2007) Medication use leading to emergency department visits for adverse drug events in older adults. Ann Intern Med 147(11):755–765
70. O'Mahony D et al (2014) STOPP/START criteria for potentially inappropriate prescribing in older people: version 2. Age Ageing 44(2):213–218
71. Wolf RS (1992) Victimization of the elderly: elder abuse and neglect. Rev Clin Gerontol 2(03):269–276
72. Lachs MS, Pillemer KA (2015) Elder abuse. N Engl J Med 373(20):1947–1956
73. Jones JS et al (1997) Elder mistreatment: national survey of emergency physicians. Ann Emerg Med 30(4):473–479

74. Nemec M et al (2010) Patients presenting to the emergency department with non-specific complaints: the Basel Non-specific Complaints (BANC) study. Acad Emerg Med 17(3):284–292
75. Griffiths R, Alper J, Beckingsale A, Goldhill D, Heyburn G, Holloway J, Wiese M, Wilson I (2012) Management of proximal femoral fractures 2011. Anaesthesia 67:85–98
76. Mason S et al (2012) A pragmatic quasi-experimental multi-site community intervention trial evaluating the impact of Emergency Care Practitioners in different UK health settings on patient pathways (NEECaP Trial). Emerg Med J 29(1):47–53
77. Vicente V et al (2014) Randomized controlled trial of a prehospital decision system by emergency medical services to ensure optimal treatment for older adults in Sweden. J Am Geriatr Soc 62(7):1281–1287
78. Carpenter CR et al (2015) Risk factors and screening instruments to predict adverse outcomes for undifferentiated older emergency department patients: a systematic review and meta-analysis. Acad Emerg Med 22(1):1–21
79. Roedersheimer KM et al (2016) Self-reported versus performance-based assessments of a simple mobility task among older adults in the emergency department. Ann Emerg Med 67(2):151–156
80. Kessler C et al (2013) Transitions of care for the geriatric patient in the emergency department. Clin Geriatr Med 29(1):49–69

Nonspecific Disease Presentation: The Emergency Department Perspective

8

Alexandra Malinovska, Christian Nickel, and Roland Bingisser

8.1 Nonspecific Disease Presentation of Older Emergency Department Patients

8.1.1 Prevalence and Outcome of Patients with Nonspecific Complaints

The diagnostic workup of older patients in emergency departments (ED) is more difficult than that of younger patients. Besides the challenges of impaired history taking, presence of multiple comorbidity and polypharmacy [1], symptom presentations of common diseases can often be atypical [2]. Such atypical or nonspecific complaints (NSCs) (e.g. weakness) do not lead straight to the underlying diseases. In contrast to specific complaints, which can be caused by a defined number of diseases, NSCs can be caused by numerous underlying conditions [3]. The fact that a complaint is not typical for a certain disease does, however, not necessarily mean it is not common. Indeed, NSCs are common, especially in older ED patients: up to 21% of older patients present to the ED with NSCs [4–6].

Some examples for NSCs are 'fatigue', 'exhaustion', and 'generalised weakness', the latter occurs most often. All these NSCs have in common that they either can be caused by multiple underlying diseases or that underlying medical conditions are absent. Nevertheless, an acute underlying disease has been found in about 50–80% of patients presenting to the ED with NSCs [7–9].

Previous studies indicated that NSCs are not just common, but are associated with increased risk of adverse outcomes: Safwenberg et al. assessed in-hospital

---

A. Malinovska (✉) • C. Nickel • R. Bingisser
Department of Emergency Medicine, University Hospital Basel, Basel, Switzerland
e-mail: alexandra.malinovska@usb.ch; christian.nickel@usb.ch; roland.bingisser@usb.ch

mortality of patients with different complaints and found the highest in-hospital mortality (27%) in the nonspecific complaint 'general disability' [4]. Elmståhl et al. obtained similar results, with a one-year mortality of 34% in a cohort with the initial diagnosis 'lack of community support'. Mortality was lower in patients if they were seen by a senior consultant suggesting that this disease presentation is challenging and experience in dissecting out the diagnosis is important [8]. Therefore, training in the presentation of disease in older people in the context of their multiple comorbidities can help the clinician dissect out key issues. Importantly, it could be shown that patients with NSCs are at high risk of adverse outcomes: in 60% of all NSCs cases, a serious outcome, defined as a potentially life-threatening condition or a condition requiring an early intervention to prevent morbidity, disability or death, was diagnosed [9]. Furthermore, NSCs were associated with a 6% 30-day mortality [10, 11].

Previously, studies indicated that patients with NSCs are associated with a high risk of hospital admission [8]. Results from the ongoing Basel nonspecific complaints (BANC) study are in line with those findings. In this cohort, it could be shown that the accuracy of disposition of patients presenting with NSCs is still in need of improvement, even after standardised workup in an observation unit [12]. Furthermore, BANC showed that causes of NSCs were not correctly recognised in 54% of patients [8, 13]. A Swedish study showed that septic patients presenting with NSCs as chief complaint received antibiotics later compared to patients with specific complaints (SC) and had higher in-hospital mortality [14]. All these observations underline that NSC diagnostic workup is complex.

8.1.2 Common Causes of NSCs

One reason for the complexity of the diagnostic workup may be the fact that causes of NSCs are numerous and cover almost all ICD-10 categories [3, 5, 15]. Although NSCs can be caused by a variety of diseases, recent studies showed that some diagnoses occur more often than others [3, 5, 7, 15]. Four studies investigated the underlying causes of NSCs [3, 5, 7, 15]. Despite the use of different inclusion criteria the results were comparable. When comparing the most common underlying conditions (excluding the merely descriptive diagnoses such as 'other malaise and fatigue' or 'functional impairment') we found a similar distribution of the common underlying medical conditions: infections, water and electrolyte disorders, heart failure, anaemia, malignancies, and cognitive impairment were consistently among the top diagnoses (see Fig. 8.1).

Though NSCs lack a common and universal definition, it is remarkable that distribution of underlying medical conditions is similar across the different study populations. In agreement with these observations, we showed that the NSC population also shares the same outcome with a high burden of morbidity and mortality [16].

Fig. 8.1 Most common causes for nonspecific complaints. (Comparison of underlying conditions for NSCs in four different studies. The study of Nickel et al. and Bhalla et al. investigate causes of 'generalised weakness', Rutschmann et al. set a focus on 'home care impossible', and Karakoumis et al. analysed NSCs in general. All studies except Nickel et al. formulated at least a top ten differential diagnosis, Nickel et al. showed only top three)

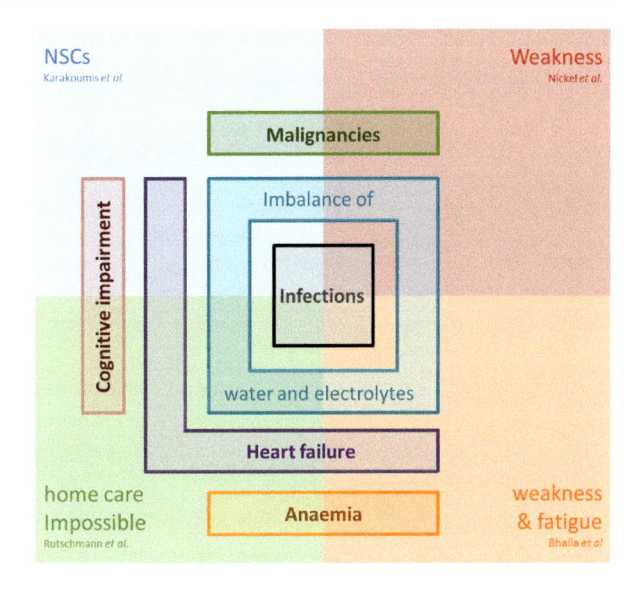

This indicates that NSCs might seem to be diffuse complaints, but patients presenting with NSC form a distinct population. Upon identification of such a population, the question arises whether there is any advice on how to perform diagnostic workup.

8.2 Diagnostic Approach for Patients Presenting to the ED with NSCs

For specific symptoms such as chest pain, standardised pathways for diagnostic workup are available and widely used. This is possible because specific symptoms tend to be caused by a small group of diseases. In contrast, for nonspecific complaints the underlying causes are numerous and therefore the establishment of management protocols is difficult. However, a broad diagnostic workup, based on established pre-test probabilities, could be helpful for the establishment of an applicable approach (see Table 8.1). In the following we provide some advice for a general approach, and cause-specific characteristics for the three most frequent groups of underlying conditions. It might appear paradoxical to apply a cause-specific approach, when in nonspecific emergency presentation any narrowing of the wide array of differential diagnoses can be problematic. However, every step of the diagnostic procedure reduces the array of differential diagnoses. Therefore it seems feasible to focus on the three most frequent groups of underlying conditions.

Table 8.1 Special considerations for diagnostic workup for NSC patients (* see text)

Diagnostic workup	
Medical history	Current complaint
	History by proxy
	Previously known malignancy
	Medication
Physical examination	Vital signs*
	Clinical indicators for dehydration*
	Overall hygiene
Laboratory test	Blood count*
	CRP*
	Urinalysis*
	Electrolyte
	Creatinine, GFR
	Serum osmolality, blood urea nitrogen-creatinine ratio
	BNP*
	Metabolic panel
	Glucose
Further tests	12-lead electrocardiogram
	Chest X-ray
	Cranial imaging
	Delirium/dementia screening test
	Neuroimaging

8.2.1 General Diagnostic Approach

8.2.1.1 History Taking

The patients' medical history, including current complaints, is generally a vital component for the evaluation of emergency patients. Yet, history taking in older patients can be difficult: it could be shown that history taking from older patients with certain comorbidities as depression or dementia was not always reliable and additional sources for medical history should always be considered [17, 18]. History taking may contribute up to 75% of the diagnostic workup to the final diagnosis in patients with specific complaints [19–22]. However in patients with NSCs, it sometimes seems to be impossible to establish working hypotheses solely based on the patients' history. This is also reflected by the fact that some studies investigating NSCs include only patients lacking a history useful for an initial working hypothesis [3].

As it is the nature of nonspecific presentation, patients describe their symptoms vaguely. For example, patients complaining about weakness may often not be able to differentiate between 'localised weakness' and 'generalised weakness'. Yet, this differentiation can be essential, because 'localised weakness' is rather specific for stroke or stroke mimics, while 'generalised weakness' is a classic NSC with an extremely broad differential diagnosis [15]. A second example is 'dizziness'. Older patients often struggle differentiating between 'vertigo' and 'dizziness'. Besides other factors such as proprioceptive failure, visual impairment or reduced cerebral perfusion pressure, (acute or chronic) cerebrovascular disease might be an explanation. Therefore, strokes are not uncommon in patients with

NSC, as neither a localisation of weakness nor the typical vertigo-complaints are helpful in these situations [3].

Besides the presenting complaint(s), the past medical history, especially the past history of cancer might help to identify the underlying conditions of NSCs. Indeed, it was shown that only 30% of cases in which malignancies caused weakness were newly diagnosed, whereas for the rest the malignancies were previously known, and the majority of these patients presented with weakness as a complication of their cancer or a deterioration of their chronic condition [15].

Another important component of history taking is medication history. It can often be obtained by proxies or family physicians, and about 11% of all underlying conditions can be attributed to medication [11]. Therefore, gathering all information on medication may be decisive in patients with NSC.

8.2.1.2 Physical Examination

Another diagnostic step is the objective measurement of patient's status via monitoring of vital signs. Thereby, the disease severity in acute settings can be classified by measurement of the four vital signs—pulse, temperature, blood pressure, and respiratory rate. These are standardised methods and have well-established normative ranges. However, reference ranges in older patients can be altered. Moreover, vital signs in older patients are less sensitive due to physiological and pathological changes occurring with age [23]. For example, older patients may have higher systolic pressures due to arterial stiffness occurring with age [23]. Unfortunately, individual baseline parameters are often unknown. If known, relative changes from individual baseline parameters are very helpful for risk stratification. It could be shown that relying on vital signs in older patients can cause undertriage of critically ill patients [24]. However, in some studies investigating NSCs, patients with severely deviating vital parameters were excluded, as hypotension, fever, and tachycardia often trigger specific workups that are standardised in many EDs [9]. Even though physical examination can be important for upgrading pre-test probabilities using, e.g. heart auscultation [25], it could be shown that in patients with NSC, only one of almost 600 cases was diagnosed by physical examination alone [26].

History taking and physical examinations generally are the main part in the diagnostic workup. Yet, this essential part of diagnostic workup in patients with SC often can be less effective in patients with NSCs. One possible approach is, to lower laboratory testing threshold and thereby complementing missing information to establish a working hypothesis (see Table 8.1).

8.2.2 Causes-Specific Approach

In the following, we describe the characteristics of the three most common groups of conditions. For the diagnostic workup in patients lacking a working hypothesis, this will allow to focus on a single group and reduce the wide diagnostic array.

8.2.2.1 Infections

The classical clinical manifestation of infections is fever. The definition of fever in older patients is still under discussion and a temperature increase by 1.1 °C from baseline is hardly feasible in emergency settings [27]. Yet, data indicate that the normative temperature range in older patients may be different from younger patients [27]. However, fever is no mandatory sign for infections and can be absent or blunted in 20–30% of the cases [27]. These alterations should be carefully taken into account when screening for infections.

To confirm the working hypothesis 'infection', laboratory examinations are a pivotal part of the diagnostic workup. The exams for infections generally include complete blood count (especially white blood count) and C-reactive protein (CRP). However, these two markers lack sensitivity and specificity [28]: leucocytosis may be absent, and CRP can increase late. Therefore measurement of Procalcitonin (Pro-CT) can be helpful [26, 29]. However, even Procalcitonin has not been shown to be as sensitive and specific as emergency physicians have hoped for [28].

Further workup should aim at the identification of the infection focus. There are multiple infections causing NSCs, but two most common infections causing NSCs are urinary tract infections (UTI) and pulmonary infections [3, 5, 7, 15]. Urinalysis is a useful tool to detect urinary tract infections only in addition to clinical symptoms *reference to UTI chapter* (see Chap. 16). Results of urine cultures may arrive too late to diagnose patients. Infectious Diseases Society of America (IDSA) guidelines presume clinical symptoms besides detection of the pathogen in the urine for the diagnosis and treatment of UTI [30]. Therefore there is no advice for antibiotic treatment of bacteriuria in older patients as long as infection is asymptomatic [31]. However, it remains challenging to define 'asymptomatic' in the case of a nonspecific presentation (such as weakness) or a patient with delirium. The second common infection is pulmonary infection: More than half of all older patients with pneumonia can have non-respiratory symptoms [32]. Another prospective multicentre study showed that patients aged 65 and older frequently have no cough (20%), no dyspnoea (35%), no fever (50%) [33]. Therefore indication for chest X-ray should be handled liberally in older patients presenting with NSC.

8.2.2.2 Water and Electrolyte Disorders

Water and electrolyte disorder includes electrolyte disorders, volume depletion, dehydration, and acute kidney injury. These disorders are difficult to assess on clinical grounds in the older people, therefore laboratory tests are pivotal for diagnosis (see Table 8.1). However, there are some characteristics in medical history and physical examination that should be considered during diagnostic workup and can increase the pre-test probability for water and electrolyte disorders:

History taking could indicate an important reason for electrolyte disorder: It could be shown that these disorders are especially common in patients on new medication, above all diuretics [34].

The physical examination has limitations in evaluating water and electrolyte disorders; thus, the clinical evaluation of hydration status in patients with NSCs should be performed carefully. In general, clinical indicators for dehydration are dry oral mucosa and skin turgor. These, however, are not reliable indicators in older adults, due to changes occurring with age [35, 36], and medication (e.g. anti-cholinergics). Therefore, the most reliable indicators for altered hydration status are serum markers like serum osmolality and blood urea nitrogen-creatinine ratio [35]. Besides incorporating physiological parameters, there are some ultrasound-guided protocols available, which might help evaluating hydration status of emergency patients [37].

8.2.2.3 Heart Failure

The clinical presentation of heart failure in older people is often atypical [38], however, biomarkers exist which can help to exclude congestive heart failure. It was shown that normal serum B-type natriuretic peptide minimises the probability of heart failure [39]. Studies showed BNP increases with age, therefore there is an ongoing discussion about adjusting the cut-off value of BNP in older patients. Suggestions for cut-offs range from 100 to 250 pg/ml [39, 40].

Conclusion
The diagnostic workup of patients presenting with NSCs is complex and to date, no guidelines exist. The standard approach of history taking and physical examination can be supplemented by focussed investigations, e.g. augmented laboratory tests.

References

1. Samaras N, Chevalley T, Samaras D, Gold G (2010) Older patients in the emergency department: a review. Ann Emerg Med 56(3):261–269
2. Aminzadeh F, Dalziel WB (2002) Older adults in the emergency department: a systematic review of patterns of use, adverse outcomes, and effectiveness of interventions. Ann Emerg Med 39(3):238–247
3. Karakoumis J, Nickel CH, Kirsch M, Rohacek M, Geigy N, Muller B et al (2015) Emergency presentations with nonspecific complaints-the burden of morbidity and the spectrum of underlying disease: nonspecific complaints and underlying disease. Medicine (Baltimore) 94(26):e840
4. Vanpee D, Swine C, Vandenbossche P, Gillet JB (2001) Epidemiological profile of geriatric patients admitted to the emergency department of a university hospital localized in a rural area. Eur J Emerg Med 8(4):301–304
5. Bhalla MC, Wilber ST, Stiffler KA, Ondrejka JE, Gerson LW (2014) Weakness and fatigue in older ED patients in the United States. Am J Emerg Med 32(11):1395–1398
6. Castren M, Kurland L, Liljegard S, Djarv T (2015) Non-specific complaints in the ambulance; predisposing structural factors. BMC Emerg Med 15:8
7. Rutschmann OT, Chevalley T, Zumwald C, Luthy C, Vermeulen B, Sarasin FP (2005) Pitfalls in the emergency department triage of frail elderly patients without specific complaints. Swiss Med Wkly 135(9–10):145–150
8. Elmståhl S, Wahlfrid C (1999) Increased medical attention needed for frail elderly initially admitted to the emergency department for lack of community support. Aging (Milan, Italy) 11(1):56–60
9. Nemec M, Koller MT, Nickel CH, Maile S, Winterhalder C, Karrer C et al (2010) Patients presenting to the emergency department with non-specific complaints: the basel non-specific complaints (BANC) study. Acad Emerg Med 17(3):284–292

10. Nickel CH, Ruedinger J, Misch F, Blume K, Maile S, Schulte J et al (2011) Copeptin and peroxiredoxin-4 independently predict mortality in patients with nonspecific complaints presenting to the emergency department. Acad Emerg Med 18(8):851–859
11. Nickel CH, Messmer AS, Geigy N, Misch F, Mueller B, Dusemund F et al (2013) Stress markers predict mortality in patients with nonspecific complaints presenting to the emergency department and may be a useful risk stratification tool to support disposition planning. Acad Emerg Med 20(7):670–679
12. Misch F, Messmer AS, Nickel CH, Gujan M, Graber A, Blume K et al (2014) Impact of observation on disposition of elderly patients presenting to emergency departments with nonspecific complaints. PLoS One 9(5):e98097
13. Peng A, Rohacek M, Ackermann S, Ilsemann-Karakoumis J, Ghanim L, Messmer AS, et al. (2015) The proportion of correct diagnoses is low in emergency patients with nonspecific complaints presenting to the emergency department. Swiss Med Wkly. 145:w14121
14. Wallgren UM, Antonsson VE, Castren MK, Kurland L (2016) Longer time to antibiotics and higher mortality among septic patients with non-specific presentations—a cross sectional study of emergency department patients indicating that a screening tool may improve identification. Scand J Trauma Resusc Emerg Med 24:1
15. Nickel CH, Nemec M, Bingisser R (2009) Weakness as presenting symptom in the emergency department. Swiss Med Wkly 139(17–18):271–272
16. Nickel CH, Malinovska A, Bingisser R. (2015) Should weakness be subsumed to nonspecific complaints?-Correspondence in response to Bhalla et al. Am J Emerg Med.;33(5):722–723
17. Wiener P, Alexopoulos GS, Kakuma T, Meyers BS, Rosenthal E, Chester J (1997) The limits of history-taking in geriatric depression. Am J Geriat Psychiat 5(2):116–125
18. Ganguli M, Du Y, Rodriguez EG, Mulsant BH, McMichael KA, Bilt JV et al (2006) Discrepancies in information provided to primary care physicians by patients with and without dementia: the steel valley seniors survey. Am J Geriat Psychiat 14(5):446–455
19. Hampton J, Harrison M, Mitchell J, Prichard J, Seymour C (1975) Relative contributions of history-taking, physical examination, and laboratory investigation to diagnosis and management of medical outpatients. BMJ 2(5969):486–489
20. Colman N, Bakker A, Linzer M, Reitsma JB, Wieling W, Wilde AA (2009) Value of history-taking in syncope patients: in whom to suspect long QT syndrome? Europace 11(7):937–943
21. Wang CS, FitzGerald JM, Schulzer M, Mak E, Ayas NT (2005) Does this dyspneic patient in the emergency department have congestive heart failure? JAMA 294(15):1944–1956
22. Kroenke K (2014) A practical and evidence-based approach to common symptoms: a narrative review. Ann Internal Med 161(8):579–586
23. Chester JG, Rudolph JL (2011) Vital signs in older patients: age-related changes. J Am Med Directors Assoc 12(5):337–343
24. LaMantia MA, Stewart PW, Platts-Mills TF, Biese KJ, Forbach C, Zamora E et al (2013) Predictive value of initial triage vital signs for critically ill older adults. Western J Emerg Med 14(5):453
25. Iversen K, Teisner A, Bay M, Kirk V, Boesgaard S, Nielsen H (2006) Heart murmur and echocardiographic findings in 2,907 non-selected patients admitted to hospital. Ugeskr Laeger 168(26–32):2551–2554
26. Patzen A, Messmer AS, Rohacek M, Keil C, Nickel CH, Bingisser R. Unpublished data
27. Norman DC (2000) Fever in the elderly. Clin Infect Dis 31(1):148–151
28. Simon L, Gauvin F, Amre DK, Saint-Louis P, Lacroix J (2004) Serum procalcitonin and C-reactive protein levels as markers of bacterial infection: a systematic review and meta-analysis. Clin Infect Dis 39(2):206–217
29. Christ-Crain M, Stolz D, Bingisser R, Müller C, Miedinger D, Huber PR et al (2006) Procalcitonin guidance of antibiotic therapy in community-acquired pneumonia: a randomized trial. Am J Respiratory Crit Care Med 174(1):84–93
30. Nicolle LE, Bradley S, Colgan R, Rice JC, Schaeffer A, Hooton TM (2005) Infectious diseases society of America guidelines for the diagnosis and treatment of asymptomatic bacteriuria in adults. Clin Infect Dis 40(5):643–654

31. Colgan R, Nicolle LE, McGlone A, Hooton TM. (2006) Asymptomatic bacteriuria in adults. Am Fam Physician 74(6):985–90
32. Venkatesan P, Gladman J, Macfarlane J, Barer D, Berman P, Kinnear W et al (1990) A hospital study of community acquired pneumonia in the elderly. Thorax 45(4):254–258
33. Metlay JP, Schulz R, Li YH, Singer DE, Marrie TJ, Coley CM et al (1997) Influence of age on symptoms at presentation in patients with community-acquired pneumonia. Arch Intern Med 157(13):1453–1459
34. Ruedinger JM, Nickel CH, Maile S, Bodmer M, Kressig RW, Bingisser R (2012) Diuretic use, RAAS blockade and morbidity in elderly patients presenting to the emergency department with non-specific complaints. Swiss Med Wkly 142:w13568
35. Mentes J (2006) Oral hydration in older adults: greater awareness is needed in preventing, recognizing, and treating dehydration. Am J Nurs 106(6):40–49
36. Weinberg AD, Minaker KL, Coble YD Jr et al (1995) Dehydration: evaluation and management in older adults. JAMA 274(19):1552–1556
37. McGee S, Abernethy IW, Simel DL (1999) IS this patient hypovolemic? JAMA 281(11):1022–1029
38. Tresch DD (1997) The clinical diagnosis of heart failure in older patients. J Am Geriat Soc 45(9):1128–1133
39. Hill SA, Booth RA, Santaguida PL, Don-Wauchope A, Brown JA, Oremus M et al (2014) Use of BNP and NT-proBNP for the diagnosis of heart failure in the emergency department: a systematic review of the evidence. Heart Fail Rev 19(4):421–438
40. Blondé-Cynober F, Morineau G, Estrugo B, Fillie E, Aussel C, Vincent JP (2011) Diagnostic and prognostic value of brain natriuretic peptide (BNP) concentrations in very elderly heart disease patients: specific geriatric cut-off and impacts of age, gender, renal dysfunction, and nutritional status. Arch Gerontol Geriat 52(1):106–110

Falls Presenting in the Emergency Department

Jay Banerjee and Anna Björg Jónsdóttir

9.1 Introduction

A fall is defined by WHO as "an event which results in a person coming to rest inadvertently on the ground or floor or other lower level" [1].

One could think of a fall as a simple thing, but it can be just the tip of the iceberg and a non-specific final presentation for many different problems in older people. Therefore, it is very important to look at falls from a biopsychosocial perspective. A multidisciplinary and holistic approach is needed in frail older people with multiple morbidities and non-specific presentations. It is also important to appreciate how to adapt traditional model of an emergency department and its pathways of care to make it suitable for older people. We need to ensure the emergency departments are well resourced with staff competent in falls management and have well-defined processes for high-quality care for older people who fall.

Every older person looks at a fall differently. The "Help the Aged" report [http://www.slips-online.co.uk/resources/dont-mention-the-f-word.pdf] described a spectrum of attitudes and behaviours in older people when it came to suffering a fall. This included ignoring the fall, thinking it would never happen again, considering it an inevitable part of ageing and even rejecting the idea of falling to avoid stigmatisation as old and frail.

A fall is a presenting symptom and not a diagnosis. It should always be taken seriously and assessed properly.

J. Banerjee (✉)
Emergency Medicine, University Hospitals of Leicester NHS Trust, Leicester, UK

Department of Health Sciences, University of Leicester, Leicester, UK
e-mail: jb234@leicester.ac.uk

A.B. Jónsdóttir
Department of Geriatric Medicine, The National University Hospital of Iceland, Landakoti, 101, Reykjavík, Iceland
e-mail: annabjon@landspitali.is

9.2 Epidemiology

Falls are a serious threat to older people. About 25–28% of community dwelling older people over 65 years of age fall each year. This increases to about 50% for those over 80 years of age although majority of older people probably do not attend healthcare settings following a fall as 90% are noninjurious [2].

It is not feasible to screen the population for falls, but the emergency department may be a good setting for targeted intervention [3, 4].

Many falls are certainly amenable to community interventions [5].

There is a long-term consequence, with falls being a factor in long-term care admissions. Forty-four percent of people are readmitted to the hospital within 1 year and have 33% 1-year mortality. Up to 52% of people experience a subsequent fall in 6 months after an index fall [6], and 49% are readmitted.

Fear of falling, a significant contributor to quality of life following a fall, is however highly prevalent among older persons, and there is a lack of uniformity in the instruments used [7].

Falls account for about 700,000 visits to the emergency department, 4 billion annual bed days and 60,000 annual hip fractures and contribute to the largest number of deaths in older people in England alone. Each year approximately 10% of the older population in Europe (65+) will be treated by a doctor for an injury, and approximately 100,000 older people in the EU27 and EEA countries will die from injury from a fall each year [8]. A comprehensive national audit of falls and bone health management across England and Wales, including emergency departments, showed that there were many missed opportunities in improving care [9]. Given that half of the patients with hip fractures have previously had a fragility fracture of another bone [10] and many had not received treatment for osteoporosis or interventions to reduce further falls, there were missed opportunities to reduce the incidence of subsequent hip fractures in this group. The clinical audit indicated that two-thirds of patients presenting with a non-hip fragility fracture missed the best or only opportunity for their falls and fracture risk to be identified in the majority of hospitals [9].

9.3 Risk Factors

Staying upright requires sensory inputs (namely, vision, proprioception and vestibular function), coordination of the information (the brain) and effector mechanisms (strength and balance). Deficits in any or all of these domains can perturb balance leading to falls. In addition, environmental factors can act as enhancers or detractors to the upright posture.

One might find it helpful to use a body map to think about the factors at play (Fig. 9.1).

Risk factors can therefore affect all the mechanisms that help us stay upright.

Having taken a detailed and comprehensive history, one will now be able to think about which factors are likely to be affecting the various systems illustrated above.

9 Falls Presenting in the Emergency Department

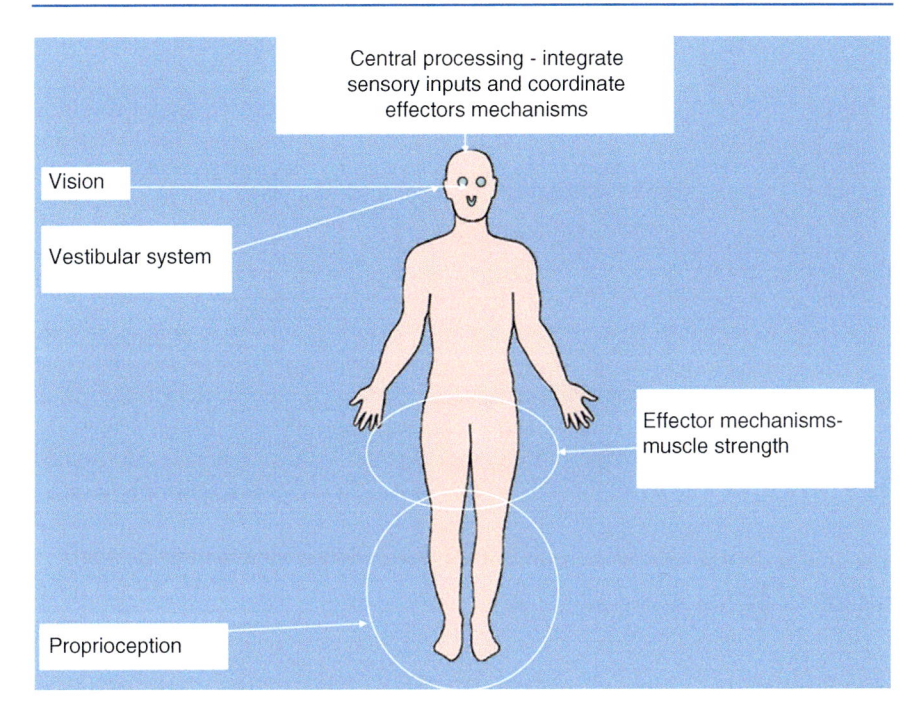

Fig. 9.1 Factors involved when staying upright

Consider someone with a non-syncopal fall with a background of diabetes, hypertension and cerebrovascular disease:

- Is there any evidence of disrupted cerebral perfusion pressure? Are there significant fluctuations in blood pressure or evidence of symptomatic and clinically correlated orthostatic hypotension?
- Has the cerebrovascular disease affected balance—either directly through motor or sensory impairment or more indirectly through disrupting cortical processing pathways?
- Is vision affected—stroke, diabetes, hypertension could all perturb vision alongside other common pathologies such as cataracts?
- Is joint position sense affected because of diabetic neuropathy or conditions such as arthritis that disrupt large joint proprioception?
- Is there a history of middle ear disease or cerebellar problems that could affect vestibular function?
- What's their strength like? It might be MRC grade 5 on formal testing, but can they "get up and go"?

One could divide risk factors into intrinsic or extrinsic as done in Fig. 9.2. Falls are often multifactorial, and the priorities in the ED are to understand the cause and circumstances of the fall, any precipitating factors and the consequences of the fall

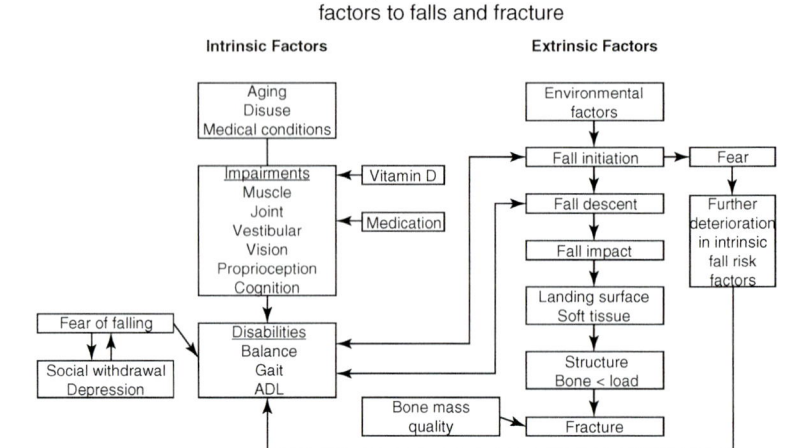

The relationship of intrinsic and extrinsic risk factors to falls and fracture

Carter ND, Kannus P, and Khan KM. Exercise in the prevention of falls in older people: a systematic literature review examining the rationale and evidence. Sports Med. 2001;31:427-438.

Fig. 9.2 Intrinsic and extrinsic risk factors

Table 9.1 Falls risk-increasing drugs and odds ratios—reproduced after Woolcott et al. [11]

Drug class	Odds ratio	95% CI
Antihypertensive	1.24	1.01–1.50
Diuretics	1.07	1.01–1.14
Beta blockers	1.01	0.86–1.17
Sedatives and hypnotics	1.47	1.35–1.62
Neuroleptics and antipsychotics	1.59	1.37–1.83
Antidepressants	1.68	1.47–1.91
Benzodiazepines	1.57	1.43–1.72
Narcotics	0.96	0.78–1.18
Non-steroidal anti-inflammatory	1.21	1.01–1.44

such as injuries or a prolonged period on the floor. It is important to be thorough with obtaining the history so as not to miss conditions such as Parkinson's disease, chronic musculoskeletal pain, knee osteoarthritis, cognitive impairment, stroke and diabetes as all increase the risk of falls.

Medications are an important risk factor. A meta-analysis from Woolcott et al. showed a correlation with nine unique drug classes; see Table 9.1. Situations where one should be especially careful include new prescriptions and polypharmacy, that is, more than four drugs with at least one in the "at-risk classes".

The patient's home circumstances are especially relevant as it may provide further clues to falling, trigger the need for a home assessment and influence disposition and rehabilitation. People with dementia are at particularly higher risk of falls and can be very difficult to manage as many have a habit of wandering at night. More than this is when the risk is compounded by inappropriate use of sedatives to reduce these wanderings which translates to increased daytime falls.

The American Geriatrics Society and the British Geriatrics Society (AGS and BGS) guideline recommends everyone aged 65 and over be screened for falls in the ED [12]; this can be carried out with minimal impact on efficiency. A positive answer to any of these puts the patient at high risk of falls.

1. Have you had two or more falls in the last 12 months?
2. Have you presented acutely with a fall?
3. Do you have problems with walking or balance (not necessarily restricting activity)?

These provide context to an unexplained fall as secondary to syncope: abnormal ECGs, heart failure, exertional syncope, family history, sudden cardiac death <40 years, new or unexplained breathlessness, heart murmur, age > 65 and no prodrome and falls irrespective of posture including while sitting.

Postprandial hypotension as a cause of fall or collapse is also increasingly described and appreciated (http://biomedgerontology.oxfordjournals.org/content/60/10/1268.full) as are postprandial reactive hypoglycaemia from ingestion of refined sugar.

9.4 Management

There are two situations when older people present to emergency departments that provide opportunities for improving management of falls and prevention of future ones.

The first scenario is where an older person presents with any complaint other than a fall. This contact with any healthcare professional presents an excellent opportunity to screen for falls by simply enquiring of any instances of falling in the preceding year. Depending on the response, further follow-up and multidisciplinary assessment of falls may be indicated.

The second scenario is when an older person presents to the ED after a fall. When that is the case, one first and foremost needs to do the primary assessment. The patient has to be examined from head to toe, looking for typical but sometimes hidden injuries such as subdural haematoma, C1/C2 fractures, rib fractures or hip fractures. There are a basic set of three questions that frame the assessment and management at this stage: why did they fall? what injuries did they suffer as a result of the fall? how to prevent future falls?

When assessing an older person with a fall, it is probably most useful to consider the fall as a signal that something has gone wrong and then proceed in an orderly manner to exclude the more serious and urgent from the less so.

First you need to identify the life-threatening and limb-threatening conditions and treat them. Then you need to take a history; this does need to be fairly detailed. Start with a wide-angled lens as a fall can be a presenting condition of pretty much any medical or surgical condition. So you need to find additional anchors to guide the history—has there been a recent illness? Is there a change from the usual state? Is this one of many falls or a completely new event? Importantly ask if there is evidence of syncope.

You could use an approach as outlined in Fig. 9.3.

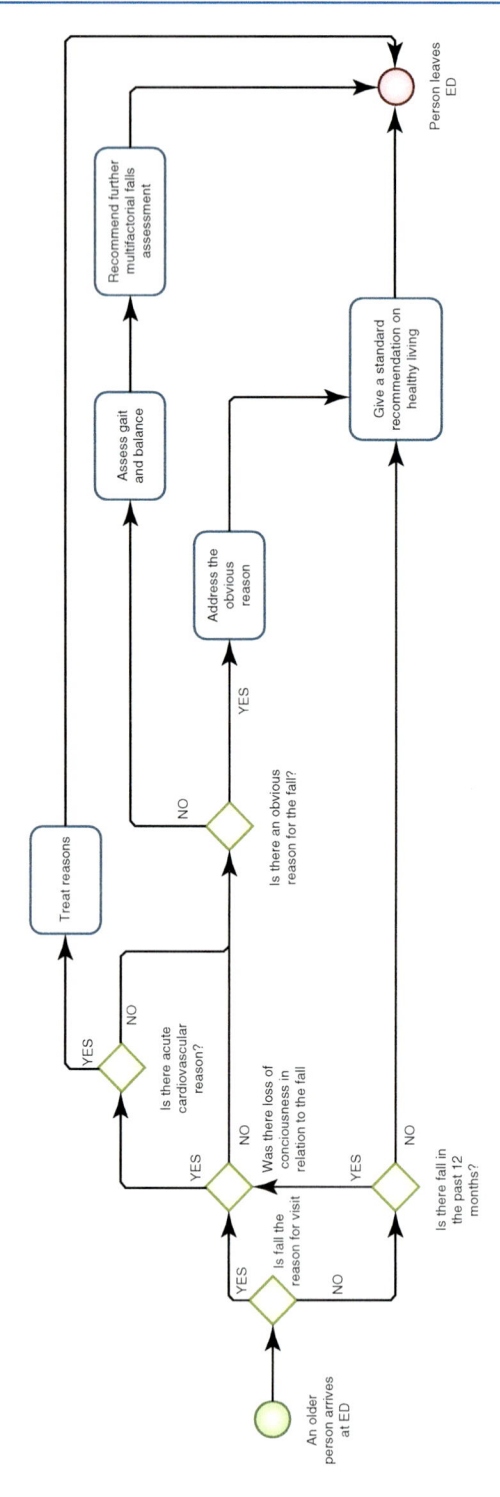

Fig. 9.3 Scheme for management of a fall patient in the ED

When it comes to assessing injuries as a result of the fall, it is important to remember that a fall from a standing position in a frail older person is akin to more serious mechanisms of injury in younger people such as being hit by a car at 30 miles per hour (50 kph). Further assessment including use of diagnostics needs to take this into consideration. Liberal use of CT scanning offers an opportunity to carry out a thorough assessment and decreases the chance of missing serious injuries. For example, the initial X-rays can be normal in hip fracture in 1–4% of patients. This justifies MRI or CT scanning of the hip in patients where strong clinical suspicion exists for a fracture [13, 14].

A recent review of the UK's national Trauma Audit Research Network (TARN) revealed serious shortcomings in management of polytrauma (ISS > 15) in older people with a significant number of missed diagnosis and poor management outside major trauma centres. Nearly half of all the patients on the UK TARN registry are older people. It is emerging how trauma in the developed world is a disease increasingly affecting older people, and trauma systems are not set up to improve outcomes.

9.5 Further Management

In the ED there is an opportunity to prevent the first fall (primary prevention), recurrent falls (secondary prevention) or injurious falls (tertiary prevention). Any person presenting with an injurious fall should be referred for a multidisciplinary falls assessment; systematic reviews indicate that falls programmes can reduce the rate of falls by 25% [5]. The theme seems to be that you need to begin the intervention soon after the initial presentation in the ED.

Medication is an important risk factor for falls. It is possible to use some aid such as STOPP/START criteria to do a structured approach to medication review. Sometimes drugs need to be stopped in the ED. That includes alpha blockers and nitrates if blood pressure is labile and diuretics if the patient is dehydrated. Benzodiazepines and diuretics usually need a tapered reduction. Warfarin or other anticoagulants are sometimes stopped because of falls; unless someone is falling weekly or more often, there is no evidence in stopping warfarin unless there are other considerations—the benefits usually outweigh the risks.

The environment is important—if going home, a home hazard assessment should be undertaken—this could be done by the community therapy teams or whatever system there is in place locally. If the older person is being admitted, then there is a need to ensure that those at high risk of falls are flagged as such and more intensively monitored.

Any history of an unexplained fall in the past year requires an observation of balance and gait deficits in older people as any impairment should trigger the offer of a multifactorial falls assessment. This would depend on the older person's ability to benefit from interventions to improve strength and balance.

When it comes to avoiding further falls, the first priority is appreciating that a person presenting with a fall is at increased risk of further falls even while an inpatient. Multifactorial intervention is effective in reducing the falls burden in cognitively intact older people presenting to the ED following a fall although the effect on the individual cannot be predicted. Comprehensive geriatric assessment has been shown to be effective in older people seen after an ED presentation following a fall. PROFET study reduced falls from 52% to 32% in 1 year [15].

It is important to remember that we cannot stop everyone from falling either. In spite of addressing risk factors and a multifactorial management programme, one can only reduce falls by 25%. This translates to someone falling three times per year from a previous tally of four falls per year. We need to ensure that we have mitigated the consequences of future falls, by ensuring that the patient has access to help if they do fall, that they know how to fall safely and get back up (the falls programme will often address this) and that the potential consequences of a fall are addressed. This means thinking about fracture risk and consider adding bone protection. Vitamin D can reduce the rate of falls by about 20%, so it is usually worth adding it to the prescription. It is also important to present the intervention in a patient-friendly way. That is to say to give a positive health message instead of "at-risk" message.

Conclusion

Falls in older people are among the commonest conditions seen in emergency departments. All these people are at risk of further falls and need comprehensive assessment to address reasons for falling, management of injuries and prevention of further falls. From a usefulness perspective, CGA and bone health management in cognitively intact older people presenting with non-syncopal, injurious fall to ED who can participate in a 6-week exercise programme will probably reduce further injurious falls.

Poor processes and lack of access to information and timely CGA are resulting in missed opportunities in improving falls care in older people in EDs.

References

1. WHO (2012) Falls, fact sheet No. 344. Secondary falls, fact sheet No. 344. http://www.who.int/mediacentre/factsheets/fs344/en/
2. National Institute for Clinical Excellence (2013) The assessment and prevention of falls in older people. NICE, London
3. Caplan GA, Williams AJ, Daly B et al (2004) A randomized, controlled trial of comprehensive geriatric assessment and multidisciplinary intervention after discharge of elderly from the emergency department—the DEED II study. J Am Geriatr Soc 52(9):1417–1423
4. Close J, Ellis M, Hooper R et al (1999) Prevention of falls in the elderly trial (PROFET): a randomised controlled trial. Lancet 353:93–97
5. Gillespie LD, Gillespie WJ, Robertson MC, Lamb SE, Cumming RG, Rowe BH (2004) Interventions for preventing falls in elderly people (Cochrane Review). Wiley, Chichester, UK
6. Close JC, Lord SR, Antonova EJ et al (2012) Older people presenting to the emergency department after a fall: a population with substantial recurrent healthcare use. Emerg Med J 29(9):742–747
7. Scheffer A, Schuurmans M, Van Dijk N et al (2008) Fear of falling: measurement strategy, prevalence, risk factors and consequences among older persons. Age Ageing 37:19–24
8. Commission E. Secondary. http://ec.europa.eu/health/data_collection/databases/idb/index_en.htm

9. Banerjee J, Benger J, Treml J et al (2012) The national falls and bone health audit: implications for UK emergency care. Emerg Med J 29(10):830–832
10. Klotzbuecher C, Ross P, Landsmann P (2005) Patients with prior fractures have an increased risk of future fractures: a summary of the literature and statistical synthesis. J Bone Miner Res 15:721e39
11. Woolcott JC, Richardson KJ, Wiens MO et al (2009) Meta-analysis of the impact of 9 medication classes on falls in elderly persons. Arch Intern Med 169(21):1952–1960
12. Panel on Prevention of Falls in Older Persons, American Geriatrics Society and British Geriatrics Society (2011) Summary of the Updated American Geriatrics Society/British Geriatrics Society clinical practice guideline for prevention of falls in older persons. J Am Geriatr Soc 59(1):148–157
13. Lubovsky O, Liebergall M, Mattan Y et al (2005) Early diagnosis of occult hip fractures MRI versus CT scan. Injury 36(6):788–792
14. Kirby MW, Spritzer C (2010) Radiographic detection of hip and pelvic fractures in the emergency department. AJR Am J Roentgenol 194(4):1054–1060
15. Close J, Patel A, Hooper R et al (2000) PROFET: improved clinical outcomes at no additional cost. Age Ageing 29(Suppl 1):48

Syncope in Older People in the Emergency Department

10

Nissa J. Ali, Laure Joly, and Shamai A. Grossman

10.1 Introduction

Although syncope is one of the most common symptoms of older patients presenting to the ED, the underlying etiology of geriatric syncope is frequently difficult to discern [1–4]. It is estimated that cardiac causes may claim up to 40% of syncopal episodes in patients aged 65 or more, whereas non-cardiac causes involve only 20% [5]. However, the diagnosis of syncope is particularly challenging in older patients as the causes are complex and often multifactorial [6]. Older people commonly have multiple medical conditions requiring numerous medications, many of which can contribute to syncope due to drug side effects and potential lack of compliance. Unfortunately, syncope is also associated with a higher level of morbidity and mortality in older patients as they are more likely to have associated comorbidities and are more prone to trauma associated with falls following syncope events [7–10]. The differential diagnosis is broad and complex in older individuals. A

N.J. Ali, MD, MEd (✉)
Department of Emergency Medicine, Mount Auburn Hospital and Harvard Medical School, Cambridge, MA, USA

Department of Emergency Medicine, Tufts Medical Center and Tufts University School of Medicine, Boston, MA, USA
e-mail: nissaali@post.harvard.edu

L. Joly, MD, PhD
Department of Geriatrics, CHRU-Nancy, Nancy F-54000, France
e-mail: l.joly@chru-nancy.fr

S.A. Grossman, MD, MS
Department of Emergency Medicine, Beth Israel Deaconess Medical Center and Harvard Medical School, Boston, MA, USA

Department of Emergency Medicine, Shaare Zedek Medical Center and Hebrew University, Jerusalem, Israel
e-mail: sgrossma@bidmc.harvard.edu

multidimensional geriatric assessment can be performed in these cases in order to provide a synthesis of the problems, leading to a specific care plan. Thus, it is important to recognize treatable etiologies not only to care for the event at hand but to prevent recurrent syncope in older adults as well.

10.2　Background and Epidemiology

Syncope, by definition, is a transient loss of consciousness, which is caused by a brief loss in generalized cerebral blood flow. Syncope produces a temporary period of unresponsiveness and a loss of postural tone, ultimately resulting in spontaneous recovery requiring no resuscitation measures [11]. It occurs in the absence of clinical features specific for other forms of transient loss of consciousness. Syncope is very common in older patients as well as in the general population, accounting for nearly 3% of all ED visits and 1–6% of all hospital admissions [8, 12, 13]. Syncope is more frequently found in older patients than in any other age group [10]. Age-related degeneration causing impairment of the heart rate, blood pressure, baroreflex sensitivity, and cerebral blood flow, combined with the higher prevalence of comorbidities and utilization of multiple medications, likely accounts for this increased incidence of syncope [10]. Furthermore, as one grows physiologically older, there may be a decrease in the body's ability to respond to hypotensive challenges, causing syncope [4]. Atypical presentations of conditions are also more likely in older patients than in the younger population [14].

Older patients frequently experience amnesia of the syncopal event. One study demonstrates amnesia after vasovagal syncope to be particularly common in older people, although not unique to older age groups, with findings of amnesia following tilt testing in 42% of people >60 years and 20% in <60 years [15]. Due to the amnesia, it is hypothesized that unexplained falls might be related to syncope or near syncope in older patients [16]. Thirty to forty percent of non-institutionalized older adults over the age of 65 years fall each year, with an estimated 20% of these falls as unexplained [16]. Of the unexplained falls, it has been suggested that 20% are due to a modifiable cardiac dysrhythmia causing syncope [17].

Despite extensive medical evaluation, 30–50% of all cases of syncope in older patients are not given a definable etiology [4, 5, 18–20]. Furthermore, most diagnoses are presumptive, cannot be confirmed by standard criterion, and may not be able to exclude a dysrhythmic cause of syncope [21]. Many of the conditions that may be responsible for producing syncope in older patients, such as cardiac conduction system disease and myocardial ischemia, may go undiscovered and have potentially life-threatening consequences as patients with cardiac syncope are at increased risk of death [20]. One study found 6.1% of patients suffered serious outcomes within 10 days of syncope, with 10% occurring within 48 h of the sentinel event. Nine percent of syncope patients have long-term severe outcomes, particularly those with the following risk factors: of age over 65, neoplasms, cerebrovascular disease, structural heart disease, and ventricular dysrhythmias [22].

Women over the age of 65, despite being less likely to have concomitant coronary artery disease or diabetes, have been shown to be significantly more likely to present to an ED with syncope, yet less likely to be discharged with a defined etiology [23]. Syncope is included as a manifestation of somatization, generalized anxiety, and substance abuse disorder [24]. Furthermore, psychiatric diagnoses were demonstrated in 22% of patients >65 and are more common in patients with syncope of unknown etiology [25]. This has prompted thought that to improve the quality of care for syncope in older patients, and for older women in particular, clinicians need to pursue a broader differential in evaluation of such patients to include sociodemographic and psychosocial contributors as well as organic causes [23].

The need for prompt risk stratification and concern for cardiac etiology may be a factor influencing ED physicians to pursue extensive evaluations and hospital admission for many older patients who present to the ED with syncope. There have been multiple scoring systems developed to guide the rationale for inpatient versus outpatient management of syncope [26–29]. However, the value and success of such evaluations has been incompletely studied, and the rationale for inpatient versus outpatient evaluation of older patients with syncope remains unproven [21, 30–32].

There is also limited information related to near syncope in older patients. It has been shown that older patients with near syncope are as likely as those with syncope to have adverse outcomes or critical interventions [33]. However, near syncope patients are less likely to be admitted [34, 35]. Although further studies on near syncope in older patients are warranted, a workup similar to that of syncope should be considered.

10.3 Etiologies

The causes of syncope in older people are diverse, ranging from the benign to the life threatening. Syncope in older patients may be grouped into cardiac and non-cardiac etiologies. In those younger than 65 years of age, 10% may be attributed to cardiac abnormalities, whereas non-cardiac causes make up approximately 40% of the remaining syncope cases in which an etiology can be defined [20, 36]. In contrast, cardiac etiologies may cause up to 40% of cases in patients aged 65 or more, and non-cardiac causes involve only 20% [5].

Cardiac syncope is commonly characterized by an absent or brief prodrome, palpitations, and a transient loss of consciousness. It is important to gather collateral or bystander history to obtain relevant information that may suggest a cardiac cause [37]. Syncope that occurs while in a sitting/supine position or during effort/exercise is also concerning for a cardiac etiology [27, 28]. Cardiac etiologies can be classified into mechanical/structural causes and dysrhythmic causes. Dysrhythmias, which induce hemodynamic impairment that can cause a critical decrease in cardiac output and cerebral blood flow, are the most common cardiac cause [27, 38]. Bradycardias are the most frequent dysrhythmias in the older population and are often caused by sinus node dysfunction, atrioventricular conduction disease, or implanted device malfunction [2, 38]. Tachycardias include supraventricular and ventricular dysrhythmias. Structural cardiovascular disease produces syncope when circulatory demands are greater than the heart's ability to increase output [38].

Structural causes may include valvular disease, obstruction of the left outflow tract, cardiac masses, tamponade, pulmonary embolism or dissection, acute coronary syndrome, and ischemic cardiopathy.

As noted, older patients often take multiple medications and, thus, are especially at risk for medication-induced syncope [39]. Nitrates and antihypertensives such as beta-blockers are often implicated, particularly if multiple medications for supine hypertension are prescribed, which is common in older adults [5]. Additional common medications to consider in older patients include but are not limited to vasodilators (alpha blockers, calcium channel blockers, ACE inhibitors), diuretics, antidysrhythmics, L-Dopa, antidepressants, and antipsychotics [5, 38]. Medications, including antidysrhythmics, which can prolong the QTc interval over 500 ms, increase the probability of dangerous dysrhythmias such as torsades de pointes. Medication side effects and patient compliance must be considered in assessing the etiology of geriatric syncope and in risk/benefit analysis when considering adding new medications to an older patient's regimen. The drug side effects may be confounded due to the pharmacokinetic and pharmacodynamic changes that occur with aging, which in turn may cause a delay in elimination and increased bioavailability of these drugs in the older population [40]. To help avoid these effects, the numerous electronic medical record systems that include specific tools for safe medication prescribing including the risk of drug interactions and potential side effects have been developed.

The most commonly identified etiology of syncope in all patients is vasovagal or sometimes called neurocardiogenic syncope. Vasovagal syncope history differs from cardiac syncope in that it is characterized by a prodrome and is commonly associated with precipitating events or stresses [41–43]. Typical prodromes include nausea, flushing, sweating, blurred vision, and light-headedness. Patients may also report provoking causes such as prolonged standing, a warm environment, a stressful event, or change in posture. Therefore, it is extremely important to obtain a detailed history by both the patient and witnesses of events prior to the syncopal event to help determine the etiology. Unfortunately, an older patient may be less likely to have the usual prodromes or provoking causes that one may expect in a younger patient with a vasovagal mechanism [44]. In addition, in younger individuals, syncope is most often associated with a single, isolated disease process [6]. Neurally mediated hypotension is often the lone culprit in this patient population [45]. In contrast, it is often difficult to find a single etiology of syncope in the older population. Lastly, a carefully obtained history is often the only way to differentiate a seizure from a syncopal event.

Orthostatic hypotension (OH) is commonly seen in older patients presenting with recurrent episodes of syncope or light-headedness. Guidelines define OH as a decrease in systolic blood pressure (SBP) $\geq$ 20 mm Hg or a diastolic blood pressure (DBP) $\geq$10 mm Hg within 3 min of standing [38]. Postural homeostasis is predominantly mediated by the autonomic nervous system [46]. The prevalence of OH increases with age, thought to be associated with reduced baroreflex responsiveness, decreased cardiac compliance, and attenuation of the vestibulosympathetic reflex in older adults [47, 48]. One study demonstrates impaired blood pressure stabilization increases from 15.6% in people >50 to 41.2% in those >80 years [47]. Studies have also suggested that the presence of OH increases the risk of mortality and cardiovascular events [46, 49]. Another type of OH, acute OH, can be observed as a consequence of fluid or blood loss or adrenal insufficiency [50]. However, OH has been shown to be present in up to 40% of asymptomatic patients older than 70 years and 6–23% of patients who are younger than 60 years, limiting its use in sorting out a diagnosis in the ED following a syncopal event in older patients [46, 51]. Novel beat-to-beat measurements show an even higher incidence, with one study demonstrating an OH prevalence of 72% in fallers and 50% in non-fallers at an older patient day center [52]. Since OH is common but not always symptomatic, it is important to correlate the finding with a patient's syncope history, examination, and laboratory findings.

Common causes of OH in older adults include medications and primary/secondary autonomic disorders such as neurodegenerative diseases (i.e., Parkinson's disease, multi-system atrophy, Lewy body dementia, pure autonomic failure) [48]. Parkinson's disease is particularly challenging as the disease itself can cause OH as well as treatment with levodopa [53]. Overtreatment of supine hypertension with beta-blockers and other antihypertensive medications may also lead to OH in older patients. One study shows beta-blocker monotherapy was associated with more than twofold increase in initial OH and more than threefold increase in sustained OH in older adults as compared to untreated grade one hypertension [54]. Older patients on bed rest are particularly susceptible to OH and appropriate precautions should be taken with any recently hospitalized patient.

Carotid sinus syndrome (CSS) should be considered in older patients who present with recurrent syncope after a negative diagnostic evaluation [5, 55]. Infrequently, patients may report a trigger such as neck turning, a tight collar, or a neck tumor; however, patients often report little or no warning prior to the event [55]. CSS is defined as syncope with reproduction of symptoms during carotid sinus massage (CSM) of 10 s [56]. One study showed the average duration of asystole to cause symptoms is 7.6 s and a decrease in systolic blood pressure of 65 mm Hg due to vasodepressive effects [57]. CSS typically presents in the older adult with a mean age of 75 years, with a male dominance and is thought to be a pathological reflex from cardioinhibition via the vagus nerve and sympathetic withdrawal. Conversely, carotid sinus hypersensitivity (CSH) is more common in younger patients and is defined as a positive response to CSM without symptoms [55].

Atypical causes of syncope should be considered more closely in older patients than in younger populations. Pulmonary embolism (PE) may present with syncope or other atypical symptoms in older patients and should be considered in populations with risk factors, unexplained hypoxia or dyspnea [58]. Less common causes of syncope, such as mesenteric steal, abdominal aortic aneurysm, and aortic dissection, are also important to consider in older patients. Syncope secondary to diffuse coronary vasospasms has been discussed in a case report as the cause of unexplained syncope [59]. The patient's risk factors, presenting history, medications, past medical history, and prior events must be taken into account when determining how aggressively to pursue these causes. Yet, once more, older patients may not present with the typical pain or dyspnea that is seen in younger groups. One retrospective study with a mean age of 66 years finds that 17% of patients with an aortic dissection have no pain on presentation, but 25% of these patients present with syncope [60]. Another retrospective study with a mean age of 73.5 years shows 23% of patients admitted with a ruptured abdominal aortic aneurysm have syncope as a symptom [61].

Sepsis is another life-threatening illness that may manifest as syncope. Realizing that older adults may be less likely to mount a fever or express a leukocytosis, syncope may also be one of the few signs of impending sepsis or severe infection developing in an older patient.

10.4 Evaluation

As delineated above, determining the etiology of a syncopal event, particularly in older adults, can be challenging. Syncope is often transient and can resolve independently, without recurrence. Often the event is not witnessed and not remembered by the patient, making it difficult to find the specific circumstances that led up to and occurred during the syncopal episode [4]. In determining whether the patient experienced a seizure, stroke, or a syncopal episode, several factors should be considered and a careful history taken. Unresponsiveness during syncope is brief, whereas generalized seizures will often have postictal confusion, and loss of consciousness from a stroke is generally not transient.

Therefore, one must first determine whether the patient had a syncopal event. Second, one must determine if this syncopal event is dangerous. If the syncopal event potentially had a worrisome cardiac etiology, one must decide what evaluation and what immediate therapy are appropriate. Lastly, if this event does not appear to be dangerous, one must determine whether the patient can be discharged home and define the appropriate follow-up.

The history, physical examination, and ECG have the greatest utility in evaluating syncope in older patients [62, 63]. To sort out the etiology, the physician must obtain the best history from the greatest number of witnesses. Similarly, all syncope patients need a thorough physical examination. The patient's medication list should be reviewed for drugs that increase the risk for syncope, including antihypertensive, cardiovascular agents, and antipsychotics, as well as recent changes to these medications that may have influenced the event.

The initial task in an older patient with syncope is to obtain vital signs and determine the need for immediate stabilization. Most syncope patients who are otherwise asymptomatic should have normal or near normal vital signs within minutes following resolution of their syncopal event. While the utility of orthostatic vital signs is controversial, orthostatics may be helpful in older adults if the syncopal event directly follows standing or in any patient thought to be volume depleted [51, 64]. To obtain orthostatics correctly, measure the blood pressure in the supine position and after 3–5 min of standing. Again, review of the patient's medication list for causative drugs and careful physical examination may help determine risk of volume depletion. Consider comparing the patient's current blood pressure to the baseline blood pressure, as older patients who appear normotensive may actually be relatively hypotensive if there is a history of hypertension. However, relative hypotension may be a false positive given the burden of vascular disease in older patients. Once more, OH findings should be linked to a patient's symptoms and syncope history to help determine relevancy.

Physical examination should include careful auscultation of the heart and lungs and palpation of the peripheral arteries. A neurological examination should be performed if there is concern for neurological symptoms or head trauma secondary to a fall. There is no clear evidence to support routine stool sampling in syncope. However, if there is concern for gastrointestinal bleeding based on history, vital signs, or a low hemoglobin/hematocrit, then further testing might be required, potentially as an inpatient, if there are signs of an acute bleed. It is also important to look at all skin areas to evaluate for trauma or skin infections that may be easily missed, particularly if considering a source for sepsis.

Evidence of trauma such as contusions, tenderness, or lacerations from tongue biting should be meticulously noted.

10.5 Testing

There is no gold standard against which the results of diagnostic tests can be measured in syncope [62, 63]. All patients should have basic tests such as an ECG and a finger stick glucose test. ECG findings that may suggest a dysrhythmic or concerning cause of syncope include intraventricular conduction abnormalities, Mobitz II second-degree or third-degree block, non-sustained VT, prolonged QT intervals, bifascicular blocks, sinus pause ≥ 3 s, or evidence of myocardial infarction. Other concerning ECG findings that may be more common in younger patients with syncope include Brugada syndrome, Wolff-Parkinson-White syndrome, hypertrophic cardiomyopathy pattern, or epsilon waves. However, studies have shown that an ECG will determine the cause of syncope in only 5% of patients [62].

Blood tests such as cardiac enzymes, electrolytes, complete blood count, lactate, blood cultures, and imaging modalities such as head CT, echocardiography, and carotid ultrasonography should be guided by history and physical examination [65]. Routine blood tests typically only confirm clinical suspicion in syncope as they only uncover an etiology in 2% of patients [62]. Specifically, cardiac enzymes are of little value if drawn routinely on older patients who are admitted with syncope. Cardiac enzymes should only be drawn if the patient has other signs or symptoms suggestive of myocardial ischemia by history such as chest pain, dyspnea, a concerning ECG, or an ECG that is uninterpretable for ischemia [66]. Similarly, it's suggested that lactate only be sent if there's concern for sepsis or mesenteric ischemia based on the history and physical examination. Urine and blood cultures should be sent if there's concern for sepsis. Additional studies such as electroencephalography and cardiac stress testing have a low diagnostic use and should not be routinely performed [21].

Studies have shown that telemetry may help determine the etiology of syncope in 3–5% of patients and most commonly from causes such as atrial fibrillation or bradycardia [67, 68]. There is neither evidence nor consensus on the duration of monitoring in the ED for intermediate-risk patients, but many experts suggest at least 3 h [31]. If a new murmur is heard on examination, then an echocardiogram may be obtained either in the ED or as an inpatient. However, if a patient doesn't have a history of a murmur or an audible murmur on examination, they are unlikely to have a valvular etiology of their syncope [26]. An echocardiogram may give a diagnosis 2–22% of the time and most often in older patients from aortic stenosis [67, 68].

Head CT scans should be limited in older adults to those presenting to the ED with syncope and concomitant signs of head trauma, neurologic deficit, or neurologic complaints [32, 69]. It is unlikely that a cerebral vascular event alone will cause syncope. However, neurological complaints may be due to head trauma that occurred during the syncopal event. All other patients presenting with syncope have a low likelihood of having abnormal findings on head CT and do not require a scan [65]. In one pilot study, limiting CT scans to patients with neurological signs or symptoms, including headache and trauma above the clavicles, or medicating with warfarin, would have reduced scans by 56% [65]. Additional studies should be used sparingly and based on the initial data, as many tests for syncope in older patients have a low diagnostic yield. Choosing tests based on history and examination and prioritizing less expensive and higher yield tests may enable a more informed and cost-effective approach to evaluating syncope in older patients [65].

A recent study on older individuals demonstrates that 50% of unexplained falls in patients with dementia and without were caused by true syncope. This supports the idea that that older patients with cognitive impairment can be evaluated in a fashion similar to those without cognitive impairments [70, 71].

Finally, a patient's social situation, coping capacity, and ability to return home safely must be considered for any older patient that presents to the ED. An older patient may need social or physical support at home, particularly if there is risk of recurrent syncope and falls. Discussions with the patient and caregivers as well as evaluation of the patient's ability to ambulate safely should be included in any workup.

10.6 Scoring Tools

There are multiple scoring systems that have been developed to guide the evaluation of syncope and rationale for inpatient versus outpatient management. Select scoring systems are reviewed below.

The consensus from the first international workshop on syncope risk stratification in the ED suggests low-risk features include age <40, report of prodrome or a trigger, syncope while standing, and prolonged history of similar syncope events [31]. The consensus advised that high-risk characteristics include syncope during exertion or while supine, chest discomfort, palpitations, concerning cardiac history or ECG, family history of sudden death, anemia, and abnormal vital signs. Indeterminate-risk patients are challenging with no clear consensus on management. For these patients, further exams and telemetry monitoring in the ED for at least 3 h to better determine disposition is suggested [31]. Events during monitoring that would indicate admission for further workup include a pause >3 s, ventricular tachycardia, high grade AV block, or bradycardia [31].

Another study used four predictors of adverse outcomes in 72 h including a history of ventricular dysrhythmia, an abnormal ECG in the ED, age older than 45 years, and a history of congestive heart failure [72]. In patients with none of these risk factors, there was no 72 h cardiac mortality, but a 0.7% risk of dysrhythmia [72]. One-year cardiac mortality and dysrhythmia rates range from 7% in those with no risk factors to 57% in those with three and 80% in those with four risk factors [72].

The San Francisco Syncope Rule (SFSR) was proposed as a tool to predict serious outcomes of patients with syncope [29]. However, multiple studies have been unable to validate this rule [73–75]. Schladenhaufen found low sensitivities and specificities of the SFSR specifically for older patients [76]. Thus, SFSR may not be applicable to the older ED population.

The Boston Syncope Criteria is an alternative rule to identify ED patients at risk for adverse outcomes at 30 days [26]. A large urban university ED study yields a sensitivity of 97%, specificity of 62% with a negative predictive value of 99% [33]. Risk factors for adverse outcomes include signs of acute coronary syndrome, a cardiac or valvular disease history, family history of sudden death, signs of conduction disease, persistent abnormal vital sign, or profound volume depletion such as with gastrointestinal bleeding [26, 33]. Admitting only patients identified by risk factors would reduce hospital admissions by 11–48% [26, 34]. Furthermore, high-risk patients who present with a benign etiology of syncope or near syncope (vasovagal or dehydration) with a normal ED workup would not benefit from hospitalization based on risk factors or older age alone [30, 33, 77]. Discharging these patients with a benign etiology and negative workup would result in an additional 19% reduction in hospital admissions [77].

Age was not used as a criterion for admission with the Boston Syncope Criteria. Adverse outcomes in older patients appeared to be related to other comorbidities and not age alone. Roussanov similarly finds that new-onset syncope is not an independent predictor of mortality in older patients [78]. As age over 65 does not appear to be an independent predictor of an adverse outcome following syncope, it is safe to discharge older adults with syncope but without other risk factors [79].

The OESIL (Osservatorio Epidemiologico sulla Sincope nel Lazio) score uses a two-step approach. The first step includes a history, examination, ECG, hemoglobin count, and blood glucose test. If the cause of syncope is inconclusive, further evaluation is recommended in the second step based on if the hypothesized cause of syncope is cardiac, neurally mediated, or psychiatric/neurological [80]. One-year mortality is predicted to increase as the score increased, with risk factors including age greater than 65 years, cardiovascular disease history, an abnormal ECG, or lack of prodromes [81].

The EGSYS is a tool to provide guidance when evaluating for cardiac syncope [28]. Risk factors include an abnormal ECG, palpitations, effort syncope, supine position, age >64, and lack of precipitating factors or prodromes [28]. Negative points are assigned for symptoms indicating non-cardiac syncope, including blurred vision, neurovegetative signs or prodromes, and precipitating factors [28].

10.7 Disposition

Successful response to treatment is difficult to predict in older patients [8]. The European Heart Rhythm Association survey suggests that there are significant management differences for patients with syncope, specifically related to hospitalization rates [82]. With concern that potentially life-threatening diseases or cardiac causes might be the etiology, older patients in particular are frequently admitted to the hospital regardless of the most likely etiology, comorbidities, or lack thereof. Potential for transient dysrhythmia is likely the most significant issue influencing physicians to pursue inpatient evaluations for those patients presenting with syncope of unknown origin. However, recommendations for hospital admission for older adults should be based on the potential for adverse outcomes if further evaluation and workup is delayed or thought to be unnecessary [22, 30, 79]. The scoring systems discussed above can help guide disposition and rationale for inpatient versus outpatient management of syncope.

A proposed stepwise approach for syncope evaluation in the ED is as follows: First, determine if syncope has occurred. Next, any serious conditions identified should be managed appropriately. If the cause is uncertain, patients should be classified into a low, indeterminate, or high risk of serious outcome [31]. Consider discharge if low risk, admission for high risk and further exams, and monitoring for indeterminate risk [31].

Syncope units (SUs) have been recommended by the European Society of Cardiology as specialized facilities providing a standardized approach to syncope diagnosis and treatment, with a goal of reducing the wide variation in syncope evaluation [83]. Anticipated benefits include accurate and efficient diagnoses, specialist opinions, shorter length of stays, reduced costs, and access to data for research. Unfortunately SUs have not been widely established in Europe, possibly due to limited resources and trained specialists, lack of awareness, and complex presentations of patients [83].

Patients should also be advised not to drive following syncope. A Danish cohort study found that the 5-year crash risk following syncope was 8.2% compared with 5.1% in the general population [84]. The risk of injury if syncope occurs during work should also be assessed. Most work accidents are classified as occurring after a slip, fall, or loss of control, and it can be theorized that occult syncope can be the cause of these accidents [85, 86]. One study reports that 6% of syncope occurs while at work, yet there are no studies to guide work in high-risk occupations [21]. Although there is limited data to suggest an appropriate length of time, our practice is to advise the patient not to drive or perform high-risk jobs at least until PCP follow-up occurs. As with any patient, discharge instructions are useless if the patient lacks the cognitive ability to understand the discharge instructions.

If an older adult is discharged from the ED, regardless of etiology, he should have close follow-up with his primary care physician (PCP) or cardiologist, ideally scheduled prior to discharge. Direct communication between the PCP and emergency team can be particularly useful. The social and home situation must be considered prior to discharging older patients with syncope. An older patient may need social support at home, particularly if there is concern for recurrent syncope and falls.

Conclusions

Assessing and managing syncope in older patients is a daunting task. The variability of presentations is numerous, the histories are often limited, and the spectrum of disease is considerable. Successful interventions center primarily on the cardiovascular disorders that cause syncope in older patients. Disposition should be based on the results of the initial evaluation as well as risk factors for adverse outcomes with associated syncope. With a growing older population worldwide, the future rests in creating more directed and expeditious protocols for evaluation and testing of syncope patients and increasing public awareness to the nuance of worrisome concurrent symptomatology [87].

References

1. Hogan TM, Constantine ST, Crain AD (2016) Evaluation of syncope in older adults. Emerg Med Clin North Am 34(3):601–627. doi:10.1016/j.emc.2016.04.010
2. Kapoor W, Snustad D, Peterson J et al (1998) Syncope in the elderly. Am J Med 80:419–428
3. Lipsitz LA (1983) Syncope in the elderly. Ann Intern Med 99:92–105
4. Lipsitz LA, Pluchino FC, Wei JY et al (1986) Syncope in institutionalized elderly: the impact of multiple pathological conditions and situational stress. J Chronic Dis 39:619–630
5. Kapoor WN (1992) Evaluation and management of the patient with syncope. J Am Med 268:2553–2560
6. Kapoor WN (1987) Evaluation of syncope in the elderly. J Am Geriatr Soc 35:826–828
7. Grossman SA (2016) Dysrhythmia and occult syncope as an explanation for falls in older patients. Heart 102(9):657. doi:10.1136/heartjnl-2016-309274
8. Kapoor WN (1990) Evaluation and outcome of patients with syncope. Medicine 69(3):160–175
9. Kapoor WN (1991) Diagnostic evaluation of syncope. Am J Med 90:91–106
10. Kenny RA (2003) Syncope in the elderly: diagnosis, evaluation, and treatment. J Cardiovasc Electrophysiol 14(Suppl. 9):S74–S77
11. Kapoor WN, Karpf M, Wieand S et al (1983) A prospective evaluation and follow-up of patients with syncope. N Engl J Med 309:197–204
12. Bhangu JS, King-Kallimanis B, Cunningham C, Kenny RA (2014) The relationship between syncope, depression and anti-depressant use in older adults. Age Ageing 43(4):502–509
13. Sun BC, Emond JA, Camargo CA Jr (2005) Direct medical costs of syncope-related hospitalizations in the United States. Am J Cardiol 1(95):668–671
14. Hood R (2007) Syncope in the elderly. Clin Geriatr Med 23:351–361
15. O'Dwyer C, Bennett K, Langan Y et al (2011) Amnesia for loss of consciousness is common in vasovagal syncope. Eur Secur 13:1040–1045

16. Davies AJ, Kenny RA (1996) Falls presenting to the accident and emergency department: types of presentation and risk factor profile. Age Ageing 25:362–366
17. Bhangu J, McMahon G, Hall P et al (2016) Long term cardiac monitoring in older adults with unexplained falls and syncope. Heart 102(9):681–686. doi:10.1136/heartjnl-2015-308706
18. Getchell WS, Larsen GC, Morris CD et al (1999) Epidemiology of syncope in hospitalized patients. J Gen Intern Med 14:677–687
19. Kapoor H, Hanusa B (1996) Is syncope a risk factor for poor outcomes? Comparison of patients with and without syncope. Am J Med 100:647–655
20. Soteriades ES, Evans JC, Martin GL (2002) Incidence and prognosis of syncope. N Engl J Med 327(12):878–885
21. Sun BC, Costantino G, Barbic F et al (2014) Priorities for emergency department syncope research. Ann Emerg Med 64:649–655
22. Costantino G, Perego F, Dipaola F et al (2008) Short and long term prognosis of syncope, risk factors, and role of hospital admission. Results from the STePS (short-term prognosis of syncope) study. JACC 51(3):276–283
23. Grossman SA, Shapiro NI, Van Epp S et al (2005) Sex differences in the emergency department evaluation of elderly patients with syncope. J Gerontol A Biol Sci Med Sci 60(9):1202–1205
24. Diagnostic and Statistical Manual of Mental Disorders, 3rd edn. (1987) American Psychiatric Association, Washington, DC
25. Kapoor WN, Fortunato M, Hanusa BH et al (1995) Psychiatric illnesses in patients with syncope. Am J Med 99:505–512
26. Grossman SA, Fischer C, Bar JL et al (2007) The yield of head CT in syncope: a pilot study. Intern Emerg Med 2:46–49
27. Kariman H, Harati S, Safari S et al (2015) Validation of EGSYS score in prediction of cardiogenic syncope. Emerg Med Int 2015:1–5. doi:10.1155/2015/515370
28. Plasek J, Doupal V, Furstova J et al (2010) The EGSYS and OESIL risk scores for classification of cardiac etiology of syncope: comparison, revaluation, and clinical implications. Biomed 154(2):169–173
29. Quinn IG, Stiell IG, Seller KA et al (2002) The San Francisco syncope rule to predict patients with serious outcomes. Acad Emerg Med 9:358
30. Costantino G, Dipaola F, Solbiati M et al (2014) Is hospital admission valuable in managing syncope? Results from the STePS study. Cardiol J 21(6):606–610
31. Costantino G, Sun BC, Barbic F et al (2015) Syncope clinical management in the emergency department: a consensus from the first international workshop on syncope risk stratification in the emergency department. Eur Heart J 37(19):1493–1498. doi:10.1093/eurheartj/ehv378
32. Grossman SA, Fischer C, Lipsitz L et al (2007) Predicting adverse outcomes in syncope. J Emerg Med 33:233–239
33. Grossman SA, Bar J, Fischer C et al (2012) Reducing admissions utilizing the Boston syncope criteria. J Emerg Med 42(3):345–352
34. Grossman SA, Babineau M, Burke L et al (2012) Do outcomes of near syncope parallel syncope? Am J Emerg Med 30:203–206
35. Grossman SA, Babineau M, Burke L et al (2012) Applying the Boston syncope criteria to near syncope. J Emerg Med 43(6):958–963
36. Mosqueda-Garcia R, Furlan R, Tank J et al (2000) The elusive pathophysiology of neurally mediated syncope. Circulation 102:2898–2906
37. Del Rosso A, Alboni P, Brignole M et al (2005) Relation of clinical presentation of syncope to the age of patients. Am J Cardiol 96:1431–1435
38. Task Force for the Diagnosis and Management of Syncope, European Society of Cardiology (ESC) (2009) Guidelines for the diagnosis and management of syncope. Eur Heart J 30:2631–2671
39. Hanlon J, Linzer M, MacMillan J et al (1990) Syncope and presyncope associated with probable adverse drug reactions. Arch Intern Med 150:2309–2312
40. Verhaeverbeke H, Mets T (1997) Drug-induced orthostatic hypotension in the elderly: avoiding its onset. Drug Saf 17(2):105–118

41. Calkins H, Shyr Y, Frumin H et al (1995) The value of the clinical history in the differentiation of syncope due to ventricular tachycardia, atrioventricular block, and neurocardiogenic syncope. Am J Med 98:365–373
42. Day SC, Cook EF, Funkenstein H et al (1982) Evaluation and outcome of emergency room patients with transient loss of consciousness. Am J Med 73:15–23
43. Martin G, Adams S, Martin H et al (1984) Prospective evaluation of syncope. Ann Emerg Med 13:499–504
44. Duncan GW, Tan MP, Newton JL et al (2010) Vasovagal syncope in the older person: differences in presentation between older and younger patients. Age Ageing 39:470–475
45. Braunwald E (ed) (1997) Heart disease: a textbook of cardiovascular medicine, 5th edn. WB Saunders, Philadelphia, pp 868–935
46. Fedorowski A, Stavenow L, Hedblad B et al (2010) Orthostatic hypotension predicts all-cause mortality and coronary events in middle-aged individuals (the Malmo preventive project). Eur Heart J 31:85–91. doi:10.1093/eurheartj/ehp329
47. Finucane C, O'Connel MDL, Fan CW et al (2014) Age-related normative changes in phasic orthostatic blood pressure in a large population study. Findings from the Irish longitudinal study on ageing (TILDA). Circulation. doi:10.1161/CIRCULATIONAHA.114.009831
48. Freeman R (2008) Neurogenic orthostatic hypotension. N Engl J Med 358:615–624
49. Rose KM, Eigenbrodt ML, Biga RL et al (2006) Orthostatic hypotension predicts mortality in middle-aged adults. The atherosclerosis risk in communities (ARIC) study. Circulation 114(51):630–636
50. Gupta V, Lipsitz LA (2007) Orthostatic hypotension in the elderly: diagnosis and treatment. Am J Med 120:841–847
51. Atkins D, Hanusa B, Sefcik T, Kapoor W (1990) Syncope and orthostatic hypotension. Am J Med 91:179–185
52. Van der Velde N, Van den Meiracker AH, Stricker BH et al (2007) Measuring orthostatic hypotension with the Finometer device: is a blood pressure drop of one heartbeat clinically relevant? Blood Press Monit 12:167–171
53. Barbic F, Perego F, Canesi M et al (2007) Abnormalities of vascular and cardiac autonomic control in Parkinson's disease without orthostatic hypotension. Hypertension 49:120–126
54. Canney M, O'Connell MDL, Murphy CM et al (2016) Single agent antihypertensive therapy and orthostatic blood pressure behaviour in older adults using beat-t-beat measurements: the Irish longitudinal study on ageing. PLoS One 11(1):e0146156. doi:10.1371/journal.pone.0146156
55. Sutton R (2014) Carotid sinus syndrome: progress in understanding and management. Glob Cardiol Sci Pract 18(2):1–8. doi:10.5339/gcsp.2014.18an
56. Task Force on cardiac pacing and resynchronization therapy, European Society of Cardiology (ESC), European Heart Rhythm Association (EHRA) (2013) ESC guidelines on cardiac pacing and cardiac resynchronization therapy. Eur Secur 15(8):1070–1118. doi:10.1093/europace/eut206. Epub 2013 Jun 24
57. Solari D, Maggi R, Oddone D et al (2014) Clinical context and outcome of carotid sinus syndrome diagnosed by means of the "method of symptoms". Europace 16(6):928–934. doi:10.1093/europace/eut283
58. Kokturk N, Oguzulgen IK, Demir N et al (2005) Differences in clinical presentation of pulmonary embolism in older vs younger patients. Circ J 69:981–986
59. Quiang L, Gao C, Liu C, Wang T, Jia R (2015) Diffuse triple-vessel coronary spasm as a cause of asystole and syncope. Am J Emerg Med 33:1546.e1–1546.e3
60. Imamura H, Sekiguchi Y, Iwashita T et al (2011) Painless acute aortic dissection. Circ J 75(1):59–66
61. Akkersdijk GJ, Van Bockel JH (1998) Ruptured abdominal aortic aneurysm: initial misdiagnosis and the effect on treatment. Eur J Surg 164:29–34
62. Linzer M, Yang EH, Estes NA III et al (1997) Diagnosing syncope. Part 1: value of history, physical examination, and electrocardiography. Clinical efficacy assessment project of the American College of Physicians. Ann Intern Med 126:989–996

63. Linzer M, Yang EH, Estes NA III et al (1997) Diagnosing syncope. Part 2: unexplained syncope: clinical efficacy assessment project of the American College of Physicians. Ann Intern Med 127:76–86
64. Ooi WL, Hossain M, Lipsitz LA (2000) The association between orthostatic hypotension and recurrent falls in nursing home residents. Am J Med 108:106–111
65. Grossman SA (2006) Testing in syncope. Intern Emerg Med 1:135–136
66. Grossman SA, Van Epp S, Arnold R et al (2003) The value of cardiac enzymes in elderly patients presenting to the emergency department with syncope. J Gerontol A Biol Sci Med Sci 58:1055–1059
67. Chiu DT, Shapiro NI, Sun BC et al (2014) Are echocardiography, telemetry, ambulatory electrocardiography monitoring and cardiac enzymes in emergency department patients presenting with syncope useful tests? A preliminary investigation. J Emerg Med 47(1):113–118. doi:10.1016/j.jemermed.2014.01.018. Epub 2014 Mar 31
68. Mendu ML, McAvay G, Lampert R et al (2009) Yield of diagnostic tests in evaluating syncopal episodes in older patients. Arch Intern Med 169:1299–1305
69. Jones PK, Gibbons CH (2014) The role of autonic testing in syncope. Auton Neurosci 184:40–45
70. Ungar A, Mussi C, Ceccofiglio A et al (2016) Etiology of syncope and unexplained falls in elderly adults with dementia: syncope and dementia (SYD) study. J Am Geriatr Soc 64(8):1567–1573. doi:10.1111/jgs.14225. [Epub ahead of print]
71. Ungar A, Rivasi G, Rafanelli M (2016) Safety and tolerability of tilt testing and carotid sinus massage in the octogenarians. Age Aging 45(2):242–248. doi:10.1093/ageing/afw004. Epub 2016 Jan 31
72. Martin TP, Hanusa BH, Kapoor WN (1997) Risk stratification of patients with syncope. Ann Emerg Med 29:459–466
73. Birnbaum A, Esses D, Biju P et al (2008) Failure to validate the San Francisco syncope rule in elderly ED patients. Am J Emerg Med 26:773–778
74. Fischer CM, Shapiro NI, Lipsitz L et al (2005) External validation of the San Francisco syncope rule. Acad Emerg Med 12:S127
75. Sun BC, Mangione CM, Merchant G et al (2007) External validation of the San Francisco syncope rule. Ann Emerg Med 49:420–427
76. Schladenhaufen R, Feilinger S, Pollack M et al (2008) Application of San Francisco syncope rule in elderly ED patients. Am J Emerg Med 26:773–778
77. Grossman SA, Fischer C, Kancharla A et al (2011) Can benign etiologies predict benign outcomes in high-risk syncope patients? J Emerg Med 40(5):592–597
78. Roussanov O, Estacio G, Capuno M et al (2007) Outcomes of unexplained syncope in the elderly. Am J Geriatr Cardiol 16:249–254
79. Grossman SA, Chiu D, Lipsitz L et al (2014) Can elderly patients without risk factors be discharged home when presenting to the emergency department with syncope? Arch Gerontol Geriatr 58:110–114
80. Ammirati F, Colivicchi F, Santini M (2000) Implementation of a simplified diagnostic algorithm in a multicentre prospective trial — the OESIL 2 study (Osservatorio Epidemiologico della Sincope nel Lazio). Eur Heart J 21:935–940
81. Colivicchi F, Ammirati F, Melina D et al (2003) Development and prospective validation of a risk stratification system for patients with syncope in the emergency department: the OESIL risk score. Eur Heart J 24:811–819
82. Dagres N, Bongiorni MG, Dobreanu D et al (2013) Current investigation and management of patients with syncope: results of the European heart rhythm association survey. Eur Secur 15:1812–1815. doi:10.1093/europace/eut354
83. Kenny RA, Brignole M, Dan GA et al (2015) Syncope unit: rationale and requirement – the European heart rhythm association position statement endorsed by the heart rhythm society. Eur Secur 17(9):1325–1340. doi:10.1093/europace/euv115

84. Nume AK, Gislason G, Christiansen CB et al (2016) Syncope and motor vehicle crash risk: a Danish Nationwide Study. JAMA Intern Med 176(4):503–510. doi:10.1001/jamainternmed.2015.8606. [Epub ahead of print]
85. Barbic F, Dipaola F, Solbiati M et al (2013) Do work accidents play any role in the increased risk of death observed in 25- to 44-year-old patients after syncope? J Am Coll Cardiol 61:2488–2489
86. EUROSTAT European Commission (2012) European Statistics on Accident at Work (ESAW). Bilbao
87. Grossman SA (2009) Assessing and managing syncope in older subjects. J Gene Med 21(4):19–22

Trauma in Older People

Nicolas Bless

11.1 Introduction

Globally, the population aged 60 or over is the fastest growing [1]. It is expected to increase by 45% globally by the middle of the century [1]. The increasing number of older individuals among the population is reflected by the increasing proportion of hospitalizations in this group [2]. Older patients have a higher absolute mortality rate following traumatic injury than younger patients [3]. Older age is associated with higher incidence rates of pre-existing comorbidities and chronic diseases [4]. The majority of older patients suffer typically from blunt trauma; falls from low height are the leading cause [3]. Despite existing triage tools, older people are often under-triaged [5, 6]. Delays in transfer of less-severely injured, older trauma patients to a regional trauma center can result in poor outcomes, including increased mortality [7]. Older adults with minor injuries have different injury patterns, higher acuity, and longer length of stay and are less often discharged home compared to younger adults [8]. The temporary loss of function of an extremity, combined with social isolation, often makes it impossible for the patient to continue an independent life. Furthermore, impaired cognition affects the capacity of older individuals to comprehend, recall, and adhere to treatment recommendations after an injury and puts them at risk for further negative health events [9].

N. Bless
Department of Emergency Medicine, University Hospital Basel,
Petersgraben 2, CH-4032 Basel, Switzerland

Department of Traumatology, University Hospital Basel,
Petersgraben 2, CH-4032 Basel, Switzerland
e-mail: Nicolas.Bless@usb.ch

© Springer International Publishing Switzerland 2018
C. Nickel et al. (eds.), *Geriatric Emergency Medicine*,
https://doi.org/10.1007/978-3-319-19318-2_11

11.2 Resuscitation

Often, physiological changes exist in the cardiovascular system of older patients such as decreased beta-adrenergic responsiveness, conduction abnormalities, arrhythmias, and hypertension. The increased afterload due to stiffened walls of the arteries leads to ventricular hypertrophy, with decreased myocardial compliance and an increased reliance on Frank-Starling mechanism for cardiac output. In the non-compliant older heart, small changes in venous return will produce large changes in ventricular preload and cardiac output [10]. The primary causes for traumatic cardiac arrest are hypovolemia, severe head injury, and hypoxia [11]. The first monitored rhythms in cardiac arrest caused by hypovolemia are pulseless electrical activity (PEA) and asystole in the majority of cases, while ventricular fibrillation dominates the mechanisms of cardiac arrest in severe head injury [11]. To stop the bleeding and to replace the blood loss are the most important steps in the treatment of hemorrhage leading to hypovolemia. High volume resuscitations with crystalloid solution though are associated with high mortality particularly in older trauma patients [12]. Excessive preclinical fluid resuscitation should therefore be avoided. Registry data suggest that a restricted preclinical volume therapy is safe in older patients [13]. However, restriction of blood transfusion on the basis of age alone cannot be supported. Survival to hospital discharge was demonstrated in older patients receiving massive transfusions post trauma, even in the presence of multiple risk factors for mortality [14]. Venous lactate-guided therapy of occult hypoperfusion with early trauma surgeon involvement is associated with significantly lower mortality [15, 16].

11.3 Airway and Breathing

In every trauma patient, blockade of the upper airway must be ruled out. Peripheral deafferentation combined with decreased central nervous system reflex activity in older people increases the risk of aspiration [17, 18]. With increasing age, a decrease in elastic tissues and an increase in collagen in the extracellular matrix lead to a loss of elasticity [19]. In the upper airway, this causes loss of pharyngeal support, which predisposes older people to upper airway obstruction [20, 21]. While loose objects in the mouth must be removed, intact dentures should be left in place for assisted ventilation because with teeth or dentures, the bag mask fits better to the face. Although limited mouth opening may occur, frail older patients are intubated with a higher success rate compared to younger patients [22]. In the lower airway, the reduction in the intrinsic elastic recoil of the lung parenchyma leads to smaller airways with a higher resistance [21]. Whereas the lung parenchyma loses elastic recoil and becomes more compliant, the chest wall becomes stiffer [21]. Older peoples' ribs are more prone to fracture but also to fracture in multiple places [23]. Instability of the chest wall may compromise the respiration by pain, lung contusion, and hematothorax/pneumothorax. While the thorax enlarges with age, the diaphragm flattens. This increases the work for respiration. The reduced vital capacity, reduced functional capacity, and reduced forced expiratory volume lead to a smaller respiratory reserve in frail older patients. As a first measure for all trauma patients, additional oxygen should be applied. Because endotracheal intubation may become necessary with the signs of inadequate ventilation, the older patient must be closely monitored for altered mental status, hypercarbia, acidosis, and respiratory distress. When rapid sequence intubation is performed, the doses of the medical drugs applied, which may cause hemodynamic compromise, should be adapted. Sedative agents such as propofol, etomidate, benzodiazepines, and barbiturates as well as opioids should be decreased by up to 20–50% [24–27]. The dose for neuromuscular blocking agent remains unchanged, but rocuronium should be applied instead of succinylcholine in case of known or suspected hyperkalemia (burn injuries, prolonged immobility). While good evidence exists for safe priming with rocuronium in younger adults, there is some evidence that priming should not be applied in older people [28, 29].

11.4 Disability

There are numerous changes with age, which affect the neurological evaluation of frail older patients. Neuroanatomical changes include, among others, neuronal shrinkage and neuronal loss (loss of brain volume, increase of ventricular size), loss of synapses, decreased vascular compliance due to atherosclerosis, and reduced number of motor units in the spinal cord (resulting in decreased reflex activity) [30, 31]. Neurochemical changes, among others, are a reduction of serotonin (linked to non-cognitive changes in behavior such as depression, aggression, and sleep disturbance) and acetylcholine (associated with memory impairment) [30, 32, 33]. Physiological changes include, among others, a decrease in cerebral blood flow (more than 25% by age 80), decreased protein synthesis (resulting in neuronal cell size shrinkage), and delays in complex pathways (decreasing processing speed) [30, 34–36]. Cranial nerve alterations are functional deficits of the olfactory nerve (possible cause for nutritional deficit), presbyopia, senile miosis, decreased lacrimal secretion, presbycusis and impaired vestibulospinal reflexes, decreased number of taste buds (possible cause for nutritional deficit), and delay in swallowing [30]. Further limitation of neurologic function in older people may occur from chronic degenerative disease, such as diabetic neuropathy, diabetic retinopathy, or macular degeneration. The prevalence of stroke is more than double in the age group of 80+ compared to the group of 60–79 [37]. Older patients who have sustained isolated severe traumatic brain injury may present with a higher Glasgow Coma Scale (GCS) than younger patients [38].

11.5 Exposure

Frailty is a common and important geriatric syndrome characterized by age-associated declines in physiologic reserve and function across multi-organ systems, leading to increased vulnerability for adverse health outcomes [39]. Older people can preserve homeostasis, when they are not stressed, but homeostatic failure occurs, when stress is induced. Frailty in older adults is associated with poor survival with a dose-responsive reduction in survival per increasing number of frailty criteria [40]. The risk of malnutrition is more than four times higher in frail older adults compared to non-frail adults [41]. The prevalence of malnutrition varies substantially depending on the diagnostic measure applied [42]. Malnutrition is an independent risk factor for increased mortality in fracture patients [43].

11.6 Clinical Assessment

A thorough history and physical examination should direct all diagnostic and therapeutic measurements. To understand the circumstances of trauma is even more important in frail older people in the light of the higher number of underlying chronic medical conditions. In respect of the sensory changes in older people, medical personnel must assure that the patient has assistive aids, such as glasses and hearing devices. For the surgical decision making, it is crucial to assess the physical ability and demands of the patient before trauma. The knowledge of and the adherence to the recent medication are notoriously bad in older patients [44, 45]. Written reports from healthcare providers (family doctors, nursing home personnel, home care providers) should be sought out. Vital signs show age-related changes. Change from an individual reference range may indicate important warning signs and thus may require additional evaluation to understand potential underlying pathological process [46]. Repeated clinical evaluation is therefore necessary. High suspicion for the presence of aggravating factors in terms of an increased perioperative risk or an impaired postoperative healing is indicated. Crucial basic decisions concerning resuscitation and end-of-life treatment should be addressed with the older patient at the very beginning of the hospitalization and documented in the hospital chart. The accuracy of surrogate substituted judgment even in the presence of an instructional advance directive is challenged by literature [47, 48].

11.7 Imaging

Poor bone quality due to altered bone metabolism and the sequelae of degenerative bone and joint diseases make the interpretation of acute changes of the skeleton in the older patient by conventional X-ray more difficult. Painful immobilization due to undetected sacral fractures or devastating neuronal damage by undetected fractures of the cervical spine are possible consequences of insufficient imaging. Liberal use of computed tomography (CT) is therefore warranted.

11.8 Head Injury

Age is a major determinant of outcome after traumatic brain injury [49]. Rate of fall-related fatal traumatic brain injury increases and rate of traffic accident-related fatal traumatic brain injury decreases with age [50]. Older fall patients who are at their baseline mental status have a low incidence of intracranial injury [51]. The best predictor of intracranial injury are physical findings of trauma to the head and history of loss of consciousness [51]. Severe head injury in older people carries a high mortality owing to associated comorbidities [52]. Preadmission GCS score bears a positive correlation to Glasgow Outcome Scale (GOS) [52]. Neurosurgical management is associated with the improvement of the prognosis and a decrease in the rate of mortality in geriatric traumatic brain injury [49]. However, surgical management was not shown to be an effective treatment in older patients with GCS scores 3–5 [49].

11.9 Neck and Spine

Frail older patients tend to sustain more upper C-spine fractures than non-frail older patients regardless of the mechanisms [53]. Ground level falls or less not only can cause isolated C-spine fracture(s) but also lead to other significant injuries with intracranial pathology as the most common one in frail older patients [53]. Extreme care is warranted in patients with advanced idiopathic skeletal hyperostosis (DISH). DISH is associated with age. The clinical outcome of patients with fractures in previously ankylosed spines, due to ankylosing spondylitis or DISH, is considerably worse compared to the general trauma population [54].

11.10 Thorax

Due to the smaller respiratory reserve in frail older people, the control of the respiratory situation by repeated clinical evaluation and monitoring and the adequate pain management are even more important. Early mobilization and active respiratory physiotherapy should be pursued. The vast majority of rib fractures can be treated nonoperatively even in the presence of flail chest [55]. The benefit from an epidural analgesia is controversial in literature [56–58]. Surgical rib fracture fixation might be indicated in a broader range of cases than is currently performed [59]. It was shown to reduce ventilation requirement and intensive care stay in a cohort of multi-trauma patients with severe flail chest injury [60]. Meta-analyses still lack an adequate number of prospectively randomized participants [61]. Since the myocardium is less protected in the older patient due to a decreased intercostal muscle mass and a weakened rib cage, blunt cardiac injury should be ruled out. Every frail older patient with blunt chest trauma should have routine electrocardiogram (ECG) on admission [62]. Normal ECG and normal serum troponin-I levels have a negative predictive value of 98% for blunt cardiac injury [63]. Advanced age is associated with higher mortality in traumatic aortic lesion [64]. Endovascular repair for descending thoracic aortic disease was shown to reduce early death, but sustained benefits on survival have not been proven [65].

11.11 Abdomen

Occult abdominal injuries as serious consequences in falls in older patients are rare [66]. Nonoperative management of blunt solid abdominal organ injury currently is the treatment modality of choice in hemodynamically stable patients, irrespective of patient age, with monitoring, serial clinical evaluation, and an operating room for urgent laparotomy being available [67, 68]. Early low molecular weight heparin-based anticoagulation was not associated with the development of bleeding complications in patients with blunt solid abdominal organ injuries undergoing nonoperative management [69].

11.12 Pelvis

Whereas the incidence of intertrochanteric and femoral neck fractures decline, the number of acetabular fractures and pelvic fractures increase in older people [70, 71]. Pubic rami fractures are frequently associated with concomitant posterior pelvic ring injuries, making these injuries more unstable than generally assumed [72]. Patients with displaced inferior pubic rami fractures warrant a detailed examination of their posterior ring to identify additional injuries and instability [73]. The clinical examination proved to be equally effective to CT in detecting posterior pelvic ring fractures [74]. Using magnetic resonance imaging (MRI) is beneficial in cases of reduced bone density [74]. Low-energy lesions without disruption of the pelvic ring may be treated nonoperatively. When pain management is unsatisfactory and/or early mobilization is not achieved, conservative treatment has failed. Percutaneous iliosacral screw fixation results in a better pain relief, less residual displacement, and better functional outcome than conservative treatment of unstable posterior ring injuries [75]. The management principles for high-energy traumas should include aggressive resuscitation and medical optimization, with surgical care focusing on survival without sacrifice of skeletal stability and early mobilization [76]. The decision for operative vs. nonoperative treatment of acetabular fractures should not be justified based upon concern for increased or decreased mortality alone [77]. The combination of open reduction and internal fixation combined with total hip arthroplasty is a valuable option for the older patient [78, 79]. There is 28% secondary conversion rate to hip arthroplasty in the literature for primary open reduction and internal fixation of acetabular fractures in older people [80].

11.13 Extremities

The three most common associated extremity injuries with fall in the older patient are fracture of the femur, radial fracture, and fracture of the humerus [81]. The number of peri- and interprosthetic fractures is increasing [82]. The rate of open fractures in patients aged ≥ 80 years is higher than the rate in the patients aged ≥ 65, and the difference is even more pronounced comparing to the patients aged < 65 [83]. The change in mechanical properties of the skin is believed to account for this increased incidence [83]. The pre-existing adverse conditions for wound healing in the older patient due to accompanying medical comorbidities may explain, for example, the high mortality associated with low-energy open ankle fractures [84]. All measures applied should aim for an early functional recovery. The proximal fracture of the femur warrants an operative treatment because otherwise the patient would have to be immobilized for a long time, and it is challenging to nurse the patient without causing pain. For the treatment of the femoral neck fracture, the patient's functional status before trauma in terms of walking capacity, tendency to fall, compliance to load removal with crutches, smoking, and degenerative diseases must be taken into consideration [85–88]. Data in the literature for the decision making of primary hip arthroplasty versus hemiarthroplasty is not conclusive [89]. Fragility fractures of the proximal humerus and distal radius are a significant burden in terms of loss of independence, inpatient hospitalizations, and prolonged nursing home or rehabilitation needs accounting for considerable healthcare costs [90]. Despite a small improvement of quality of life, surgical treatment for displaced proximal humeral fracture with osteosynthesis or hemiarthroplasty does not significantly improve the functional outcomes including Constant score and DASH (disabilities of the arm, shoulder, and hand) [91]. Reverse total shoulder arthroplasty taking in account the often present degenerative changes in shoulders may change this situation both in terms of function and costs [92]. In the treatment of intra-articular distal radius fractures in older patients, there is marginal and inconsistent evidence for the superiority of volar angle-stable plate osteosynthesis over closed reduction and casting with respect to mobility, functionality, and quality of life at 12 months [93]. Every older patient with a fracture should be evaluated and treated for musculoskeletal frailty including osteoporosis, depending on recent status and risk factors [94, 95]. A high burden of subsequent fracture in individuals with normal bone mineral density and osteopenia and excess mortality particularly for those with osteopenia (and osteoporosis) is reflected in the literature [96].

11.14 Special Considerations: Abuse and Neglect

Elder abuse or mistreatment includes psychological, physical, and sexual abuse, neglect (caregiver neglect and self-neglect), and financial exploitation [97]. Physical signs of intentional actions that cause harm or failure to satisfy the older person's needs include decubital ulcers, skin bruises, or burns [98, 99]. Poor hygiene, bad nutritional status, delayed presentation with results from trauma (organized hematoma over fracture site), inconsistency of trauma history, or dominant behavior of accompanying persons should raise the awareness in the medical personnel about a potentially hazardous situation. Caregivers involved should have access to specialized social healthcare providers and should be familiar with the local legal regulations.

11.15 Summary

Older and frail patients have an age-associated decline in physiologic reserve and function across multi-organ systems, leading to increased vulnerability for adverse health outcomes like trauma. In the assessment of the older patient, special allowance must be made for the often impaired ability to communicate and age-related changes in vital signs. For imaging, liberal use of computed tomography is warranted. The surgical decision making should be based on patient's needs rather than on feasibility.

References

1. World population prospects the 2012 revision, United Nations, New York, 2013
2. Hill AD, Pinto R, Nathens AB, Fowler RA (2014) Age-related trends in severe injury hospitalization in Canda. J Trauma Acute Care Surg 77(4):608–613
3. O'Neill S, Brady RR, Kerssens JJ, Parks RW (2012) Mortality associated with traumatic injuries in the elderly: a population based study. Arch Gerontol 54:e426–e430
4. Rau C, Lin T, Wu S, Yang J, Hsu S, Cho T, Hsieh C (2014) Geriatric hospitalizations in fall-related injuries. Scand J Trauma Resusc Emerg Med 22:63
5. Lehmann R, Beekley A, Casey L et al (2009) The impact of advanced age on trauma triage decisions and outcomes: a statewide analysis. Am J Surg 197:571–574
6. Grossmann FF, Zumbrunn T, Frauchiger A, Delport K, Bingisser R, Nickel C (2012) At risk of undertriage? Testing the performance and accuracy of the emergency severity index in older emergency department patients. Ann Emerg Med 60(3):317–325
7. Fischer PE, Colavita PD, Fleming GP, Huynh TT, Christmas AB, Sing RF (2014) Delays in transfer of elderly less-injured trauma patients can have deadly consequences. Am Surg 80(11):1132–1135
8. Lutze M, Fry M, Gallagher R (2014) Minor injuries in older adults have different characteristics, injury patterns, and outcomes when compared with younger adults: an emergency department correlation study. Int Emerg Nurs
9. Ouellet MC, Sirois MJ, Beaulieu-Bonneau S, Morin J, Perry J, Daoust R, Wilding L, Provencher V, Camden S, Allain-Boulé N, Emond M (2014) Is cognitive function a concern in independent elderly adults discharged home from the emergency Department in Canada after a minor injury? J Am Geriatr Soc 62(11):2130–2135
10. Kanonidou Z, Karystianou G (2007) Anesthesia for the elderly. Hippokratia 11(4):175–177
11. Georgescu V, Tudorache O, Strambu V (2014) Traumatic cardiac arrest in the emergency department – overview upon primary causes. J Med Life 7(2):287–290
12. Ley EJ, Clond MA, Srour MK, Barnajian M, Mirocha J, Margulies DR, Salim A (2011) Emergency department crystalloid resuscitation of 1.5 L or more is associated with increased mortality in elderly and nonelderly trauma patients. J Trauma 70(2):398–400
13. Leenen M, Scholz A, Lefering R, Flohé S (2014) Limited volume resuscitation in hypotensive elderly multiple trauma is safe and prevents early clinical dilutive coagulopathy – a matched pair analyses from Trauma Registry DGU. Injury 45:59–63
14. Mitra B, Olaussen A, Cameron PA, O'Donohoe T, Fitzgerald M (2014) Massive blood transfusions post trauma in the elderly compared to younger patients. Injury 45(9):1296–1300
15. Bar-Or D, Salottolo KM, Orlando A, Mains CW, Bourg P, Offner PJ (2013) Association between a geriatric trauma resuscitation protocol using venous lactate measurements and early trauma surgeon involvement and mortality risk. J Am Geriatr Soc 61(8):1358–1364
16. Salottolo KM, Mains CW, Offner PJ, Bourg PW, Bar-Or D (2013) Retrospective analysis of geriatric trauma patients: venous lactate is a better predictor of mortality than traditional vital signs. Scand J Trauma Resusc Emerg Med 21:7

17. Aviv J (1997) Effects of aging on sensitivity of the pharyngeal and supraglottic area. Am J Med 103(5A):74S–76S
18. Marik P (2001) Aspiration pneumonitis and aspiration pneumonia. N Engl J Med 334(9): 665–671
19. Sell D, Lane MA, Johnson WA, Masoro EJ, Mock OB, Reiser KM, Fogarty JF, Cutler RG, Ingram DK, Roth GS, Monnier VM (1996) Longevity and the genetic determination of collagen glycoxidation kinetics in mammalian senescence. Proc Natl Acad Sci U S A 93(1):485–490
20. Zaugg M, Lucchinetti E (2000) Respiratory function in the elderly. Anesthesiol Clin North Am 18(1):47–58
21. Bergman SA, Coletti D (2006) Perioperative management of the geriatric patient. Part I: respiratory system. Oral Surg Oral Med Oral Pathol Oral Radiol Endod 102:e1–e6
22. Imamura T, Brown CA, Ofuchi H, Yamagami H, Branch J, Hagiwara Y, Brown DFM, Hasegawa K (2013) Emergency airway management in geriatric and younger patients: analysis of a multicenter prospective observational study. Am J Emerg Med 31(1):190–196
23. Agnew AM, Schafman M, Moorhouse K, White SE, Kang YS (2015) The effect of age on the structural properties of human ribs. J Mech Behav Biomed Mater 41:302–314
24. Alrayashi W (2014) Anesthesia for the geriatric trauma patient. In: Anesthesia for trauma. Springer + Business Media, New York
25. Arden JR, Holley FO, Stanski DR (1986) Increased sensitivity to etomidate in the elderly: initial distribution versus altered brain response. Anesthesiology 65(1):9–27
26. Homer TD, Stanski DR (1985) The effect of increasing age on thiopental disposition and anesthetic requirement. Anesthesiology 62(6):714–724
27. Reves JG, Fragen RJ, Vinik HR, Greenblatt DJ (1985) Midazolam: pharmacology and uses. Anesthesiology 62(3):310–324
28. Rao MH, Venkatraman A, Mallleswari R (2011) Comparison of intubating conditions between rocuronium with priming and without priming: randomized and double-blind study. Indian J Anaesth 55(5):494–498
29. Aziz L, Jahangir SM, Choudhury SNS, Rahman K, Ohta Y, Hirakawa M (1997) The effect of priming with vecuronium and rocuronium on young and elderly patients. Anesth Analg 85:663–666
30. American Association of Neuroscience Nurses (2007) AANN clinical practice guideline series. Retrieved March 10th, 2015, from www.aann.org/pdf/cpg/aannneuroassessmentolderadult.pdf
31. Love S (2006) Neuropathology of aging. In: Pathy MSJ, Sinclair AJ, Morley JE (eds) Principles and practice of geriatric medicine, 4th edn. Wiley, Hoboken, pp 69–84
32. Keck BJ, Lakoski JM (2001) Neurochemistry of receptor dynamics in the aging brain. In: Hof PR, Mobbs CV (eds) Functional neurobiology of aging. Academic Press, San Diego, pp 21–29
33. Agins AP, Kelly JF (2006) Assessment, pharmacotherapy and clinical management of depression, dementia and delirium in geriatric patients [computer DVD]. American Association of Neuroscience Nurses, Glenview
34. Meyer JS, Kawamura J, Terayama Y (1994) Cerebral blood flow and metabolism with normal and abnormal aging. In: Albert ML, Knoefel JF (eds) Clinical neurology og aging, 2nd edn. Oxford University Press, New York, pp 214–234
35. Mobbs C (2006) Aging of the brain. In: Pathy MSJ, Sinclair AJ, Morley JE (eds) Principles and practice of geriatric medicine, 4th edn. Wiley, Hoboken, pp 59–67
36. Gilmore R (1995) Evoked potentials in the elderly. J Clin Neurophysiol 12(2):132–138
37. Mozaffarian D, Benjamin EJ, Go AS, Arnett DK, Blaha MJ, Cushman M, de Ferranti S, Després JP, Fullerton HJ, Howard VJ, Huffman MD, Judd SE, Kissela BM, Lackland DT, Lichtman JH, Lisabeth LD, Liu S, Mackey RH, Matchar DB, McGuire DK, Mohler ER 3rd, Moy CS, Muntner P, Mussolino ME, Nasir K, Neumar RW, Nichol G, Palaniappan L, Pandey DK, Reeves MJ, Rodriguez CJ, Sorlie PD, Stein J, Towfighi A, Turan TN, Virani SS, Willey JZ, Woo D, Yeh RW, Turner MB (2015) Heart disease and stroke statistics-2015 update: a report from the American Heart Association. Circulation 131(4):e29–e322

38. Kehoe A, Rennie S, Smith JE (2014) Glasgow coma scale is unreliable for the prediction of severe head injury in elderly trauma patients. Emerg Med J:1–3
39. Chen X, Mao G, Leng SX (2014) Frailty syndrome: an overview. Clin Interv Aging 19(9):433–441
40. Shamliyan T, Talley KM, Ramakrishnan R, Kane RL (2013) Association of frailty with survival: a systematic literature review. Ageing Res Rev 12(2):719–736
41. Toussaint N, de Roon M, van Campen JP, Kremer S, Boesveldt S (2015) Loss of olfactory function and nutritional status in vital older adults and geriatric patients. Chem Senses 40(3):197–203
42. Bell JJ, Bauer JD, Capra S, Pulle RC (2014) Concurrent and predictive evaluation of malnutrition diagnostic measures in hip fracture inpatients: a diagnostic accuracy study. Eur J Clin Nutr 68(3):358–362
43. Gosch M, Druml T, Nicholas JA, Hoffmann-Weltin Y, Roth T, Zegg M, Blauth M, Kammerlander C (2015) Fragility non-hip fracture patients are at risk. Arch Orthop Trauma Surg 135(1):69–77
44. Cline CMJ, Björck-Linné AK, Israelsson BYA, Willenheimer RB, Erhardt LR (1999) Non-compliance and knowledge of prescribed medication in elderly patients with heart failure. Eur J Heart Fail 1(2):145–149
45. Pasina L, Brucato AL, Falcone C, Cucchi E, Bresciani A, Sottocorno M, Taddei GC, Casati M, Franchi C, Djade CD, Nobili A (2014) Medication non-adherence among elderly patients newly discharged and receiving polypharmacy. Drugs Aging 31(4):283–289
46. Chester JG, Rudolph JL (2011) Vital signs in older patients: age-related changes. J Am Med Dir Assoc 12(5):337–343
47. Dritto PH, Danks JH, Smucker WD, Bookwala J, Coppola KM, Dresser R, Fagerlin A, Gready RM, Houts RM, Lockhart LK, Zyzanski S (2001) Advance directives as acts of communication: a randomized controlled trial. Arch Intern Med 161(3):421–430
48. Shapiro SP (2015) Do advance directives direct? J Health Polit Policy Law
49. Shimoda K, Maeda T, Tado M, Yoshino A, Katayama Y, Bullock MR (2014) Outcome and surgical management for geriatric traumatic brain injury: analysis of 888 cases registered in the Japan Neurotrauma Data Bank. World Neurosurg 82(6):1300–1306
50. Brazinova A, Mauritz W, Majdan M, Rehorcikova V, Leitgeb J (2014) Fatal traumatic brain injury in older adults in Austria 1980 – 2012: an analysis of 33 years. Age Ageing 44(3):502–506. pii: afu 194
51. Hamden K, Agresti D, Jeanmonod R, Woods D, Reiter M, Jeanmonod D (2014) Characteristics of elderly fall patients with baseline mental status: high-risk features for intracranial injury. Am J Emerg Med 32(8):890–894
52. Borkar SA, Sinha S, Agrawal D, Satyarthee GD, Gupta D, Mahapatra AK (2011) Severe head injury in the elderly: risk factor assessment and outcome analysis in a series of 100 consecutive patients at a level 1 trauma centre. Indian J Neurotrauma 8(2):77–82
53. Wang H, Coppola M, Robinson RD, Scribner JT, Vithalani V, de Moor CE, Gandhi RR, Burton M, Delaney KA (2013) Geriatric trauma patients with cervical spine fractures due to ground level fall: five years experience in a level one trauma center. J Clin Med Res 5(2):75–83
54. Westerveld LA, Verlaan JJ, Oner FC (2009) Spinal fractures in patients with ankylosing spinal disorders: a systematic review of the literature on treatment, neurological status and complications. Eur Spine J 18(2):145–156
55. Deghan N, de Mestral C, McKee MD, Schemtisch EH, Nathens A (2014) Flail chest injuries: a review of outcomes and treatment practices from the national trauma data bank. J Trauma Acute Care Surg 76(2):462–468
56. Bulger EM, Edwards T, Klotz P, Jurkovich GJ (2004) Epidural analgesia improves outcome after multiple rib fractures. Surgery 136(2):426–430
57. Yeh DD, Kutcher ME, Knudson MM, Tang JF (2012) Epidural analgesia for blunt thoracic injury – which patients benefit most? Injury 43(10):1667–1671

58. Carrier FM, Turgeon AF, Nicole PC, Trépanier CA, Fergusson DA, Thauvette D, Lessard MR (2009) Effect of epidural analgesia in patients with traumatic rib fractures: a systematic review and meta-analysis of randomized controlled trials. Can J Anaesth 56(3):230–242
59. De Jong MB, Kokke MC, Hietbrink F, Leenen LPH (2014) Surgical management of rib fractures: strategies and literature review. Scand J Surg 103(2):120–125
60. Marasco SF, Davies AR, Cooper J, Varma D, Bennett V, Nevill R, Lee G, Bailey M, Fitzgerald M (2013) Prospective randomized controlled trial of operative rib fixation in traumatic flail chest
61. Slobogean GP, MacPherson CA, Sun T, Pelletier ME, Hameed M (2013) Surgical fixation vs nonoperative management of flail chest: a meta-analysis. J Am Coll Surg 216(2):302–311
62. Clancy K, Velopulos C, Bilaniuk JW, Collier B, Crowley W, Kurek S, Lui F, Nayduch D, Sangosanya A, Tucker B, Haut ER (2012) Screening for blunt cardiac injury: an eastern association for the surgery of trauma practice management guideline. J Trauma Acute Care Surg 73(5 Suppl 4):301–306
63. Velmahos GC, Karaiskakis M, Salim A, Toutouzas KG, Murray J, Asensio J, Demetriades D (2003) Normal electrocardiography and serum troponin I levels preclude the presence of clinically significant blunt cardiac injury. J Trauma 54(1):45–50
64. Naughton PA, Park MS, Morasch MD, Rodriguez HE, Garcia-Toca M, Wang CE, Eskandari MK (2012) Emergent repair of acute thoracic aortic catastrophes. Arch Surg 147(3):243–249
65. Cheng D, Martin J, Shennib H, Dunning J, Muneretto C, Schueler S, Von Segesser L, Sergeant P, Turina M (2010) Endovascular aortic repair versus open surgical repair for descending thoracic aortic disease. J Am Coll Cardiol 55(10):986–1001
66. Schattner A, Mavor E, Adi M (2014) Unsuspected serious abdominal trauma after falls among community-dwelling older adults. QJM 107(8):649–653
67. Strassen NA, Bhullar I, Cheng JD, Crandall M, Friese R, Guillamondegui O, Jawa R, Maung A, Rohs TJ Jr, Sangosanya A, Schuster K, Seamon M, Tchorz KM, Zarzuar BL, Kerwin A (2012) Nonoperative management of blunt hepatic injury: an eastern association for the surgery of trauma practice management guideline. J Trauma Acute Care Surg 73(5 Suppl 4):288–293
68. Strassen NA, Bhullar I, Cheng JD, Crandall M, Friese R, Guillamondegui OD, Jawa RS, Maung AA, Rohs TJ Jr, Sangosanya A, Schuster KM, Seamon MJ, Tchorz KM, Zarzuar BL, Kerwin AJ (2012) Selective nonoperative management of blunt splenic injury: an eastern association for the surgery of trauma practice management guideline. J Trauma Acute Care Surg 73(5 Suppl 4):294–300
69. Bellal J, Pandit V, Harrison C, Lubin D, Kulvatunyou N, Zangbar B, Tang A, O'Keeffe T, Green DJ, Gries L, Friese RS, Rhee P (2015) Early thromboembolic prophylaxis in patients with blunt solid abdominal injuries undergoing nonoperative management: is it safe? Am J Surg 209(1):194–198
70. Sullivan MP, Baldwin KD, Donegan DJ, Mehta S, Ahn J (2014) Geriatric fractures about the hip: divergent patterns in the proximal femur, acetabulum, and pelvis. Orthopedics 37(3):151–157
71. Clement ND, Court-Brown CM (2014) Elderly pelvic fractures: the incidence is increasing and patient demographics can be used to predict the outcome. Eur J Orthop Surg Traumatol 24(8):1431–1437
72. Studer P, Suhm N, Zappe B, Bless N, Jakob M (2013) Pubic rami fractures in the elderly – a neglected injury? Swiss Med Wkly 143:w13859
73. Courtney PM, Taylor R, Scolaro J, Donegan D, Mehta S (2014) Displaced inferior ramus fractures as a marker of posterior pelvic injury. Arch Orthop Trauma Surg 134(7):935–939
74. Nüchtern JV, Hartel MJ, Henes FO, Groth M, Jauch SY, Haegele J, Briem D, Hoffmann M, Lehmann W, Rueger JM, Grossterlinden LG (2015) Significance of clinical examination, CT and MRI scan in the diagnosis of posterior pelvic ring fractures. Injury 46(2):315–319
75. Chen PH, Hsu WH, Li YY, Huang TW, Huang TJ, Peng KT (2013) Outcome analysis of unstable posterior ring injury of the pelvis: comparison between percutaneous iliosacral screw fixation and conservative treatment. Biomed J 36(6):289–294

76. Hill BW, Switzer JA, Cole PA (2012) Management of high-energy acetabular fractures in the elderly individuals: a current review. Geriatr Orthop Surg Rehabil 3(3):95–106
77. Gary JL, Paryavi E, Gibbons SD, Weaver MJ, Morgan JH, Ryan SP, Starr AJ, O'Toole RV (2015) The effect of surgical treatment on mortality after acetabular fracture in the elderly: a multicenter study on 454 patients. J Orthop Trauma 29(4):202–208
78. Herscovici D, Lindvall E, Bolhofner B, Scaduto JM (2010) The combined hip procedure: open reduction internal fixation combined with total hip arthroplasty for the management of acetabular fractures in the elderly. J Orthop Trauma 24(5):291–296
79. Jakob M, Droeser R, Zobrist R, Messmer P, Regazzoni P (2006) A less invasive anterior intrapelvic approach for the treatment of acetabular fractures and pelvic ring injuries. J Trauma 60(6):1364–1370
80. O'Toole RV, Hui E, Chandra A, Nascone JW (2014) How often does open reduction and internal fixation of geriatric acetabular fractures lead to hip arthroplasty? J Orthop Trauma 28(3):148–153
81. Rau CS, Lin TS, Wu SC, Yang J, Hsu SY, Cho TY, Hsieh CH (2014) Geriatric hospitalizations in fall-related injuries. Scand J Trauma Resusc Emerg Med 22(1):63
82. Lindahl H, Malchau H, Herberts P, Garellick G (2005) Periprosthetic femoral fractures classification and demographics of 1049 periprosthetic femoral fractures from the Swedish national hip arthroplasty register. J Arthroplast 20(7):857–865
83. Court-Brown CM, Biant LC, Clement ND, Bugler KE, Duckworth AD, McQueen MM (2015) Open fractures in the elderly. The importance of skin ageing. Injury 46(2):189–194
84. Toole WP, Elliott M, Hankins D, Rosenbaum C, Harris A, Perkins C (2014) Are low-energy open ankle fractures in the elderly the new geriatric hip fracture? J Foot Ankle Surg 54(2):203–206
85. Charlson ME, Pompei P, Ales KL, MacKenzie CR (1987) A new method of classifying prognostic comorbidity in longitudinal studies: development and validation. J Chronic Dis 40(5):373–383
86. Parker MJ, Palmer CR (1993) A new mobility score for predicting mortality after hip fracture. J Bone Joint Surg Br 75(5):797–798
87. Maxwell MJ, Moran CG, Moppett IK (2008) Development and validation of a preoperative scoring system to predict 30 day mortality in patients undergoing hip fracture surgery. Br J Anaesth 101(4):511–517
88. Penrod JD, Litke A, Hawkes WG, Magaziner J, Koval KJ, Doucette JT, Silberzweig SB, Siu AL (2007) Heterogeneity in hip fracture patients: age, functional status, and comorbidity. J Am Geriatr Soc 55(3):407–413
89. Hopley C, Stengel D, Ekkernkamp A, Wich M (2010) Primary total hip arthroplasty versus hemiarthroplasty for displaced intracapsular hip fractures in older patients: systematic review. BMJ 340:c2332
90. Sabesan VJ, Valikodath T, Childs A, Sharma VK (2015) Economic and social impact of upper extremity fragility fractures in elderly patients. Aging Clin Exp Res 27(4):539–546
91. Fu T, Xia C, Li Z, Wu H (2014) Surgical versus conservative treatment for displaced proximal humeral fractures in elderly patients: a meta-analysis. Int J Clin Exp Med 7(12):4607–4615
92. Chalmers PN, Slikker W, Mall NA, Gupta AK, Rahman Z, Enriquez D, Nicholson GP (2014) Reverse total shoulder arthroplasty for acute proximal humerla fracture: comparison to open reduction-internal fixation and hemiarthroplasty. J Shoulder Elb Surg 23(2):197–204
93. Salzmann GM, Strohm P, Südkamp NP, Morawski M, Spranger A, Ekkernkamp A, Dietz S, Rothenbach E, Roomens PM, Müller-Pongratz F, Siebert N, Kirschner M, Wagner M, Siebenlist S, Stöckle U, Kallasch E, Ockert B, Kessler M, Mutschler W, Schulz A, Borninger N, Wilde E, Schlottau S, Schreiber T, Grützner PA, Veiel T, Sarkar MR, Obermaier S, Ramsayer B, Scheiderer B, Scola A, Buhl K, Erni B, Büchler MW, Napp M, Gondert M, Bachmann S, Probst C, Gaulke R, Krettek C (2014) The treatment of displaced intra-articular distal radius fractures in elderly patients. Dtsch Arztebl Int 111(46):779–787

94. Gielen E, Verschueren S, O'Neill TW, Pye SR, O'Connell MD, Lee DM, Ravindrarajah R, Claessens F, Laurent M, Milisen K, Tournoy J, Dejaeger M, Wu FC, Vanderschueren D, Boonen S (2012) Muskuloskeletal frailty: a geriatric syndrome at the core of fracture occurrence in older age. Calcif Tissue Int 91(3):161–177
95. Harper CM, Fitzpatrick SK, Zurakowski D, Rozental TD (2014) Distal radius fractures in older men: a missed opportunity? J Bone Joint Surg Am 96(21):1820–1827
96. Bliuc D, Alarkawi D, Nguyen TV, Eisman JA, Center JR (2014) Risk of subsequent fractures and mortality in elderly women and men with fragility fractures with and without osteoporotic bone density: the dubbo osteoporosis epidemiology study. J Bone Miner Res
97. Dong X (2012) Advancing the field of elder abuse: future directions and policy implications. J Am Geriatr Soc 60(11):2151–2156
98. Bonnie RJ, Wallace RB (eds) 2003 Elder mistreatment: abuse, neglect, and exploitation in an aging America. Panel to review risk and prevalence of elder abuse and neglect. Committee on National Statistics and Committee on Law and Justice, Division of Behavioral and Social Sciences and Education. The National Academics Press, Washington
99. Rinker AG Jr (2009) Recognition and perception of elder abuse by prehospital and hospital-based care providers. Arch Gerontol Geriatr 48(1):110–115

Management of Sepsis in Older Patients in the Emergency Department

12

Abdelouahab Bellou and Hubert Blain

12.1 Introduction and Definition of Sepsis

Sepsis and septic shock are common causes of intensive care unit (ICU) admission for patients of all ages. The incidence of sepsis in the USA has been estimated at 751,000 cases per year with overall mortality rates of 28.6% and up to 50% of patients developing septic shock [1]. The overall frequency of septic shock was 8.2 per 100 admissions, and crude mortality in the ICU was 60.1%, declining from 62.1% in 1993 to 55.9% in 2000 [1].

Detecting sepsis is a challenge in older patients. It has been estimated that up to 65% of patients who develop sepsis are older patients (defined as age 65 years or more) [2]. In a recent ICU cohort study in Europe of 1448 septic shock patients, 45.9% were aged 70 to more than 80 years (70–<80 years = 29.4%, ≥80 = 16.5%) and 58.5% came from nursing homes [3]. Data from the ED are rare and approximately 1 of every 33 adult patients with an infection had a suspected severe sepsis [4]. Wang et al. showed in a national survey in the USA that older patients with suspected severe sepsis represent 51.6% (65–74 years = 19.8%, ≥75 years = 31.8%) among all severe sepsis patient visits in the ED and 16.6% came from nursing home residence [4].

Sepsis is a common disease in the older population, defined as an inflammatory response to infection; severe sepsis and septic shock were the more severe clinical presentation [5]. In 2016, a group of international experts proposed a new definition

---

A. Bellou, MD, PhD (✉)
Department of Emergency Medicine, Beth Israel Deaconess Medical Center,
Harvard Medical School, Boston, MA, USA
e-mail: abellou@bidmc.harvard.edu

H. Blain, MD
Department of Geriatrics, University Hospital of Montpellier, University of Montpellier,
Montpellier, France
e-mail: h-blain@chu-montpellier.fr

© Springer International Publishing Switzerland 2018
C. Nickel et al. (eds.), *Geriatric Emergency Medicine*,
https://doi.org/10.1007/978-3-319-19318-2_12

named the Sepsis-3 definition [6]: Sepsis was defined as a life-threatening organ dysfunction caused by a dysregulated host response to infection. Organ dysfunction can be represented by an increase in the sequential [sepsis-related] organ failure assessment (SOFA) score of 2 points or more (Table 12.1), which is associated with in-hospital mortality greater than 10%. Septic shock should be defined as a subset of sepsis in which particularly profound circulatory, cellular, and metabolic abnormalities are associated with a greater risk of mortality than with sepsis alone. Patients with septic shock can be clinically identified by a vasopressor requirement to maintain a mean arterial pressure of 65 mmHg or greater and serum lactate level greater than 2 mmol/L (>18 mg/dL) in the absence of hypovolemia. This combination is associated with hospital mortality rates greater than 40% [8]. In the context of sepsis, arterial lactate is higher in non-survivors who are older (65–81 years) and is an independent predictor of mortality [9].

In pre-hospital, emergency department, or general hospital ward settings, adult patients with suspected infection can be rapidly identified as being more likely to have poor outcomes typical of sepsis if they have at least two of the following clinical criteria that together constitute a new bedside clinical score termed quickSOFA

Table 12.1 Sequential organ failure assessment score (SOFA score)

System	Score 0	Score 1	Score 2	Score 3	Score 4
Respiration PaO2/FiO2 mmHg (kPa)	≥400	<400	<300	<200 with respiratory support	<100 with respiratory support
Coagulation platelets (× 10³/μL)	≥150	<150	<100	<50	<20
Liver bilirubin, mg/dL (μmol/L)	<1.2	1.2–1.9	2.0–5.9	6.0–11.9	>12
Cardiovascular	MAP ≥ 70 mmHg	MAP < 70 mmHg	Dopamine < 5 or dobutamine (any dose)	Dopamine 5.1–15 or epinephrine ≤ 0.1[b] or norepinephrine ≤ 0.1	Dopamine >15 or epinephrine > 0.1[b] or norepinephrine > 0.1
CNS Glasgow Coma Scale score[a]	15	13–14	10–12	6–9	<6
Renal creatinine, mg/dL (mol/L), urine output, mL/d	<1.2	1.2–1.9	2.0–3.4	3.5–4.9 (300–440); <500	>5; <200

Adapted from Singer et al. [6], Vincent et al. [7]
FIO2 fraction of inspired oxygen, *MAP* mean arterial pressure, *PaO2* partial pressure of oxygen, *CNS* central nervous system
[a]Glasgow Coma Scale scores range from 3 to 15; higher score indicates better neurological function
[b]Catecholamine doses are given as μg/kg/min for at least 1 h

(qSOFA): respiratory rate of 22/min or greater, altered mentation (defined by a Glasgow score < 15), or systolic blood pressure of 100 mmHg or less [6, 8].

However, recently, Shurpek et al. showed that early warning scores like Modified Early Warning Score (MEWS) and the National Early Warning Score (NEWS) seem to be more accurate than the qSOFA score for predicting death and ICU transfer in non-ICU patients (Shurpek et al. 2016). These results suggest that the qSOFA score should not replace general early warning scores when risk-stratifying patients with suspected infection. April et al. showed in a retrospective cohort chart review study of ED patients admitted to an ICU with suspected infection that among ED patients admitted to an ICU, the SIRS and qSOFA criteria had comparable prognostic value for predicting in-hospital mortality [10]. Moreover, Giamarellos-Bourboulis et al. showed that qSOFA score has a low sensitivity for early prediction of death as compared to three and more SIRS criteria [11]. Recently, Freund et al. in a European ED prospective study showed that qSOFA in patients visiting the ED with suspected infection, has a high prognostic accuracy for in-hospital mortality as compared to SIRS or severe sepsis [12].

Nevertheless, these recent controversies emphasize the need for prospective and multicentric clinical trials, especially in the older population to evaluate qSOFA performance. Nevertheless, the qSOFA score might be helpful in non-ICU settings (e.g., ED and geriatric units) for recognizing sepsis in a quicker manner, leading to more timely treatment, and potentially better outcomes [8].

It has been considered that the older patients have clinical manifestations different from the ones observed in middle-age adults during sepsis. The behavior of most clinical and laboratory variables suggests a less pronounced response of patients above 65 years of age who died 28 days after being diagnosed with sepsis [13, 14]. These special considerations must be taken into account when sepsis is suspected in older patients. Comorbidity and frailty will certainly impact the diagnostic process and the prognosis.

12.2 Epidemiology

There are few data on the epidemiology of sepsis in older people. Angus et al. reported an annual incidence of severe sepsis of 3 cases/1000 population, which is more than 100 times greater than the incidence among those between 5 and 14 years of age (0.2/1000 in children to 5.3/1000 in patients aged 60–64 years and 26.2/1000 in patients ≥85) and that mortality increased from 10% in children to 26% in patients 60–64 and 38% in those ≥85 [1, 15]. Martin et al. reported a similar annual incidence of sepsis (2,4 cases/1000 population) and found that incidence of sepsis (all cases, not limited to severe sepsis) likewise increased exponentially across all adult ages, and this increased incidence was around 20% more in older population as compared to younger patients, with a case fatality rate of 27.7% for those >65 versus 17.7% for those <65 (Martin et al. 2006).

European countries have similar rates of sepsis [3, 16]. Two thirds of septic patients hospitalized are represented by older patients (Martin et al. 2006, [17–21]) and 84% of those who were managed in the ED will be hospitalized with only 12% admitted in the ICU [22].

12.3 Causes of Sepsis

Pneumonia is the most common cause of infection in all ages, followed by intra-abdominal and urinary tract infections [1, 23–25]. In older patients, the most frequent infection site is respiratory tract, followed by genitourinary infections (Martin et al. 2006, [4, 6, 26, 27]). Blood and site cultures are negative in one third of cases [1, 24, 28, 29].

Classically, *Staphylococcus aureus* and *Streptococcus pneumoniae* are the most frequent Gram-positive pathogen isolated from cultures, and *Escherichia coli*, *Klebsiella species*, and *Pseudomonas aeruginosa* predominate among Gram-negative isolates [24, 29–31]. Gram-negative pathogens are more frequently isolated in older patients probably because of frequent hospitalizations and procedures, which lead to antibiotic resistance (Martin et al. 2006, [26, 32, 33]).

12.4 Pathophysiology

The pathophysiologic mechanisms that underlie the process of aging on the immune system are complex and multifactorial. The immune system in the older population is in a state called immunosenescence, characterized by impairment of cell-mediated and humoral immune responses [35]. However, aging does not necessarily lead to an unavoidable decline in immune function. Some authors think that it is better to use the concept of "senescent immune remodeling" (Dewan 2012).

Aging is characterized by a chronic inflammatory status with increased pro-inflammatory cytokines, such as IL-6 and TNFα, which create oxidative stress and decrease cellular antioxidant capacity. So, alterations of inflammatory responses that occur in aging are responsible for the increased susceptibility of older people to infectious diseases. Sepsis is composed by hyperinflammation in the acute phase followed by immunosuppression.

There are functional changes in both cell-mediated immunity and humoral immune responses with age, which contribute to the increased incidence of infection in older patients. Within the adaptive immune system, B cell and plasma cell populations and generation of naïve T cells gradually decrease with aging [34]. It was recently found that older patients with a decreased IgM production might be more susceptible to infection by Gram-negative bacteria and fungi [37]. Impaired humoral immunity with increased exhausted B cells and insufficient immunoglobulin M production may be a critical immunological change in sepsis [37].

Older patients have decreased number of immunocompetent T cells [38], which are mostly represented by memory T cells [35, 39, 40]. In response to antigens, these memory cells cannot proliferate normally with low expression of co-stimulatory molecules, which reduce the activation of mitogen-activated protein kinase [35, 39].

Serum IL-6 levels in septic older patients are persistently high as compared to young patients [38]. This excessive inflammation continues during the early phase of sepsis, and it was observed a persistent inflammation and T-cell exhaustion in older patients after sepsis with a high mortality compared to younger patients [35, 38–44]. Severe sepsis and mortality are associated with higher levels of pro-inflammatory markers; however, few clinical studies have compared sepsis-induced cytokine responses in young and older patients. Kale et al. reported no age-related difference in inflammatory markers IL-6, TNFα, or IL-10 at admission or over the first week of hospitalization in patients with community-acquired pneumonia; however, IL-6 levels at discharge were significantly higher in older patients suggesting an age-dependent delay in resolution of inflammation [45].

Genomic studies have detected several genes whose expression could be used to differentiate immune responses of the older patients from those of young people, including genes related to oxidative phosphorylation, mitochondrial dysfunction, and TGF-β signaling. These studies identified major molecular pathways that are affected in older patients during sepsis and could play a role in worsening outcomes compared with young people with sepsis [46].

During sepsis, there is a hyperactivation of the coagulation cascade inducing microvascular thrombosis responsible of hypoperfusion [47, 48]. Coagulation abnormalities play an important role in the pathophysiology of sepsis. Kale et al. suggested older patients might have a more exaggerated response to similar levels of inflammatory and thrombotic factors, which influences the development of organ dysfunction [45].

Finally, the severe myocardial depression observed in sepsis and induced by mediators released during the inflammation phase increases mortality [49–51].

12.5 Risk Factors of Sepsis in Older Patients

Sepsis awareness is essential and includes identification of population-focused risk factors, recognition of clinical signs and symptoms, and timely implementation of interventions. Previous comorbid conditions are commonly associated with increased susceptibility to sepsis and organ dysfunction [1, 18, 32, 44, 52]. Other factors are involved such as poor functional status, frailty, polypharmacy, malnutrition, and nursing home residence [53].

Recurrent hospitalizations with exposure to instrumentation and procedures, such as urinary catheterizations and a higher rate of complications throughout their hospital course, are also identified as a risk factor for sepsis, particularly in the presence of compromised immunity [54–56].

Old age itself is an independent risk factor for predisposition to sepsis by increased colonization by Gram-negative organisms, which may be multidrug resistant (Martin et al. 2006, [52]). In the USA, up to one third of patients at 80 years of age reside in long-term care facilities where bacterial flora demonstrates a level of resistance higher than that seen in the community [32]. In the UK, Marwick et al. found that residence in a long-term care facility was associated with a higher prevalence of resistant organisms [57]. However, to live in a residence place was not an independent factor of 30-day mortality. Marwick et al. recommend that antibiotic therapies active against resistant organisms, guided by local resistance patterns, should be considered for all older patients admitted with sepsis regardless of their place of residence [57].

It is recommended that assessment of older patients should include functional status (see Chap. 6). Preadmission functional status is much more important than comorbid illness and has been found to be an independent predictor of poor outcome in older patients [58, 52]. Wester et al. noted that non-specific functional deterioration, such as reduced ability to complete daily tasks, might be the only symptom of sepsis [54]. Additional evidence reported by Nasa et al. [52] identified preadmission functional status as an independent predictor of outcome in older patients [54, 59].

Older people present unique pathophysiological characteristics that confer a great complexity, so in the face of any stressful event, injury, or a critical illness as sepsis, they are less able to meet the increased physiological demands because there is a reduction or a delay in the implementation of compensatory mechanisms, due to a reduction of organic functional reserve. The concept of frailty, as a state of vulnerability to adverse outcomes in which multiple body systems gradually lose their built-in reserves is becoming more and more essential in the management of older patients in the ED and should be assessed during disease conditions. Frailty is common in critically ill older patients and is independently associated with increased mortality and greater disability [60, 62]. Future studies should explore routine screening for clinical frailty in critically ill older patients.

A reliable biomarker for the prognosis of sepsis is critical. Thus far, there are no such biomarkers available for sepsis [61]. SOFA and abbMEDS (abbreviated mortality in emergency department sepsis) scores were effective in predicting ICU admissions and the death of older sepsis patients in the ED, but biomarkers such as procalcitonin, IL-10, IL-6, and IL-5 although effective in predicting ICU admission were not effective in predicting death of older patients [63].

Recently, it was shown that the GYM (Glasgow < 15, tachypnea > 20, comorbidity charlson index $\geq$ 3) score showed better capacity than the classic and the modified sepsis criteria to predict 30-day mortality in older patients attended for infection in the ED [64].

12.6 Clinical Presentation and Diagnosis

Although sepsis is a serious life-threatening disease its recognition is often difficult. In addition to the difficulties of the diagnosis of sepsis in older patients, a clear history may not be available in many patients because of pre-existing dementia or prevalent delirium. It could be also difficult to obtain samples of blood, sputum, body fluids, or tissue from patients who are cognitively impaired, debilitated, dehydrated, or frail [65].

12 Management of Sepsis in Older Patients in the Emergency Department

The decrease in the acuity of symptoms and delay in presentation can make the diagnosis of sepsis difficult. The clinical presentation in older patients is different than in younger patients. The initial inflammatory response of infection, which normally produces symptoms and signs of sepsis, are blunted or may be absent in older patients, while later presentation may be very severe [67] with rapid progression to septic shock [29, 32, 35, 43]. Unfortunately, the findings reported in Table 12.2 can also be present in noninfectious diseases making the diagnosis difficult ([32, 65, 66, 67, 69, 70]) (see Chap. 8).

It has been shown that the febrile response may be blunted in up to 47% of older septic patients [71]. Although, fever is a cardinal sign of infection, its absence in older patients is frequent and may delay the diagnosis and the initiation of appropriate antimicrobial therapy [71]. However, 40% of the afebrile nosocomial bacteremias of older patients occurred in those who were receiving antibiotics [71, 72]. Neither chills are always observed and are reported in only 35% of older patients, with a lower prevalence than younger patients [73]. Site of measurement of temperature can influence the results, sublingual temperature readings detect one third of fevers, and rectal temperature measurement will detect fever in up to 86% of infected patients [74]. Another explanation could be that in older patients, pathways involved in thermoregulation are impaired (Yoshikawa and [68, 75]). Hypothermia,

Table 12.2 Clinical presentation of sepsis in older patients

Possible chief complaints found in any infection[a]	Findings with specific infections[b]
Change in cognition (e.g., delirium/agitation)	**Bacteremia**
	Dyspnea, confusion, falls, hypotension
Falls	May be afebrile
Lethargy	**Pneumonia**
Anorexia	Tachypnea
Failure to thrive	May be afebrile
Change in baseline body temperature	Cough and sputum production may be absent
	Intraabdominal infection
	Anorexia
	May be afebrile
	Peritoneal signs may be absent
	Meningitis
	Confusion, altered consciousness
	Stiff neck may be absent
	Tuberculosis
	Weight loss, lethargy
	Failure to thrive
	May be afebrile
	Urinary tract infection
	May occur without dysuria, frequency, flank pain, or fever

Adapted from Norman [68]
[a]The first column shows chief complaints that could be observed in any infection
[b]The second column shows symptoms and signs that could be observed during specific infections

which can be observed during the first 24 h of presentation, independently predicts hospital mortality in older septic patients [76].

The cardiovascular system may have a limited or absent compensatory response to inflammation after an infectious insult, and the febrile response and recruitment of white blood cells may be blunted because of immunosenescence in aging. Older patients are more likely than young patients to present with polymorphonuclear lymphocyte counts of <2000 lymphocytes/mm^3. In the presence of serious infections, approximately 60% of older patients will exhibit leukocytosis; however, its absence does not rule out an infection [77]. Three of the four hallmark responses (temperature, heart rate, and white blood cell count) to systemic inflammation may be diminished in older adults as compared with younger adults [2]. Recently, Valencia et al. showed that the course of most clinical and laboratory variables suggests a less pronounced response of patients above 65 years of age who died 28 days after being diagnosed with sepsis [13, 14]. Finally, most studies evaluate the ability of an isolated biomarker result to predict infection, whereas biomarkers probably will have the most value if combined with data from history, physical examination, imaging, and other laboratory testing.

In a model to predict bacteremia in emergency room patients, both PCT and CRP were included along with other clinical variables, and in doing so, the area under the curve was improved from 0.639 (CRP) and 0.737 (PCT) to 0.854 when biomarkers and clinical variables were combined [78].

Table 12.3 summaries the classical criteria for the diagnosis of sepsis [79, 80]. The major limitation is the absence of criteria for the specific subpopulation of older patients.

12.7 Management of Sepsis in Older Patients in the ED

The Surviving Sepsis Campaign (SSC) includes special guidelines for adults and pediatric patients on the basis of physiologic differences, but there are no special considerations on physiologic differences in older patients. Nevertheless, the management of sepsis and septic shock in older patients should follow the recommendations of the SSC guidelines [80], although they are not very specific for the older population as they fail to take the physiology of aging into consideration. Sepsis resuscitation and management bundles should be started early and have been shown to improve survival.

The SSC emphasizes two bundles of care. The initial bundle is focused on resuscitation to restore the impaired tissue perfusion and oxygenation. This is to be accomplished in the first 6 h of presentation. The second bundle is focused on further management and is to be accomplished in the ICU. Although excellent, the Surviving Sepsis Campaign guidelines are not very specific for older patients with sepsis and septic shock. The principles of management used in younger adults are used in older patients, including early antimicrobial therapy and source control,

Table 12.3 Diagnostic criteria for sepsis

Infection, documented or suspected, and some of the following:
General variables
Fever (>38.3 °C)
Hypothermia (core temperature < 36 °C)
Heart rate > 90/min or more than two SD above the normal value for age
Tachypnea
Altered mental status
Significant edema or positive fluid balance (>20 mL/kg over 24 h)
Hyperglycemia (plasma glucose >140 mg/dL or 7.7 mmol/L) in the absence of diabetes
Inflammatory variables
Leukocytosis (WBC count >12,000 μL^{-1}), leukopenia (WBC count <4000 μL^{-1}), normal WBC count with greater than 10% immature forms
Plasma C-reactive protein more than two SD above the normal value
Plasma procalcitonin more than two SD above the normal value
Hemodynamic variables
Arterial hypotension (SBP <90 mmHg, MAP <70 mmHg, or an SBP decrease >40 mmHg in adults or less than two SD below normal for age). In older patients, arterial hypotension could not follow guidelines criteria because of chronic hypertension
Organ dysfunction variables
Arterial hypoxemia (PaO2/FiO2 < 300)
Acute oliguria (urine output <0.5 mL/kg/h for at least 2 h despite adequate fluid resuscitation)
Creatinine increase >0.5 mg/dL or 44.2 μmol/L
Coagulation abnormalities (INR >1.5 or aPTT >60 s)
Ileus (absent bowel sounds)
Thrombocytopenia (platelet count <100,000 μL)
Hyperbilirubinemia (plasma total bilirubin >4 mg/dL or 70 μmol/L)
Tissue perfusion variables
Hyperlactatemia (≥2 mmol/L)
Decreased capillary refill or mottling

Adapted from Dellinger et al. [79] and Rhodes et al. [80]

early resuscitation, and the use of low tidal volume during mechanical ventilation. Clinical conundrums that complicate clinical course of sepsis in older patients such as cardiac heart failure/atrial fibrillation, antibiotic resistance, chronic kidney disease/acute kidney injury, dysglycemia, malnutrition, ambulatory dysfunction, delirium, dementia, and polypharmacy need to be addressed [81].

Hepner et al. showed in a pre-/post-intervention study conducted in older patients that the implementation of SSC guidelines decreases the ED length of stay, mortality, and improved initial appropriate therapy [82]. Moreover, an international multicentric study from 62 countries with severe sepsis (now termed "sepsis" after the Sepsis-3 definition or septic shock) showed a 36–40% reduction of in-hospital mortality with compliance with either the 3- or 6-h SSC bundles [83]. The SSC strongly recommends the implementation of a continuous performance improvement strategy of sepsis care.

Palomba et al. showed recently that early resuscitation in older patients compared to younger patients was not associated with increased in-hospital mortality [84].

12.7.1 Initial Resuscitation in the ED

Administration of fluids can be a challenge in older patients with systolic and diastolic dysfunction. Chronic heart failure and chronic kidney disease are usually coexistent in older patients thus exacerbating the electrolyte imbalance [81]. One of the challenges of treating septic shock is the measurement of intravascular volume and oxygen delivery during fluid bolus therapy. This is of particular importance in older patients with sepsis, who are at high risk of fluid overload. Lung ultrasound is routinely used in the ED and can be helpful in detecting pulmonary edema during fluid resuscitation. Protocol-based fluid resuscitation of patients with severe sepsis and septic shock with the noninvasive cardiac output monitor and passive leg-raising maneuver did not result in better outcomes compared with usual care [3].

The SSC guidelines 2017 recommend at least 30 mL/kg of IV crystalloid fluid be given within the first 3 h [80]. Many patients will probably require more fluid than this, and for this group, further fluid could be given in accordance with functional hemodynamic measurements. Detailed initial assessment and ongoing reevaluation of physiologic variables describing the patient's clinical state (heart rate, blood pressure, arterial oxygen saturation, respiratory rate, temperature, urine output, and others as available) are essential. These parameters could be a challenge in older patients who show physiological changes at the baseline. Echocardiography has become more and more available in the ED and allows a more detailed assessment of the causes of the hemodynamic issues in older patients.

Previous SSC guidelines have recommended a protocolized quantitative resuscitation known as the early goal-directed therapy (EGDT), which was based on the protocol published by Rivers [85]. EGDT was recommended as the gold standard of the resuscitation bundle in the management of severe sepsis and septic shock in both young adults and older patients [79]. This recommendation described the use of a series of "goals" that included central venous pressure (CVP) and central venous oxygen saturation (ScvO2). It was shown that EGDT was effective in older patients [86]. Recently, this approach has been challenged following the failure to demonstrate a mortality reduction in three randomized clinical trials published in 2014 and 2015 showing that the application of a strict EGDT protocol did not lead to an improvement in mortality and is not superior to usual care [87–89].

The addition of continuous ScvO2 monitoring and strict protocols did not improve outcomes in the EGDT group [87]. Insertion of central vein catheters became not systematically required in all patients with sepsis including older patients. Because of these recent data, the SSC guidelines 2017 don't recommend EGDT in the management of sepsis and septic shock. It was previously proposed that the monitoring of the ScVO2 should be replaced by the monitoring of lactate and lactate clearance [90–92]. Because lactate is a standard laboratory test, it may serve as a more objective marker for tissue perfusion as compared with physical examination or urine output. In addition to being a non-specific test and produced from different source, lactate may not be as sensitive test as is commonly thought. In mesenteric ischemia and sepsis, a normal lactate level could be interpreted as reassuring, but it could be a false reassurance. Dugas et al. showed that 45% of patients in vasopressor-dependent septic shock did not increase lactic acid level initially, but the mortality remained high [93].

Regardless of the source and its performance, increased lactate levels are associated with worse outcomes. Jones et al. showed that high clearance of lactic acid is an independent factor for survival in sepsis [91]. A reduction of the clearance of the lactate >10% in 2 h is considered to be comparable to achieving or maintaining a ScvO2 > 70% [92]. Five RCTs showed a significant reduction in mortality in lactate-guided resuscitation compared to resuscitation without lactate monitoring [91, 94, 95, 96, 97]. In a recent meta-analysis, EGDT was associated with a higher mortality rate as compared to the early lactate clearance group [98]. Serial lactate monitoring is associated with an increase in crystalloid administration, resuscitation interventions, and improved clinical outcomes in ED patients with sepsis, and septic shock suggesting that serial lactate monitoring, targeting a reduction in lactate levels to normal, is a generalizable resuscitation target in the ED [99]. However, two meta-analyses demonstrate moderate evidence for reduction in mortality when an early lactate clearance strategy was used, compared with either usual care or with a ScvO2 normalization strategy [100, 101].

Nevertheless, del Portal et al. showed that higher ED lactate values are associated with increased mortality in ED-admitted older patients, in the presence or absence of infection [9, 102, 103].

Finally, if despite an adequate fluid resuscitation and a lactate $\geq$ 2 mmol/L, which define septic shock according to the Sepsis-3 definition, vasopressors are needed. Norepinephrine is recommended as a first choice because of its vasoconstrictive effects, and little change in heart rate with less increase of stroke volume compared with dopamine [80]. In some patients with persistent hypoperfusion, other vasopressors, e.g., vasopressin, epinephrine, or dobutamine, can be added to norepinephrine.

Once again, the SSC guidelines don't give special considerations on vasopressors use in older sepsis patients.

12.7.2 Source Control and Antimicrobial Treatment

Early source control of infection and appropriate antimicrobial treatments are the two vital components of the management bundle of the surviving sepsis guidelines [80]. Pharmacokinetic and pharmacodynamic parameters (e.g., renal function, body mass) should be well documented when starting antimicrobial drugs [104, 105]. The initial bolus dose should be kept to get maximal therapeutic dose [104, 106]. Inadequate initial antibiotic therapy is independently associated with increase mortality [106, 107]. The early institution of antibiotics decreases significantly mortality, also in older patients [106–114].

Empirical antibiotic therapy should be initiated within 1 h of the recognition of sepsis, after sample collections of blood and other suspected sites of infection are obtained for culture. The SSC guidelines 2017 give all details on the antimicrobial therapeutic strategy (e.g., type of antibiotics, type of combination, duration, etc.) (see [80]).

12.7.3 Glycemic Control

The risk of hypoglycemia is common in older septic patients, and therefore, the target of an upper blood glucose ≤180 mg/dL seems to be safe [80].

Aggressive hyperglycemia control is more a focus in the ICU rather than in the ED. But severe hyperglycemia must be treated as soon as it was observed. Hyperglycemia is an independent risk factor for death in sepsis. During the management in the ED, glycemia must be controlled to detect hyperglycemia and hypoglycemia.

12.7.4 Other Treatments

The other issues concerning the care of older patients with sepsis and septic shock may include the use of corticosteroids, mechanical ventilation, sedation and analgesia, prophylaxis for deep vein thrombosis, and stress ulcer prophylaxis are more ICU considerations or geriatric and medicine wards (see [80]).

12.7.5 In Summary

The SSC guidelines 2017 recommend the following principles for the management of sepsis and septic shock in adult patients:

1. To identify sepsis and septic shock according to the new Sepsis-3 definition.
2. To start antimicrobial therapy within 1 h after the suspicion of sepsis or septic shock. It is recommended that appropriate routine microbiologic cultures (including blood) should be obtained before starting antimicrobial therapy. It is also recommended that the source control should be done without delay.
3. To start fluid resuscitation with 30 mL/kg of IV crystalloid fluid administered within the first 3 h.
4. EGDT is not recommended, but blood lactate should be monitored as a marker of hypoperfusion for the evaluation of the treatment efficiency.
5. If the fluid resuscitation is not efficient, vasopressors should be used and norepinephrine is the first choice recommended with a target of 65 mmHg mean arterial blood pressure.
6. If mechanical ventilation is needed a target tidal volume of 6 mL/kg is recommended in patients with sepsis-induced acute respiratory distress syndrome.

Figure 12.1 shows a suggested algorithm for the management of sepsis for older patients in the ED.

12 Management of Sepsis in Older Patients in the Emergency Department

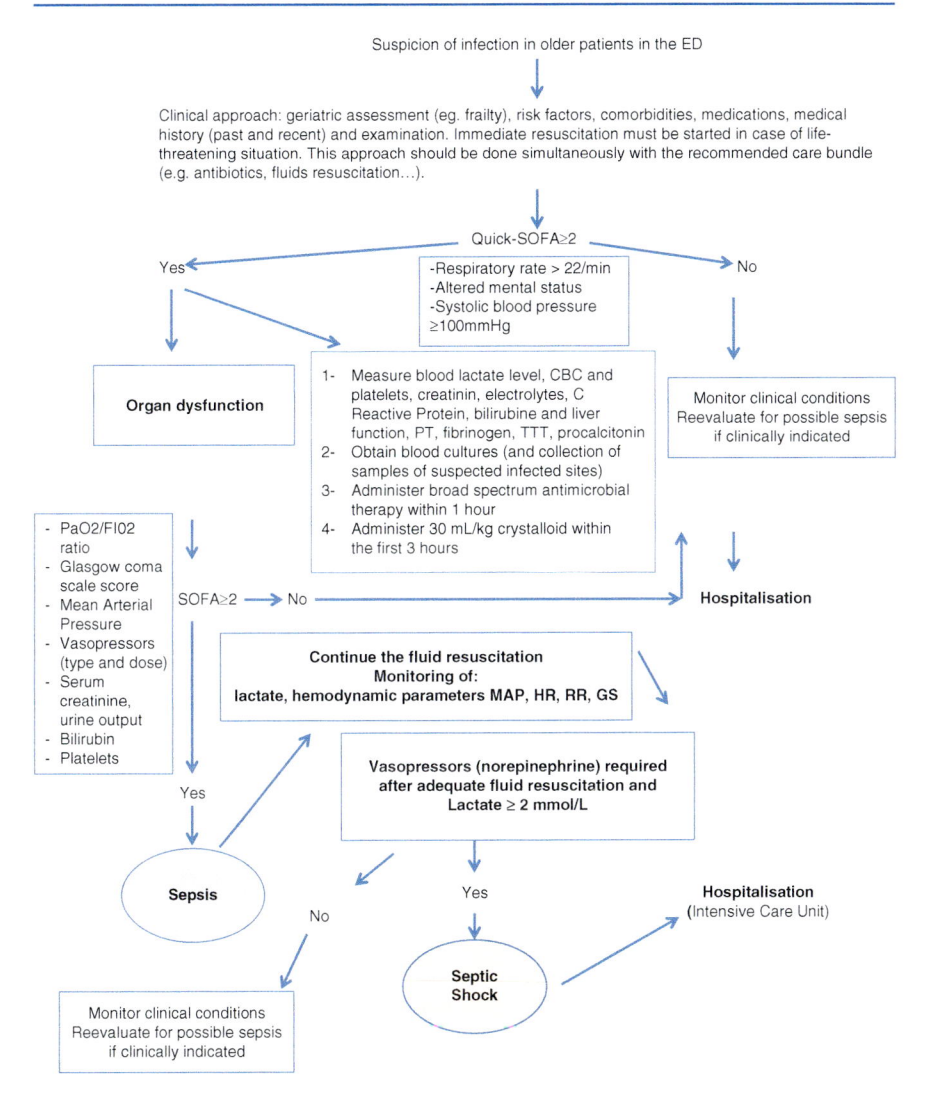

Fig. 12.1 Suggested algorithm for the management of sepsis in older patients in the ED. The new revision of the definition of sepsis is included. *MAP* mean arterial blood pressure, *HR* heart rate, *RR* respiratory rate, *GS* Glasgow score

12.8 Prognosis and Outcomes

When compared with younger patients with a diagnosis of sepsis, those older than 65 years were 13 times more likely to develop sepsis and had a twofold risk of death from sepsis [113]. Mortality increases with increasing age and the highest mortality is observed in older patients more than 85 years of age [19, 67, 115, 116].

Older patients with sepsis and septic shock have a high mortality from 50% to 60%, 1.3–1.5 times higher than younger patients (Martin et al. 2006, [19, 117]). In addition to increased mortality rates, older sepsis patients die earlier during hospitalization (Martin et al. 2006, [1, 19, 21, 54]).

Poor prognosis factors have been identified as the presence of shock, elevated serum lactate levels, and presence of organ failure [117]. In a study evaluating long-term mortality in older sepsis patients surviving at 3 months post-sepsis, an overall mortality rate of 55% with a 30.6% 1-year morality rate and a 43% 2-year mortality rate were observed [118]. It was noted that congestive heart failure, peripheral vascular disease, dementia, and diabetes were most associated with long-term mortality in older patients with post-sepsis [118]. Detection and early efficient treatment of associated diseases could improve survival in sepsis in older patients.

Older sepsis survivors often require additional care in long-term nursing facilities or rehabilitation after hospitalization to regain functional status. It was shown that 76% of those that survive were less likely to return home after hospital discharge and require continued care [118]. A larger study by Iwashyna et al. [119] found that older patients who survived severe sepsis were more likely to have new cognitive impairment and functional decline compared with those with non-sepsis admissions. However, Meurer et al. showed that among survivors, functional status measured by ADL and IADL deteriorated in these activities in some patients, and in others, they were not altered [120].

The impact of the SSC guidelines on older adults with sepsis and septic shock has not been extensively evaluated. Data on prognosis factors and outcomes in older patients are still needed.

12.9 Conclusion and Key Points

Sepsis is a frequent medical condition diagnosed in older patients managed in the ED, and the incidence is continuously increasing. This is related to the increase of older population, the specific immunosenescence state combined with the increase of frailty, and comorbidity.

The majority of ED older patients with sepsis will be hospitalized, and mortality is significantly higher than young sepsis patients. Aging is accompanied by a reduced tolerance to physiological stress, which contributes to increased vulnerability to critical illnesses in old age.

Given the limited functional reserve in older patients, it is even more essential to identify sepsis promptly and implement appropriate interventions (early antimicrobial treatments, infection source control, fluid resuscitation) in this population.

Early management time in the ED is critical for the administration of the appropriate and empirical antimicrobial treatment within 1 h and the start of the initial resuscitation and the care bundle. This target objective could be difficult to obtain because of the atypical clinical presentation of older patients with sepsis and the absence of specific markers.

The SIRS was removed from the definition of sepsis and replaced by the quick-SOFA and the SOFA scores, which are easy to use in the ED and can help to identify sepsis and septic shock patients. However, prospective multicentric studies are needed to confirm the accuracy of these scores in the ED.

The monitoring of the ScVO2 is not recommended in the ED, and the monitoring of blood lactic acid level and the clearance of lactic acid can be used for the measurement of the effect of the treatment in older patients.

Despite the tremendous efforts made by the Surviving Sepsis Campaign, the mortality of sepsis remains high in older patients, and there is a need for new strategies of prevention and treatment of infections and early detection of sepsis. Implementation of sepsis guidelines has proven effective for younger and older adults [80, 82, 86, 121], although geriatric considerations and age-related adjustments may be necessary.

Best practice protocols require a comprehensive knowledge of age-related changes and atypical presentations of illness in sepsis, which represent a new and exciting area of research.

References

1. Angus DC, Linde-Zwirble WT, Lidicker J, Clermont G, Carcillo J, Pinsky MR (2001) Epidemiology of severe sepsis in the United States: analysis of incidence, outcome, and associated costs of care. Crit Care Med 29:1303–1310
2. Umberger R, Callen B, Brown ML (2015) Severe sepsis in older adults. Crit Care Nurs Q 38(3):259–270
3. Quenot JP, Binquet C, Kara F, Martinet O, Ganster F, Navellou JC, Castelain V, Barraud D, Cousson J, Louis G, Perez P, Kuteifan K, Noirot A, Badie J, Mezher C, Lessire H, Pavon A (2013) The epidemiology of septic shock in French intensive care units: the prospective multicenter cohort EPISS study. Crit Care 17(2):R65. doi:10.1186/cc12598
4. Wang HE, Shapiro NI, Angus DC, Yealy DM (2007) National estimates of severe sepsis in United States emergency departments. Crit Care Med 35(8):1928–1936
5. Levy MM, Fink MP, Marshall JC, Abraham E, Angus D, Cook D, Cohen J, Opal SM, Vincent JL, Ramsay G (2003) 2001 SCCM/ESICM/ACCP/ATS/SIS international sepsis definitions conference. Crit Care Med 31:1250–1256
6. Singer M, Deutschman CS, Seymour CW et al (2016) JAMA 315(8):801–810. doi:10.1001/jama.2016.0287
7. Vincent JL, Moreno R, Takala J, Willatts S, De Mendonça A, Bruining H, Reinhart CK, Suter PM, Thijs LG (1996) The SOFA (Sepsis-related Organ Failure Assessment) score to describe organ dysfunction/failure. On behalf of the working group on sepsis-related problems of the European society of intensive care medicine. Intensive Care Med 22(7):707–710
8. Seymour CW, Liu VX VX, Iwashyna TJ et al (2016) Assessment of clinical criteria for sepsis for the third international consensus definitions for sepsis and septic shock (Sepsis-3). JAMA 315(8):762–774. doi:10.1001/jama.2016.0288
9. Chen YX, Li CS (2014) Arterial lactate improves the prognostic performance of severity score systems in septic patients in the ED. Am J Emerg Med 32(9):982–986. doi:10.1016/j.ajem.2014.05.025. Epub 2014 May 24
10. April MD, Aguirre J, Tannenbaum LI, Moore T, Pingree A, Thaxton RE, Sessions DJ, Md, Lantry JH (2016) Sepsis clinical criteria in emergency department patients admitted to an intensive care unit: an external validation study of quick sequential organ failure assessment. J Emerg Med. pii: S0736-4679(16)30887-3. doi:10.1016/j.jemermed.2016.10.012

11. Giamarellos-Bourboulis EJ, Tsaganos T, Tsangaris I, et al, Hellenic Sepsis Study Group (2016) Validation of the new Sepsis-3 definitions: proposal for improvement in early risk identification. Clin Microbiol Infect. pii: S1198-743X(16)30558-4. [Epub ahead of print]. doi:10.1016/j.cmi.2016.11.003
12. Freund Y, Lemachatti N, Krastinova E, Van Laer M, Claessens YE, Avondo A, Occelli C, Feral-Pierssens AL, Truchot J, Ortega M, Carneiro B, Pernet J, Claret PG, Dami F, Bloom B, Riou B, Beaune S, French Society of Emergency Medicine Collaborators Group (2017) Prognostic accuracy of sepsis-3 criteria for in-hospital mortality among patients with suspected infection presenting to the emergency department. JAMA 317(3):301–308. doi:10.1001/jama.2016.20329
13. Valencia AM, Vallejo CE, Alvarez AL, Jaimes FA (2016) Attenuation of the physiological response to infection on adults over 65 years old admitted to the emergency room (ER). Aging Clin Exp Res. doi:10.1007/s40520-016-0679-2
14. Valencia AM, Vallejo CE, Alvarez AL, Jaimes FA (2016) Attenuation of the physiological response to infection on adults over 65 years old admitted to the emergency room (ER). Aging Clin Exp Res Nov 16
15. Adhikari NK, Fowler RA, Bhagwanjee S, Rubenfeld GD (2010) Critical care and the global burden of critical illness in adults. Lancet 376:1339–1346
16. Linde-Zwirble WT, Angus DC (2004) Severe sepsis epidemiology: sampling, selection, and society. Crit Care 8:222–226
17. Brun-Buisson C, Meshaka P, Pinton P et al (2004) EPISEPSIS: a reappraisal of the epidemiology and outcome of severe sepsis in French intensive care units. Intensive Care Med 30:580–588
18. Dombrovskiy VY, Martin AA, Sunderram J, Paz HL (2007) Rapid increase in hospitalization and mortality rates for severe sepsis in the United States: a trend analysis from 1993 to 2003. Crit Care Med 35:1244–1250
19. Nasa P, Juneja D, Singh O, Dang R, Arora V (2011) Severe sepsis and its impact on outcome in elderly and very elderly patients admitted in intensive care unit. J Intensive Care Med 27(3):179–183. Epub ahead of print
20. Padkin A, Goldfrad C, Brady AR et al (2003) Epidemiology of severe sepsis occurring in the first 24 hrs in intensive care units in England, Wales, and Northern Ireland. Crit Care Med 31:2332–2338
21. Yang Y, Yang KS, Hsann YM, Lim V, Ong BC (2010) The effect of comorbidity and age on hospital mortality and length of stay in patients with sepsis. J Crit Care 25:398–405
22. Strehlow MC, Emond SD, Shapiro NI, Pelletier AJ, Camargo CA Jr (2006) National study of emergency department visits for sepsis, 1992 to 2001. Ann Emerg Med 48:326–331
23. Lagu T, Rothberg MB, Shieh MS, Pekow PS, Steingrub JS, Lindenauer PK (2012) Hospitalizations, costs, and outcomes of severe sepsis in the United States 2003 to 2007. Crit Care Med 40:754–756. [Erratum, Crit Care Med 2012;40:2932]
24. Ranieri VM, Thompson BT, Barie PS et al (2012) Drotrecogin alfa (activated) in adults with septic shock. N Engl J Med 366:2055–2064
25. Vincent JL, Rello J, Marshall J et al (2009) International study of the prevalence and outcomes of infection in intensive care units. JAMA 302:2323–2329
26. Dieckema DJ, Pfaller MA, Jones RN (2002) Age-related trends in pathogen frequency and antimicrobial susceptibility of bloodstream isolates in North America: SENTRY antimicrobial surveillance program, 1997–2000. Int J Antimicrobial Agents 20:412–418
27. Rowe T, Araujo KLB, Van Ness PH, Pisani MA, Juthani-Mehta M (2016) Outcomes of older adults with sepsis at admission to an intensive care unit. Open Forum Infectious Diseases 1–6
28. Abraham E, Reinhart K, Opal S et al (2003) Efficacy and safety of tifacogin (recombinant tissue factor pathway inhibitor) in severe sepsis: a randomized controlled trial. JAMA 290:238–247
29. Opal SM, Garber GE, LaRosa SP et al (2003) Systemic host responses in severe sepsis analyzed by causative microorganism and treatment effects of drotrecogin alfa (activated). Clin Infect Dis 37:50–58

30. Martin GS, Mannino DM, Eaton S, Moss M (2003a) The epidemiology of sepsis in the United States from 1979 through 2000. N Engl J Med 348:1546–1554
31. Martin GS, Mannino DM, Moss M (2003b) Effect of age on the development and outcome with sepsis. Am J Respir Crit Care Med 167:A837
32. Girard TD, Opal SM, Ely EW (2005) Insights into severe sepsis in older patients: from epidemiology to evidence-based management. Clin Infect Dis 40:719–727
33. Kirby JT, Fritsche TR, Jones RN (2006) Influence of patient age on the frequency of occurrence and antimicrobial resistance patterns of isolates from hematology/oncology patients: report from the chemotherapy alliance for neutropenics and the control of emerging resistance program (north America). Diagn Microbiol Infect Dis 56:75–82
34. Weksler ME (2000) Changes in the B-cell repertoire with age. Vaccine 18:1624–1628
35. Opal SM, Girard TD, Ely EW (2005) The immunopathogenesis of sepsis in elderly patients. Clin Infect Dis 41(Suppl 7):S504–S512
36. Dewan SK1, Zheng SB, Xia SJ, Bill K (2012) Senescent remodeling of the immune system and its contribution to the predisposition of the elderly to infections. Chin Med J (Engl) 125(18):3325–3331
37. Suzuki K, Inoue S, Kametani Y, Komori Y, Chiba S, Sato T, Inokuchi S, Ogura S (2016) Reduced immunocompetent B cells and increased secondary infection in elderly patients with severe sepsis. Shock 46(3):270–278. doi:10.1097/SHK.0000000000000619
38. Inoue S, Suzuki K, Komori Y, Morishita Y, Suzuki-Utsunomiya K, Hozumi K, Inokuchi S, Takehito ST (2014) Persistent inflammation and T cell exhaustion in severe sepsis in the elderly. Crit Care 18:R130
39. Sánchez M, Lindroth K, Sverremark E, González Fernández A, Fernández C (2001) The response in old mice: positive and negative immune memory after priming in early age. Int Immunol 13:1213–1221
40. Sandmand M, Bruunsgaard H, Kemp K, Andersen-Ranberg K, Pedersen AN, Skinhøj P, Pedersen BK (2002) Is ageing associated with a shift in the balance between Type 1 and Type 2 cytokines in humans? Clin Exp Immunol 127:107–114
41. De Gaudio AR, Rinaldi S, Chelazzi C, Borracci T (2009) Pathophysiology of sepsis in the elderly: clinical impact and therapeutic considerations. Curr Drug Targets 10:60–70
42. Haynes L, Eaton SM, Swain SL (2002) Effect of age on naive CD4 responses: impact on effector generation and memory development. Springer Semin Immunopathol 24:53–60
43. Renshaw M, Rockwell J, Engleman C, Gewirtz A, Katz J, Sambhara S (2002) Cutting edge: impaired toll-like receptor expression and function in aging. J Immunol 169:4697–4701
44. Walter LC, Brand RJ, Counsell SR, Palmer RM, Landefeld CS, Fortinsky RH, Covinsky KE (2001) Development and validation of a prognostic index for 1-year mortality in older adults after hospitalization. JAMA 285(285):2987–2994
45. Kale S, Yende S, Kong L, Perkins A, Kellum JA, Newman AB, Vallejo AN, Angus DC, GenIMS Investigators (2010) The effects of age on inflammatory and coagulation-fibrinolysis response in patients hospitalized for pneumonia. PLoS One 5(11):e13852. doi:10.1371/journal.pone.0013852
46. Vieira da Silva Pellegrina D, Severino P, Vieira Barbeiro H, Maziero Andreghetto F, Tadeu Velasco I, Possolo de Souza H, Machado MC, Reis EM, Pinheiro da Silva F (2015) Septic shock in advanced age: transcriptome analysis reveals altered molecular signatures in neutrophil granulocytes. PLoS One 10(6):e0128341. doi:10.1371/journal.pone.0128341. eCollection 2015
47. Angus DC, van der Poll T (2013) Severe sepsis and septic shock. N Engl J Med 369:840–851. doi:10.1056/NEJMra1208623
48. Bernard GR, Vincent JL, Laterre PF, SP LR, Dhainaut JF, Lopez-Rodriguez A, Steingrub JS, Garber GE, Helterbrand JD, Ely EW, Fisher CJ (2001) Efficacy and safety of recombinant human activated protein C for severe sepsis. N Engl J Med 344:699–709
49. Kumar A, Thota V, Dee L, Olson J, Uretz E, Parrillo JE (1996) Tumor necrosis factor alpha and interleukin 1beta are responsible for in vitro myocardial cell depression induced by human septic shock serum. J Exp Med 183:949–958

50. Rozenberg S, Besse S, Brisson H, Jozefowicz E, Kandoussi A, Mebazaa A, Riou B, Vallet B, Tavernier B (2006) Endotoxin-induced myocardial dysfunction in senescent rats. Crit Care 10:R124
51. Saito H, Papaconstantinou J (2001) Age-associated differences in cardiovascular inflammatory gene induction during endotoxic stress. J Biol Chem 276:29307–29312
52. Nasa P et al (2012) Severe sepsis and septic shock in the elderly: an overview. World J Crit Care Med 1(1):23–30
53. Ruiz M, Bottle A, Long S, Aylin P (2015) Multi-morbidity in hospitalised older patients: who are the complex elderly? PLoS One 10(12):e0145372. doi:10.1371/journal.pone.0145372
54. Englert NC, Ross C (2015) The older adult experiencing sepsis. Crit Care Nurs Q 38(2):175–181
55. Rudman D, Hontanosas A, Cohen Z, Mattson DE (1988) Clinical correlates of bacteremia in a veterans administration extended care facility. J Am Geriatr Soc 36:726–732
56. Vardi M, Ghanem-Zoubi NO, Bitterman H, Abo-helo N, Yurin V, Weber G, Laor A (2013) Sepsis in nonagenarians admitted to internal medicine departments: a comparative study of outcomes. Q J Med 106:261–266
57. Marwick C, Santiago VH, McCowan C, Broomhall J, Davey P (2013) Community acquired infections in older patients admitted to hospital from care homes versus the community: cohort study of microbiology and outcomes. BMC Geriatr 13:12. doi:10.1186/1471-2318-13-12
58. Jensen GL, McGee M, Binkley J (2001) Nutrition in the elderly. Gastroenterol Clin N Am 30:313–334
59. Carpenter CR, Shelton E, Fowler S, Suffoletto B, Platts-Mills TF, Rothman RE, Hogan TM (2015) Risk factors and screening instruments to predict adverse outcomes for undifferentiated older emergency department patients: a systematic review and meta-analysis. Acad Emerg Med 22:1–21
60. Brummel NE, Bell SP, Girard TD, Pandharipande PP, Jackson JC, Morandi A, Thompson JL, Chandrasekhar R, Bernard GR, Dittus RS, Gill TM, Ely EW (2016) Frailty and subsequent disability and mortality among patients with critical illness. Am J Respir Crit Care Med. Published on 06-December-2016 as 10.1164/rccm.201605-0939OC
61. Chaudry H et al (2013) Role of cytokines as a double-edged sword in sepsis. In Vivo 27:669–684
62. Rockwood K, Mitnitski A (2011) Frailty defined by deficit accumulation and geriatric medicine defined by frailty. Clin Geriatr Med 27:17–26
63. Lee WJ et al (2016) Are prognostic scores and biomarkers such a procalcitonin the appropriate prognostic precursors for elderly patients with sepsis in the emergency department? 2015. Aging Clin Exp Res 28(5):917–924
64. González Del Castillo J, Escobar-Curbelo L, Martínez-Ortíz de Zárate M, Llopis-Roca F, García-Lamberechts J, Moreno-Cuervo Á, Fernández C, Martín-Sánchez FJ (2015) Representing the infectious disease group of spanish emergency medicine society. GYM score: 30-day mortality predictive model in elderly patients attended in the emergency department with infection. Eur J Emerg Med
65. Rajagopalan S, Yoshikawa TT (2001) Antimicrobial therapy in the elderly. Med Clin North Am 85:133–147
66. Wester AL, Dunlop O, Melby KK, Dahle UR, Wyller TB (2013) Age-related differences in symptoms, diagnosis and prognosis of bacteremia. BMC Infect Dis 13:346. doi:10.1186/1471-2334-13-346
67. Gavazzi G, Krause KH (2002) Ageing and infection. Lancet Infect Dis 2:659–666
68. Norman DC (2009) Factors predisposing to infection. In: Yoshikawa T, Norman DC (eds) Infectious disease in the aging – a clinical handbook, 2nd edn. Humana Press, New York, pp 11–18
69. Gauer RL (2013) Early recognition and management of sepsis in adults: the first six hours. Am Fam Physician 88(1):44–53

70. Iberti TJ, Bone RC, Balk R, Fein A, Perl TM, Wenzel RP (1993) Are the criteria used to determine sepsis applicable for patients 75 years of age? Crit Care Med 21:S130
71. Gleckman R, Hibert D (1982) Afebrile bacteremia: a phenomenon in geriatric patients. JAMA 248:1478–1481
72. Hernandez C, Feher C, Soriano A, Marco F, Almela M, Cobos-Trigueros N, De La Calle C, Morata L, Mensa J, Martinez JA (2015) Clinical characteristics and outcome of elderly patients with community-onset bacteremia. J Infect 70(2):135–143. doi:10.1016/j.jinf.2014.09.002. PMID:25224642
73. Yahav D, Schlesinger A, Daitch V, Akayzen Y, Farbman L, Abu-Ghanem Y, Paul M, Leibovici L (2015) Presentation of infection in older patients–a prospective study. Ann Med 47(4):354–358. doi:10.3109/07853890.2015.1019915
74. Niven DJ, Gaudet JE, Laupland KB, Mrklas KJ, Roberts DJ, Stelfox HT (2015) Accuracy of peripheral thermometers for estimating temperature. A systematic review and meta-analysis. Ann Intern Med 163:768–777. doi:10.7326/M15-1150
75. Lu SH, Leasure AR, Dai YT (2010) A systematic review of body temperature variations in older people. J Clin Nurs 1(2):4–16
76. Tiruvoipati R, Ong K, Gangopadhyay H et al (2010) Hypothermia predicts mortality in critically ill elderly patients with sepsis. BCM Geriat 10:70
77. Mouton CP, Pierce B, Espino DV (2001) Common infections in older adults. Am Fam Physician 63(2):257–269
78. Su CP, Chen TH, Chen SY et al (2011) Predictive model for bacteremia in adult patients with blood cultures performed at the emergency department: a preliminary report. J Microbiol Immunol Infect 44:449–455
79. Dellinger RP, Levy MM, Rodhes A et al (2012) Surviving sepsis campaign: international guidelines for management of severe sepsis and septic shock, 2012. Intensive Care Med 39(2):165–228. doi:10.1007/s00134-012-2769-8
80. Rhodes A, Evans LE, Alhazzani W et al (2017) Surviving sepsis campaign: international guidelines for management of sepsis and septic shock: 2016. Crit Care Med 43(3):304–377. doi:10.1097/CCM.0000000000002255. [Epub ahead of print]
81. Sehgal V, Bajwa SJ, Consalvo JA, Bajaj A (2015) Clinical conundrums in management of sepsis in the elderly. J Transl Int Med 3(3):106–112. Epub 2015 Sep 30
82. Heppner HJ, Singler K, Kwetkat A, Popp S, Esslinger AS, Bahrmann P, Kaiser M, Bertsch T, Sieber CC, Christ M (2012) Do clinical guidelines improve management of sepsis in critically ill elderly patients? A before-and-after study of the implementation of a sepsis protocol. Wien Klin Wochenschr 124(8):692–698. doi:10.1007/s00508-012-0229-7. Epub 2012 Sep 5
83. Rhodes A, Phillips G, Beale R et al (2015) The surviving sepsis campaign bundles and outcome: results from the international multicentre prevalence study on sepsis (the IMPreSS study). Intensive Care Med 41(9):1620–1628
84. Palomba H, Corrêa TD, Silva E, Pardini A, Assuncao MS (2015) Comparative analysis of survival between elderly and non-elderly severe sepsis and septic shock resuscitated patients. Einstein (Sao Paulo) 13(3):357–363. doi:10.1590/S1679-45082015AO3313. Epub 2015 Aug 21
85. Rivers E, Nguyen B, Havstad S, Ressler J, Muzzin A, Knoblich B, Peterson E, Tomlanovich M (2001) Early Goal-Directed Therapy Collaborative Group. Early goal-directed therapy in the treatment of severe sepsis and septic shock. N Engl J Med 345(19):1368–77
86. El Solh AA, Akinnusi ME, Alsawalha LN, Pineda LA (2008) Outcome of septic shock in older adults after implementation of the sepsis "bundle". J Am Geriatr Soc 56:272–278
87. Mouncey PR, Osborn TM, Power GS et al (2015) Trial of early, goal-directed resuscitation for septic shock. N Engl J Med 372:1301–1311. doi:10.1056/NEJMoa1500896
88. The ARISE Investigators and the ANZICS Clinical Trials Group (2014) Goal-directed resuscitation for patients with early septic shock. N Engl J Med 371:1496–1506. doi:10.1056/NEJMoa1404380
89. The ProCESS Investigators (2014) A randomized trial of protocol-based care for early septic shock. N Engl J Med 370:1683–1693. doi:10.1056/NEJMoa1401602

90. Jones AE (2013) Lactate clearance for assessing response to resuscitation in severe sepsis. Acad Emerg Med 20:844–847
91. Jones AE, Shapiro NI, Trzeciak S et al (2010) Lactate clearance vs central venous oxygen saturation as goals of early sepsis therapy: a randomized clinical trial. JAMA 303:739–746
92. Jones AE (2011) Point: should lactate clearance be substituted for central venous oxygen saturation as goals of early severe sepsis and septic shock therapy? Yes. Chest 140:1406–1408
93. Dugas AF, Mackenhauer J, Salcicciolli JD, Cocchi MN, Gautam S, Donnino MW (2012) Prevalence and characteristics of nonlactate and lactate expressors in septic shock. J Crit Care 27(4):344–350
94. Jansen TC, van Bommel J, Schoonderbeek FJ et al (2010) Early lactate-guided therapy in intensive care unit patients: a multicenter, open-label, randomized controlled trial. Am J Respir Crit Care Med 182(6):752–761
95. Lyu X, Xu Q, Cai G, Yan J, Yan M (2015) Efficacies of fluid resuscitation as guided by lactate clearance rate and central venous oxygen saturation in patients with septic shock. Zhonghua Yi Xue Za Zhi 95(7):496–500
96. Yu B, Tian HY, Hu ZJ et al (2013) Comparison of the effect of fluid resuscitation as guided either by lactate clearance rate or by central venous oxygen saturation in patients with sepsis. Zhonghua Wei Zhong Bing Ji Jiu Yi Xue 25(10):578–583
97. Tian HH, Han SS, Lv CJ et al (2012) The effect of early goal lactate clearance rate on the outcome of septic shock patients with severe pneumonia. Zhongguo Wei Zhong Bing Ji Jiu Yi Xue 24(1):42–45
98. Zhang L, Zhu G, Han L, Fu P (2015) Early goal-directed therapy in the management of severe sepsis or septic shock in adults: a meta-analysis of randomized controlled trials. BMC Med 13:71. doi:10.1186/s12916-015-0312-9
99. Dettmer M, Holthaus CV, Fuller BM (2015) The impact of serial lactate monitoring on emergency department resuscitation interventions and clinical outcomes in severe sepsis and septic shock: an observational cohort study. Shock 43(1):55–61. doi:10.1097/SHK.0000000000000260
100. Gu WJ, Zhang Z, Bakker J (2015) Early lactate clearance-guided therapy in patients with sepsis: a meta-analysis with trial sequential analysis of randomized controlled trials. Intensive Care Med 41(10):1862–1863
101. Simpson SQ, Gaines M, Hussein Y, Badgett RG (2016) Early goal-directed therapy for severe sepsis and septic shock: a living systematic review. J Crit Care 36:43–48
102. Chen YX, Li CS (2015) Lactate on emergency department arrival as a predictor of mortality and site-of-care in pneumonia patients: a cohort study. Thorax 70:404–410. doi:10.1136/thoraxjnl-2014-20646
103. del Portal DA, Shofer F, Mikkelsen ME, Dorsey PJ Jr, Gaieski DF, Goyal M, Synnestvedt M, Weiner MG, Pines JM (2010) Emergency department lactate is associated with mortality in older adults admitted with and without infections. Acad Emerg Med 17(3):260–268. doi:10.1111/j.1553-2712.2010.00681.x
104. Stalam M, Kaye D (2004) Antibiotic agents in the elderly. Infect Dis Clin N Am 18:533–549
105. Wu WC, Rathore SS, Wang Y, Radford MJ, Krumholz HM (2001) Blood transfusion in elderly patients with acute myocardial infarction. N Engl J Med 345:1230–1236
106. Herring AR, Williamson JC (2007) Principles of antimicrobial use in older adults. Clin Geriatr Med 23:481–497
107. Garnacho-Montero J, Garcia-Garmendia JL, Barrero-Almodovar A, Jimenez-Jimenez FJ, Perez-Paredes C, Ortiz-Leyba C (2003) Impact of adequate empirical antibiotic therapy on the outcome of patients admitted to the intensive care unit with sepsis. Crit Care Med 31:2742–2751
108. Gaieski DF, Mikkelsen ME, Band RA, Pines JM, Massone R, Furia FF et al (2010) Impact of time to antibiotics on survival in patients with severe sepsis or septic shock in whom early goal-directed therapy was initiated in the emergency department. Crit Care Med 38:1045–1053

109. Harbarth S, Garbino J, Pugin J, Romand JA, Lew D, Pittet D (2003) Inappropriate initial antimicrobial therapy and its effect on survival in a clinical trial of immunomodulating therapy for severe sepsis. Am J Med 115:529–535
110. Houck PM, Bratzler DW, Nsa W, Ma A, Bartlett JG (2004) Timing of antibiotic administration and outcomes for Medicare patients hospitalized with community-acquired pneumonia. Arch Intern Med 164:637–644
111. Iregui M, Ward S, Sherman G, Fraser VJ, Kollef MH (2002) Clinical importance of delays in the initiation of appropriate anti-biotic treatment for ventilator-associated pneumonia. Chest 122:262–268
112. Kumar A, Roberts D, Wood KE, Light B, Parrillo JE, Sharma S et al (2006) Duration of hypotension prior to initiation of effective antimicrobial therapy is the critical determinant of survival in human septic shock. Crit Care Med 34:1589–1596
113. Martin GS, Mannino DM, Moss M (2006) The effect of age on the development and outcome of adult sepsis. Crit Care Med 34(1):15–21
114. Luna CM, Aruj P, Niederman MS, Garzón J, Violi D, Prignoni A, Ríos F, Baquero S, Gando S (2006) Appropriateness and delay to initiate therapy in ventilator-associated pneumonia. Eur Respir J 27:158–164
115. Curns AT, Holman RC, Sejvar JJ, Owings MF, Schonberger LB (2005) Infectious disease hospitalizations among older adults in the United States from 1990 through 2002. Arch Intern Med 165:2514–2520
116. Ely EW, Angus DC, Williams MD, Bates B, Qualy R, Bernard GR (2003) Drotrecogin alfa (activated) treatment of older patients with severe sepsis. Clin Infect Dis 37:187–195
117. Vosylius S, Sipylaite J, Ivaskevicius J (2005) Determinants of outcome in elderly patients admitted to the intensive care unit. Age Ageing 34:157–162
118. Starr ME, Saito H (2014) Sepsis in old age: review in human and animal studies. Aging Dis 5(2):126–136
119. Iwashyna TJ, Ely EW, Smith DM, Langa KM (2010) Long-term cognitive impairment and functional disability among survivors of severe sepsis. JAMA 304:1787–1794
120. Meurer WJ, Losman ED, Smith BL, Malani PN, Younger JG (2011) Short-term functional decline of older adults admitted for suspected sepsis. Am J Emerg Med 29(8):936–942. doi:10.1016/j.ajem.2010.04.003. Epub 2010 Jul 13
121. Nguyen HB, Corbett SW, Steele R et al (2007) Implementation of a bundle of quality indicators for the early management of severe sepsis and septic shock is associated with decreased mortality. Crit Care Med 35:1105–1112
122. Goodwin N, Sonola L, Thiel V, Kodner DL (2013) Co-ordinated care for people with complex chronic conditions. Key lessons and markers for success. Available at: www.kingsfund.org.uk/.../co-ordinated-care-for-people-with-complex-chronic-conditions-kingsfund-oct13.pdf. Accessed 24 June 2015
123. Kuan WS, Ibrahim I, Leong BSH, Jain S, Lu Q, Cheung YB, Mahadevan M (2016) Emergency department management of sepsis patients: a randomized, goal-oriented, noninvasive sepsis trial. Ann Emerg Med 67:367–378
124. Churpek MM, Edelson DP (2016) Moving beyond single parameter early warning scores for rapid response system activation. Crit Care Med 44(12):2283–2285

Cognitive Impairment in Older People Presenting to ED

Chris Miller, Elizabeth Teale, and Jay Banerjee

13.1 What Is Cognitive Impairment?

Cognitive impairment (CI) is an umbrella term to describe acquired conditions affecting memory, attention, arousal, executive functioning, language and perception. Dementia is 'a syndrome due to disease of the brain, usually of a chronic or progressive nature, in which there is disturbance of multiple higher cortical functions, including memory, thinking, orientation, comprehension, calculation, learning capacity, language, and judgement', whilst delirium is 'an aetiologically non-specific organic cerebral syndrome characterized by concurrent disturbances of consciousness and attention, perception, thinking, memory, psychomotor behaviour, emotion, and the sleep-wake schedule'. Delirium primarily affects consciousness (arousal and attention) with additional deficits in other cognitive domains. Although they commonly co-exist, delirium and dementia are distinct conditions. Patients who have a pre-existing diagnosis of dementia are at particularly high risk of developing delirium during times of physiological stress, as are those with older age, co-morbid illness, severity of medical illness, infection, 'high-risk' medication use (such as anticholinergic drugs), diminished activities of daily living, immobility, sensory impairment, urinary catheterisation, urea and electrolyte imbalance and malnutrition.

C. Miller (✉)
Department of Geriatric Medicine, University Hospitals of Leicester NHS Trust, Leicester, UK
e-mail: christopher.miller@uhl-tr.nhs.uk

E. Teale
Emergency Medicine, University Hospitals of Leicester NHS Trust, Leicester, UK

J. Banerjee
Emergency Medicine, University Hospitals of Leicester NHS Trust, Leicester, UK

Department of Health Sciences, University of Leicester, Leicester, UK

Delirium, either alone or in conjunction with a pre-existing dementia, may result in the common emergency department presentation of 'increased confusion'. Delirium has been shown to be an independent predictor of morbidity and mortality associated with poor outcomes in respect of increased rates of institutionalisation, development of dementia, functional decline, prolonged hospitalisation and higher healthcare expenditures. It is important to distinguish between delirium, dementia and delirium superimposed on dementia as early as possible in the patient pathway to ensure that investigation and management is patient centred, appropriate and timely. This process should begin in the Emergency Department.

13.2 Why Is It Important to Detect Cognitive Impairment in the ED?

Missing cognitive impairment in the ED is associated with poor outcomes [1, 2]. It represents a missed opportunity to trigger community assessment processes and access to support services. This may impact on ability to manage safely at home. People with cognitive impairment may be unable to communicate need, and this makes for a poor patient experience. There is a clinical need to identify the precipitating factors that could be addressed and lead to the development of an appropriate plans or update existing plans. It is important to distinguish delirium from dementia or delirium on dementia and not to assume all cognitive impairment is chronic. However, this requires access to information and can be challenging during out of hours in unaccompanied older people attending EDs.

13.3 Epidemiology

On average, between 7 and 20% of patients presenting to EDs over the age of 65 years do so with a delirious episode [3]. However, studies report delirium is a commonly missed diagnosis in this setting (over 43–75% of cases undetected). Unfortunately, delirium under detection is not limited to the ED; up to 94% of patients presenting with delirium not recognised in ED will remain undiagnosed or unrecognised throughout a patient's admission [4].

Hypoactive delirium is particularly poorly detected, and despite the high coprevalence of delirium and dementia (50% of cases of delirium have coexisting dementia), detection of delirium superimposed on dementia is particularly challenging. This contributes to inadequate diagnostic workups, inappropriate dispositions and delays in the diagnosis of underlying medical illness.

Patients admitted with a delirium have a mortality rate of 10–26%, and if a patient develops delirium during their hospital stay, this rate increases to 22–76% [5], with high rates of mortality also observed post discharge. Up to 25% of delirious patients are discharged home from ED, and due to the delirium, these patients are less likely to understand their discharge instructions. Discharge from the ED with undiagnosed delirium is associated with excess adjusted mortality at 6 months (HR = 8.22 95%CI = 1.69–39.89) when compared with non-delirious patients [6]. Moreover, survival is attenuated in patients with undiagnosed delirium when compared with patients with a delirium diagnosis. For every 48 h period, a patient's delirium goes unrecognised, and mortality increases on average by 11% [5]. Improved detection of delirium in the ED is therefore essential to optimise the care of older people, yet by way of example, a UK audit in older people aged over 75 years conveyed by ambulance to EDs in 2014–2015 revealed that only 11% (range 4–19%) were being assessed for cognitive impairment and there is no national requirement for ED screening.

13.4 Some Definitions

The DSM-5 criteria distinguish between delirium and neurocognitive disorders (termed dementias in previous editions). Neurocognitive disorders are further classified as major (where impairments interfere with daily function) or mild (where executive and social functioning is maintained, albeit with adaptation or compensatory strategies). Mild neurocognitive disorders are alternatively termed mild cognitive impairment (MCI).

13.5 Delirium Diagnostic Criteria

The DSM-5 has five diagnostic criteria for delirium. These are:

- Disturbance in attention or awareness.
- Acute or subacute onset (over hours or days) of changes representing a change from baseline attention or awareness, with a tendency to fluctuations in severity over the course of the day.
- Additional cognitive disturbance (e.g. memory, disorientation, language, perception).
- Disturbances are not better explained by another cognitive disorder and do not occur in the context of severely reduced arousal (e.g. coma).
- Evidence from the history, examination or investigation results that the disturbance is due to a physiological disturbance (e.g. medical condition, substance intoxication or withdrawal, toxin exposure or multiple aetiologies).

Attention and arousal are hierarchical concepts: first arousal and then attention are required for clear consciousness. In the context of reduced arousal, testing for impaired attention may be impossible or impracticable (e.g. for patients who are drowsy and non-communicative). These patients should be assumed to meet the first diagnostic criterion for delirium as to exclude them as untestable results in a significant risk that patients with the hypoactive delirium subtype are missed (see below).

13.6 Delirium Subtypes

There are three subtypes of delirium. Hypoactive delirium is characterised by reduced arousal or awareness. Patients are typically drowsy, disinterested in their environment, poorly (or non-) communicative and may even be stuporose. In hyperactive delirium, patients are agitated, hypervigilant and may be wandersome. The third subtype is mixed delirium where there is either no change to arousal (although impaired attention would be required to make a diagnosis of delirium) or where there are fluctuations between hyper- and hypoactive subtypes. Mixed delirium, although the most common subtype, may be harder to recognise in an emergency department setting given the time constraints and possible slow fluctuations between hyper- and hypoactive states.

Delirium usually lasts between a few days and a week. In about one third of cases, delirium persists for up to 3 months or longer. This is persistent delirium and is associated with a particularly poor prognosis. Outcomes for patients worsen as their duration of delirium increases from 1 to 6 months following discharge from hospital [7]. Patients who have had an episode of delirium may never return to their cognitive baseline, and there is an association between delirium and lasting or subsequent cognitive decline and dementia.

13.7 Detecting Delirium in the ED

The key to the detection of delirium in the ED is screening for its presence. This needs to be followed by establishing the acuity of onset of symptoms and whether behaviours reflect a change from baseline. A reliable way to determine this is to speak to someone that knows the patient well (a relative, friend, carer, healthcare professional).

There are a number of brief screening tests for delirium: most commonly used are the Single Question in Delirium (SQiD), the Abbreviated Mental Test-10 (AMT10), the Abbreviated Mental Test-4 (AMT4), the 4AT, the brief Confusion Assessment Method (bCAM) and the Months of the Year Backwards (MOTYB).

The Single Question in Delirium (SQiD) asks of a knowledgeable informant (e.g. friend, relative, carer) whether the patient has been more confused lately. Sensitivity for the detection of delirium is good although specificity is low (61–71%) [8]. It has high negative predictive value, and the SQiD is therefore a useful quick and simple screening test to prompt further testing for delirium. It also has the great advantage of being culturally sensitive as translation into other languages does not change the context and can be performed by anyone regardless or training without impacting upon its accuracy. Other short tests for delirium have similar sensitivities for detecting delirium, but specificities of these brief tests for delirium are generally low. Table 13.1 below has pooled data including [8].

The 4 As Test (4AT) [9] is a four-item assessment to identify individuals with the cardinal features of delirium. It includes an assessment of alertness, cognition (**A**MT4), attention (MOTYB) and acuity of onset/fluctuating course (arising within

13 Cognitive Impairment in Older People Presenting to ED

Table 13.1 Delirium screening tests commonly used in the ED

Test	Time to complete	Training required?	Sensitivity (95% CIs) (%)	Specificity (95% CIs) (%)
AMT10	Minutes	Yes	86.6	63.5
AMT4	Seconds	No	92.7	53.7
MOTYB	Seconds	No	91.3	49.7
4AT	Minutes	Yes	86.7–89.7	69.5–84.1
SQiD	Seconds	No	91.4	61.3
DTS	Seconds	No	98.0	55.0
CAM	Minutes	Yes	94.0	89.0
bCAM	Minutes	Yes	70.3, 78.0–84.0	91.4, 95.8–96.9

the last two weeks and still evident within the last 24 h). The 4AT can be completed in under 2 min and does not require specialist training. The sensitivity and specificity in English-/non-English-speaking patients are 89.7/84.1% and 91/71%, respectively. Validation studies for the emergency department are currently underway.

In contrast to the other screening tests for delirium, the brief CAM (bCAM) is a two-step screening tool, developed from the CAM and CAM-ICU instruments. It is designed to be used in the ED setting, with brevity as a core feature. It may therefore be helpful to identify from the patients with positive delirium screening questions. It is supposed to be used combined with the Delirium Triage Screen (spell the word 'lunch' backwards and/or the feature of altered level of consciousness). DTS has a very good negative likelihood ratio of 0.04 and the bCAM a positive likelihood ratio of 20.0 when used in series and can be easily used in the ED [10].

More formal diagnosis of delirium requires the criteria of the DSM to be met. Where some, but not all features are present, a sub-syndromal delirium may be present. Delirium diagnostic tools operationalise the DSM diagnostic criteria into algorithms (e.g. Confusion Assessment Method long form) or questionnaires (e.g. DRS-R-98) and are based on more lengthy interviews with patients and informants. Sensitivity of the CAM is dependent on the training of the user, and in untrained hands, sensitivity as low as 40% has been reported. The authors of the CAM [11] stress the importance of training in the use of the instrument according to the CAM manual. The requirement for specific training and the duration to administer these definitive delirium diagnostic assessments limit their feasibility in the ED setting.

13.8 Risk Factors for Delirium

There are several risk factors for the development of delirium. Some of these are fixed (e.g. coexisting dementia and frailty), whilst some are modifiable. Modifiable risk factors are highlighted in Fig. 13.1. Identification (and minimisation) of these may help to prevent an episode of delirium. Once delirium is established, there is no specific treatment other than identification and removal of the contributing factors.

Typically, predisposing non-modifiable factors (dementia, serious illness, frailty) interact with precipitating, modifiable factors (sedatives, infections, surgery, electrolyte abnormalities) for delirium to develop. The commonest risk factors for

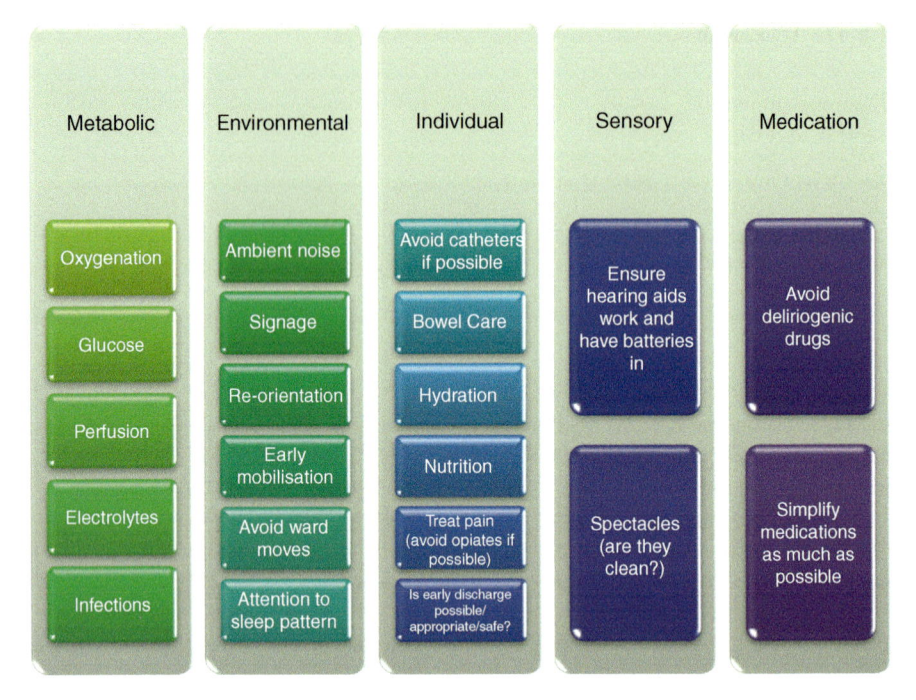

Metabolic	Environmental	Individual	Sensory	Medication
Oxygenation	Ambient noise	Avoid catheters if possible	Ensure hearing aids work and have batteries in	Avoid deliriogenic drugs
Glucose	Signage	Bowel Care		
	Re-orientation	Hydration		
Perfusion	Early mobilisation	Nutrition		
Electrolytes	Avoid ward moves	Treat pain (avoid opiates if possible)	Spectacles (are they clean?)	Simplify medications as much as possible
Infections	Attention to sleep pattern	Is early discharge possible/ appropriate/safe?		

Fig. 13.1 Modifiable risk factors for the development of delirium

delirium include age 65 years or older (who constitute 50–60% of all non-ambulatory patients in typical EDs), cognitive impairment (past or present) and/or dementia, current hip fracture (10% present with delirium, with 16–62% incidence postoperatively) [12] and any severe illness (a clinical condition that is deteriorating or is at risk of deterioration). Other important precipitating agents for delirium include anticholinergic and antiparkinsonian drugs; inflammation from trauma, infection or surgery; any acute stress mediated by increased cortisol levels; hypoxia, hypoglycaemia, fluid, electrolyte and other metabolic derangements; and hypotension and hypothermia.

13.9 Management of Delirium

There are no 'routine' investigations for delirium in the ED, and based on a thorough history, collateral information, clinical presentation and physical examination, the following investigations may be employed as needed: haemoglobin, cell count and differential, urea, creatinine and electrolytes, bone profile, chest X-ray, urine dipstick and culture (can be helpful to exclude UTI—see Chap. 16) and CT brain (2–7% pickup rate for a significant neurological lesion) [13].

Once delirium has been detected, management is directed towards addressing the underlying precipitating factors as described in Fig. 13.1.

13.10 Prevention of Delirium in Those at Risk

The most important step in the ED to improve delirium recognition and management is to institute routine screening for the condition and support it by appropriate processes that prevent its development. For example, avoidance of benzodiazepines or anticholinergics may help prevent an episode of delirium in susceptible older people. Medicines with anticholinergic effects are a frequent cause of delirium in older people, and 'anticholinergic burden' is a good means of understanding this risk [14]. Other considerations such as maintaining orientation to surroundings, meeting needs for nutrition and fluids, promoting mobility within the limitations of physical condition and providing visual and hearing adaptations for patients with sensory impairments have been shown to reduce the incidence of delirium in hospital settings (Hospital Elder Life Programme; OR 0.6, CI 0.39–0.92) [15]. These principles could be applied as feasible in the ED although there are no related studies. Appropriate management of pain, constipation, retention of urine and avoiding 'lines and tubes' that restrict mobility also benefits the older person. Environmental considerations include noise insulation, natural lighting, sympathetic décor, signage and low trolley.

13.11 Dementia

Dementia is a progressive disorder of acquired cognitive decline over several months or years. Arousal is not typically affected, although individuals may become agitated in unfamiliar surroundings or situations. Dementia typically affects the whole spectrum of cognitive domains: complex attention, executive functioning (e.g. planning or decision-making), new learning and memory, language (fluency, syntax), perception and emotional/behaviour regulation. Progressive decline in one or more of these domains (usually identified by the individual or a close informant) that is significant enough to affect day-to-day functioning is usually sufficient to make the diagnosis. Impairments in the same cognitive domains that are detectable or reported but that do not unduly impact function are termed mild cognitive impairment (MCI).

13.12 Dementia Subtypes

The pattern of decline and affected cognitive domains can help to determine the underlying aetiology in dementia. For example, the most common form of dementia (Alzheimer's disease) typically follows a smooth but relentless deterioration, whilst the deterioration in vascular dementia is classically stepwise. In practice, distinguishing between the two, which share common aetiologies, is difficult. Prominent personality changes, social disinhibition or emotional lability tend to occur with frontotemporal dementias. Development of Parkinsonian features after the onset of dementia may indicate dementia with Lewy bodies (LBD)—this is often associated with prominent and detailed visual hallucinations early during the disease and marked fluctuations in arousal. Dementia can also occur because of Parkinson's disease (PD); here, the onset of cognitive symptoms is after the onset of PD. Both LBD and dementia of PD are very sensitive to the extrapyramidal side effects of the antipsychotics, and these should be avoided. Rarer causes of dementia (to be considered particularly in early onset disease) include those associated with prion or HIV infections.

13.13 Diagnosis and Management in ED

The diagnosis of dementia should not be made in the context of delirium, ideally not in the acute setting, but by a specialist within a specialist service (e.g. a memory clinic) in the convalescent period. However, the suspicion of an underlying dementia may be raised in the emergency department and should trigger onward referral to the appropriate specialist service (directly or via primary care).

Many patients with a pre-existing diagnosis of dementia will carry hand-held documents (e.g. care plans) which will indicate their baseline cognitive and physical function and offer insight into whether findings are new, as well as useful information about likes, dislikes and potential behavioural triggers. Informant history on duration of memory issues (over the previous 5 years) is an ED friendly way to identify existing, undiagnosed dementia.

All patients with new diagnosis of probable dementia in the ED should be communicated with their family and primary care providers for further assessment and definitive diagnosis.

Patients with dementia may become distressed or agitated in unfamiliar surroundings such as the emergency department. It is important to remember that busy acute hospital settings are a confusing environment for people with dementia. Steps should be taken to minimise the distress caused. Where possible and safe to do so, early discharge or management in the community rather than admission should be considered.

13.14 Service Reconfiguration for the Management of Patients with Cognitive Impairment in ED

The following are useful considerations for delirium care in the ED. They may support structural and process changes which if combined with a measurement framework will offer a programme for delivering quality care in older people with cognitive impairment attending the ED.

- The presence of established policies for the management of people with cognitive impairment, for their support persons/families, for assessment of behavioural disturbances, for in-ED delirium prevention and for pain assessment [16].
- Screen all 75+ for cognitive impairment and delirium as the prevalence starts rising significantly in this age.

- Review the resources to develop a plan for improving care of people with delirium to offer a good experience to patients and families, address patient and service reported outcomes.
- Bring together the multidisciplinary team and ensure communication with information sharing and integrated policies.

References

1. Fong T, Tulebaev S, Inouye S (2009) Delirium in elderly adults: diagnosis, prevention and treatment. Nat Rev Neurol 5:210–220
2. Han J, Shintani A, Eden S, Morandi A, Solberg L, Schnelle J, Dittus R, Storrow A, Ely E (2010) Delirium in the emergency department: an independent predictor of death within six months. Ann Emerg Med 56:244–252
3. Barron E, Holmes J (2013) Delirium within the emergency care setting, occurrence and detection: a systematic review. Emerg Med J 30:263–268
4. Han JH, Zimmerman EE, Cutler N, Schnelle J, Morandi A, Dittus RS, Storrow AB, Ely EW (2009) Delirium in older emergency department patients: recognition, risk factors, and psychomotor subtypes. Acad Emerg Med 16:193–200
5. Mccusker J, Cole M, Abrahamowicz M, Primeau F, Belzile E (2002) Delirium predicts 12-month mortality. Arch Intern Med 162:457–463
6. Kakuma R, du Fort G, Arsenault L, Perrault A, Platt R, Monette J, Moride Y, Wolfson C (2003) Delirium in older emergency department patients discharged home: effect on survival. J Am Geriatr Soc 51:443–450
7. Cole M, Ciampi A, Belzile E, Zhong L (2009) Persistent delirium in older hospital patients: a systematic review of frequency and prognosis. Age Ageing 38:19–26
8. Hendry K, Quinn TJ, Evans JJ, Stott DJ (2015) Informant single screening questions for delirium and dementia in acute care—a cross-sectional test accuracy pilot study. BMC Geriatr 15:17
9. Maclullich A, Ryan T, Cash H (2014) 4AT-Rapid assessment test for delirium [online]. www.the4at.com. Accessed Oct 2014
10. Han JH, Wilson A, Vasilevskis EE, Shintani A, Schnelle JF, Dittus RS, Graves AJ, Storrow AB, Shuster J, Ely EW (2013) Diagnosing delirium in older emergency department patients: validity and reliability of the delirium triage screen and the brief confusion assessment method. Ann Emerg Med 62:457–465
11. Inouye SK, Westendorp RGJ, Saczynski JS (2014) Delirium in elderly people. Lancet 383:911–922
12. Dyer C, Ashton C, Teasdale T (1995) Postoperative delirium. A review of 80 primary data-collection studies. Arch Intern Med 155:461–465
13. Han JH, Wilson A, Ely EW (2010b) Delirium in the older emergency department patient—a quiet epidemic. Emerg Med Clin North Am 28:611–631
14. Fox C, Richardson K, Maidment ID, Savva GM, Matthews FE, Smithard D, Coulton S, Katona C, Boustani MA, Brayne C (2011) Anticholinergic medication use and cognitive impairment in the older population: The Medical Research Council Cognitive Function and Ageing Study. J Am Geriatr Soc 59:1477–1483
15. Inouye SK, Bogardus ST, Charpentier PA, Leo-Summers L, Acampora D, Holford TR, Cooney LM (1999) A Multicomponent intervention to prevent delirium in hospitalized older patients. N Engl J Med 340:669–676
16. Schnitker L, Martin-Khan M, Beattie E, Gray L (2013) What is the evidence to guide best practice for the management of older people with cognitive impairment presenting to emergency departments? A systematic review. Adv Emerg Nurs J 35:154–169

Depression in Acute Geriatric Care

14

R. Prettyman and J. Banerjee

14.1 Introduction and Epidemiology

Depression is the most common mental disorder in late life with overall prevalence estimates ranging from 0.4 to 35% amongst adults over 55 years old [1]. This wide variation in apparent prevalence is accounted for by the different study methodologies used, the wide range of clinical settings studied and the differing thresholds employed for defining cases of depression. However, it is important to remember that depression is a treatable medical condition and not a part of ageing [2].

Large population surveys report cross-sectional prevalence rates for major depression of around 5% in people aged over 65 [3]. However, when milder but clinically significant depressive syndromes are studied, much higher rates are found in the older people in the community (3.6–16.8%), amongst acute medical patients in hospital (7.9–18.2%) in long-term care settings (8.2–16.8%) [4] and in the emergency department (17%). Moreover, older people form a significant proportion of visits to emergency departments by people with mental health disorders (MHDs). In a study in North Carolina [5], those patients aged over 65 years with MHDs accounted for 27.3% of all MHD emergency department visits, and 51.2% were admitted. The most common MHD diagnoses for this age group were psychosis, and stress/anxiety/depression.

Apart from being a source of distress and disability in its own right, depression is a condition of importance for clinicians because of the important associations

---

R. Prettyman (✉)
Consultant Old Age Psychiatrist, Leicester Royal Infirmary, Leicester, UK
e-mail: Richard.Prettyman@leicspart.nhs.uk

J. Banerjee
Emergency Medicine, University Hospitals of Leicester NHS Trust, Leicester, UK

Department of Health Sciences, University of Leicester, Leicester, UK
e-mail: jb234@leicester.ac.uk

with physical illness and disability [6], and the way in which depressed older patients are more likely to experience more adverse overall health outcomes, poorer quality of life and increased utilisation of health and social care resources [7, 8]. Despite being a treatable disorder, there is clear evidence that depression in older people is both under-recognised and then undertreated even when it is recognised.

14.2 Diagnosing Depression in the Acute and Emergency Care Setting

The diagnosis of depression in physically ill older adults must take account of the differences in presentation between younger and older patients and the likely confounding effects of concurrent physical ill health or disability. Studies of detection rates have indicated that correct identification of depression in older adults is associated with significant problems of both false-positive and false-negative ascertainment. There is evidence that as few as 18% of patients suspected of having depression by clinicians actually meet the diagnostic criteria for major depression [9], whilst other studies have highlighted that as many as 100% of older acutely ill patients with significant depressive symptoms may have their mood disorder overlooked [10]. Shah et al. [11] observed significant variability in testing for depression and cognitive impairment in emergency departments, and a two week follow-up revealed a marked decrease in the number of people who originally tested positive. This underlines the complexities in clinical presentation of depression, the multiple comorbidities and the validity of screening tools in the emergency department seen in other studies [11].

Depression rating scales may be helpful screening tools for non-specialists in a physical healthcare setting, but for the reason already alluded to, patients who screen positive will often need more detailed diagnostic review by a clinician with appropriate expertise. In selecting a rating instrument, the clinician needs to be aware that many scales that were originally designed for rating symptoms severity in diagnosed cases are sometimes used as screening tools, a purpose for which they were never originally intended.

Clinicians also need to understand that many rating scales are heavily weighting towards items assessing 'melancholic' somatic symptoms such as sleep and appetite disturbance and reduced energy levels, which will be greatly confounded by the presence of physical comorbidity. The Geriatric Depression Scale [12], available in 30-, 15-, 10- and 4-item forms, has been shown to have good acceptability and performance in assessing depressive symptoms in physically ill and frail older people. The four-item version (see Table 14.3) is very quick and convenient to complete, and if a threshold score of 0/1 is used, it has a sensitivity of 72% and specificity of 90% in acute geriatric inpatients making it a reasonable choice for a screening instrument if time and resources would not permit the use of a longer version [13]. This scale remains the most validated of all screening tools for the geriatric population. Other rating scales that were specifically designed to be used in the context of ongoing and potentially confounding physical symptoms such as the Edinburgh Postnatal Depression Scale [14] and the Hospital Anxiety and Depression (HAD)

14 Depression in Acute Geriatric Care

Table 14.1 Symptoms of depression (ICD-10)

'Typical' core symptoms	• Pervasive and continuous low mood • Loss of interest and enjoyment • Reduced energy/increased fatiguability/tiredness after slight effort
Other common symptoms	• Reduced concentration and attention • Reduced self-esteem and self-confidence • Ideas of guilt and unworthiness (even in a mild type of episode) • Bleak and pessimistic views of the future • Ideas or acts of self-harm or suicide • Disturbed sleep • Diminished appetite

scale [15] may also be useful due to their consequent lower reliance on physical symptomatology.

Whether or not a rating scale is used, the core features that need to be elicited to diagnose depression confidently are (a) pervasive and continuous low mood, (b) an inability to experience pleasure and enjoyment (anhedonia) and (c) tiredness and effort intolerance (see Table 14.1) [WHO—ICD10]. The first two of these in particular are of great value in diagnosing depression in the context of frailty and acute ill health as they are less likely to be confounded by concurrent symptoms of physical disease. As a key fact to be established is whether there has been change relative a previous baseline, it is often easier for the patient to answer a question about such symptoms on a relative rather than an absolute scale. For example, rather than asking the patient if they find life 'pleasurable and enjoyable', the clinician could ask the patient, '…if you think about the things you used to enjoy doing a year ago, do you get as much pleasure from them now?' In most clinically significant depressive disorders, it would be expected that the symptoms would have been present for at least two weeks.

The issue of whether the phenotype of depression in older adults is distinctive from that in younger adults has now been the subject of much descriptive research. It seems that allowing for differences in presentation conferred by different health and social contexts, the symptoms of the mood disorder itself are actually quite similar in adults of all ages; a recent meta-analysis [16] concluded that older depressed patients may experience more agitation and somatic symptoms, whereas feelings of guilt and loss of sexual function may be more prevalent in younger patients.

Depression often coexists with other common mental disorders found in older patients including dementia, delirium and alcohol misuse with which there may be a coincidental or causal association and the clinician needs to be aware that the presence of any of the latter conditions does not exclude the former.

14.3 Risk Assessment in the Depressed Patient

The starkest risk faced by a patient with depression is that of intentional self-harm and suicide. Careful consideration of this risk is essential in all older patients

Table 14.2 Factors associated with highest risk of completed suicide

- Alcohol and substance abuse
- Barriers to accessing mental health care
- Cultural and religious beliefs (e.g. belief that suicide is noble route to resolving personal difficulties)
- **Depression (and other mental disorders)**
- Easy access to lethal methods
- Family history of suicide and self-harm
- Family history of abuse
- Feelings of hopelessness
- Impulsive or aggressive tendencies
- Isolation, a feeling of being cut off from other people
- Local epidemics of suicide
- Loss (relational, social, work, or financial)
- Physical illness
- Previous suicide attempt(s)
- Unwillingness to seek help because of the stigma associated with mental health or with suicidal thoughts

Adapted from WHO Preventing suicide: a global imperative [18]

presenting with depression in whom the absolute risk of suicide has traditionally been greater than for any other age group. Particularly in the case of intentional overdose, a relative lack of medical seriousness should never be taken to indicate a lack of serious intent, and as a rule, all such cases whether 'serious' or not should be referred to the acute liaison or deliberate self-harm team where one is available. Self-harm in these cases should be taken to be evidence of suicidal intent until proven otherwise [17]. The factors associated with the greatest risk of completed suicide are summarised in Table 14.2 [18].

Less dramatic but also potentially life-threatening and easier to overlook are risks of self-neglect, poor nutrition and dehydration, and these areas should be given special attention in the care plan of older patients with suspected depression. Complex management situations can frequently arise where a depressed and acutely physically ill patient is disengaged from therapeutic intervention either due to depressive anergia, lack of motivation or nihilistic thinking in which they may feel they are beyond hope and assistance. Distinguishing patients who are gravely ill and have a realistic appreciation of their prognosis with the understandable effect on their emotional state from those patient who may be physically ill but have a distorted view of their prognosis caused by low mood can be highly challenging, and the advice of a specialist psychiatric liaison team may be helpful if uncertainty persists. In the complex setting of an emergency department, it may be extremely difficult to make this distinction without access to specialists in mental health disorders in older people.

14.4 Therapeutic Intervention in Later Life Depression

A systematic review of the prognosis and treatment outcomes for older versus middle-aged depressed patients [19] found that in older patients, depression was equally responsive to initial treatment as depression in younger adults but that there was a more adverse long-term outcome with higher likelihood of relapse; this is probably due to medical comorbidity, emergent dementia and the larger number of previous episodes of depression in the older patients. The approach to treating depression with psychosocial interventions and medication should therefore be broadly similar in older compared with younger adults. As in many areas of therapeutics, the interpretation of evidence from treatment trials of antidepressants in older people is not straightforward owing to unresolved questions over whether the conditions in such trials (subjects' age, general health status, treatment duration etc.) are generalisable to cases seen in everyday clinical practice. This challenge is arguably greatest for older patients as on any physiological measure, older people tend to exhibit more diversity and heterogeneity than younger adults. The most recent NICE guidance on the treatment of depression in adults acknowledged the limitation of evidence available but reinforces the importance of a stepped care model, and that to be most effective at all ages, antidepressant drug treatment needs to be embedded in a package of support and psychosocial interventions including guided self-help programmes, supervised physical activity programmes and brief focussed psychotherapies such as cognitive behavioural therapy and interpersonal therapy.

14.5 Practical Issues in the Selection, Initiation and Monitoring of Antidepressant Treatment in Acutely Ill Older Patients

In the context of emergency geriatric care, there will be circumstances where it is opportune and clinically highly desirable to initiate antidepressant treatment during the presenting episode of acute illness rather than awaiting illness stabilisation or resolution and discharge from hospital. Moreover, as already noted in many cases, the persistence of significant depressive symptoms will have an adverse impact on the acute outcomes of the patient's physical care and treatment making antidepressant treatment an immediate priority. Nearly all currently licensed antidepressant drugs have broadly similar efficacy, so the choice of treatment will be largely determined by consideration of the drugs' tolerability profiles, secondary effect profiles (e.g. sedating versus non sedating), pharmacokinetic properties and the potential for drug interactions. In most cases, this will lead to the consideration of a selective serotonin reuptake inhibitor drug as first-line treatment or alternatively a well-tolerated sedative antidepressant such as mirtazapine if this particular property is desirable. Although tricyclic and related antidepressants are initiated much less frequently nowadays in all age groups, it is not uncommon to find older patients with long-term recurrent depressive disorders who have been prescribed with these drugs for many years and are taking them at the time of presentation to hospital with an acute health problem. In addition, tricyclic drugs are very commonly used in low doses as an adjunct to pain management. The comparative properties of some of the most commonly prescribed antidepressant drugs together with selected first-generation drugs are summarised in Table 14.3.

Table 14.3 Four-item geriatric depression scale (GDS-4)

Are you basically satisfied with your life?	NO	Yes
Do you feel that your life is empty?	No	YES
Are you afraid that something bad is going to happen to you?	No	YES
Do you feel happy most of the time?	NO	Yes

Scoring—1 point for each capitalized answer: ≥1 = depression or possible depression (see text)

Occasionally, it will be appropriate to consider electroconvulsive therapy (ECT) for severe life-threatening depression in the context of an acute admission to hospital as this is generally the most potent and rapidly affective intervention for the severest forms of depression characterised by psychotic symptoms of profound melancholic disturbance to the point of stupor. Although such patients, especially if frail and acutely physically ill may be high-risk candidates for general anaesthesia, this risk needs to be balanced against the grave risks of non-treatment and the different risks associated which may be associated with antidepressant drug therapy [20]. Safe provision of ECT to patients in a general hospital setting will require close collaboration between physicians, psychiatrists and anaesthetists and, where feasible, transfer of the patient to a psychiatric inpatient unit when physically stable.

References

1. Beekman ATF, Copeland JRM, Prince MJ (1999) Review of community prevalence of depression in later life. Br J Psychiatry 174:307–311
2. Centers for Disease Control and Prevention (2015) http://www.cdc.gov/aging/mentalhealth/depression.htm. Accessed 14 June 2016
3. Byers AL, Yaffe K, Covinsky KE, Friedman MB, Bruce ML (2010) Arch gen psychiatry. High occurrence of mood and anxiety disorders among older adults: the national comorbidity survey replication. Arch Gen Psychiatry 67(5):489–496
4. Polyakova M, Sonnabend N, Sander C, Mergl R, Schroeter ML, Schroeder J, Schönknecht P (2014) Prevalence of minor depression in elderly persons with and without mild cognitive impairment: a systematic review. J Affect Disord 152-154:28–38
5. Hakenewerth AM, Tintinalli JE, Waller AE, Ising A (2015) Emergency department visits by older adults with mental illness in North Carolina. West J Emerg Med 16(7):1142–1145
6. Bradshaw LE, Goldberg SE, Lewis SA, Whittamore K, Gladman JRF, Jones RG, Harwood R (2013) Six-month outcomes following an emergency hospital admission for older adults with co-morbid mental health problems indicate complexity of care needs. Age Ageing 42:582–588
7. Fiske A, Wetherell JL, Gatz M (2009) Depression in older adults. Ann Rev Clin Psychol 5:363–389
8. Prina AM, Huisman M, Yeap BB, Hankey GJ, Flicker L, Brayne C, Almeida OP (2013) Association between depression and hospital outcomes among older men. Can Med Assoc J 185(2):117–123
9. Mojtabai R (2014) Diagnosing depression in older adults in primary care. N Engl J Med 370(13):1180–1182
10. Meldon SW, Emerman CL, Schubert DSP, Moffa DA, Etheart RG (1997) Depression in geriatric ED patients: prevalence and recognition. Ann Emerg Med 30(2):141–145

11. Shah MN, Richardson TM, Jones CMC, Swanson PA, Schneider SM, Katz P, Conwell Y (2011) Depression and cognitive impairment in older adult emergency department patients: changes over two weeks. J Am Geriatr Soc 59(2):321–326
12. Yesavage JA, Brink TL, Rose TL et al (1982) Development and validation of a geriatric depression screening scale: a preliminary report. J Psychiatr Res 17(1):37–49
13. Shah A, Herbert R, Lewis S, Mahendran R, Platt J, Bhattacharya B (1997) Screening for depression among acutely ill geriatric inpatients with a short geriatric depression scale. Age Ageing 26:217–221
14. Cox JL, Holden JM, Sagovsky R (1987) Detection of postnatal depression: development of the 10-item Edinburgh postnatal depression scale. Br J Psychiatry 150:782–786
15. Zigmond AS, Snaith RP (1983) The hospital anxiety and depression scale. Acta Psychiatr Scand 67(6):361–370
16. Hegeman JM, Kok RM, van der Mast RC, Giltay EJ (2012) Phenomenology of depression in older compared with younger adults: meta-analysis. Br J Psychiatry 200(4):275–281. doi:10.1192/bjp.bp.111.095950
17. National Institute for Clinical Excellence (2004) Self-harm: NICE guideline CG16
18. World Health Organisation (2014) Preventing suicide: a global imperative. WHO, Geneva
19. Mitchell AJ, Subramaniam H (2005) Prognosis of depression in old age compared to middle age: a systematic review of comparative studies. Am J Psychiatry 162(9):1588–1601
20. National Institute for Clinical Excellence (2009) Guidance on the use of electroconvulsive therapy: NICE technical appraisal guideline TA59

Abdominal Pain in Older Patients

15

Zerrin Defne Dündar, A. Bulent Dogrul, Mehmet Ergin, and R. Tuna Dogrul

15.1 Introduction

Acute abdominal pain (AAP) is a common complaint in older patients and represents a diagnostic challenge for emergency physicians (EPs). The term of AAP refers to pain with sudden and unexpected onset with duration less than 24 h. It can be accompanied by other gastrointestinal symptoms. An early and accurate diagnosis is critical in older patients with AAP.

Many diseases can be the cause of AAP, which can be atypically expressed in older patients as compared to younger patients. The evaluation of AAP is different than younger patients because of physiologic, pharmacologic, and psychosocial aspects, specific to older patients. Current comorbidities and polypharmacy can change signs and findings of the physical examination. Late presentation to the emergency department (ED) is frequent. All of these factors lead to decrease the

---

Z.D. Dündar, MD
Department of Emergency Medicine, Necmettin Erbakan University Meram School of Medicine, Konya, Turkey
e-mail: zerdef@hotmail.com

A.B. Dogrul, MD
Department of General Surgery, Hacettepe University School of Medicine, Ankara, Turkey
e-mail: adogrul@hacettepe.edu.tr

M. Ergin, MD (✉)
Department of Emergency Medicine, Yıldırım Beyazıt University School of Medicine, Ankara, Turkey
e-mail: drmehmetergin@gmail.com

R.T. Dogrul, MD
Division of Geriatrics, Department of Internal Medicine, Hacettepe University School of Medicine, Ankara, Turkey
e-mail: Rana_tuna@hotmail.com

diagnostic accuracy with higher rate of mortality in older patients as compared to younger patients.

Age-related physiological changes that can affect every organ systems result in occurrence of the disease causing the abdominal pain with atypical clinical presentation and different response to interventions. Perception of pain is often suppressed in older patients due to decrease in immune response and changes in neurological system. Patients with bacteremia often do not develop fever, and even hypothermia could be observed.

A wide range of differential diagnosis, delayed admissions to the ED, and atypical presentations leads to misdiagnosis and poor outcomes in older patients with AAP.

15.2 Epidemiology

Although the epidemiology of AAP depends on geographical and ethnic origin of older patients, complaints related to gastrointestinal system are the most frequent cause of visits to the ED. Diagnoses related to the gastrointestinal system are ranked number two after cardiovascular chief complaints [1]. Diagnostic challenge in the management of AAP in the ED is related to physiological changes due to age and the weakening of inflammatory responses. Gastrointestinal changes with aging include decreased emptying time and fundal compliance, increased acid secretion, increased diverticula in the bowel, and increased colonic transit time [2–4].

As compared to younger patients, older patients have worse clinical outcomes, greater hospitalization rates, and longer length of stay in the ED and in the hospital [5]. It has been reported that about 60% of older patients visiting the ED with AAP are hospitalized, 20% require surgical or invasive interventions, and about 10% return to the ED with the same complaint [6, 7]. While mortality rates differ depending on the underlying pathology and comorbidities, total mortality ranges between 5 and 10% in older patients, which represents tenfold of the mortality rate in younger patients [5]. Again, it has been reported that delays in diagnosis increase mortality rate twofold in advanced age, particularly after 80 years of age [8]. It was also reported that there are no differences between male and female with regard to the number of tests done, surgical diagnosis, and hospitalization [6].

15.3 General Approach

15.3.1 History and Physical Examination

Obtaining a detailed history of AAP from older patients can be difficult. Cognitive and physical incompetency associated with advancing age must be carefully evaluated, and EPs must be sure of the reliability of the medical history. Older patients with a history of previous strokes, dementia, or Alzheimer's disease may be unable to express their subjective symptoms accurately. EPs must consider the functional loss in hearing, speaking, and visual capacity of their patients. Furthermore, older patients or their caregivers may accept the symptoms as the natural consequences of advanced age and can have a tendency of erroneous perception [5]. History of older patients must therefore be obtained both from the patient and from the caregiver, which will provide more comprehensive details. Finally, the caregiver must always be interviewed about the basic status of the patient.

It must be remembered that abuse is more frequent in the older population than the other age groups. If any inconsistencies that might lead to a suspicion of abuse must be taken into consideration, the history and physical examination must be detailed in suspicion of sexual abuse findings, which can be expressed by acute abdominal pain [9].

As with all other age groups, information that must be obtained from older patients in relation with AAP must include the following:

- When did AAP start, and for how long has it been present?
- How did the AAP start? Suddenly or gradually?
- What is the localization of the AAP? Upper right quadrant, diffuse, lower left quadrant, etc.
- What is the quality of the pain? Colic, continuous, with intervals, severe, gradually increasing, etc.
- Does the course of pain change during the day?
- Does the pain refer to another anatomical area? Back, retrosternal area, inguinal area, etc.
- Are there factors that increase or decrease the pain? Eating, drugs, position or exposure to cold, etc.
- Has she/he experienced similar pain previously?
- When were the last meal, last defecation, and emission of gas?
- Does the color or consistency of stool change?
- Are there any accompanying symptoms? Nausea, vomiting, anorexia, fever, dysuria, tenesmus, diarrhea, vertigo, syncope, black stool, red stool, dyspnea, etc.
- Has she/he undergone any abdominal surgery previously?
- Has the patient undergone any abdominal diseases including pancreatitis, cholecystitis, or diverticulitis?
- What is the personal past medical history? Are there any comorbidities including diabetes mellitus, coronary artery disease, chronic heart failure, atrial fibrillation, hypertension, chronic liver disease, atherosclerosis, or peripheral vascular disease?
- What are the drugs used? Nonsteroidal anti-inflammatory drugs (NSAIDs), steroids, anticoagulants, digoxin, etc.
- Has the patient started any new medications?
- Does the patient have trauma in his/her history?

Physical examination of patients with AAP requires a deep and complete evaluation in the ED. Like all patients in the ED, physical examination starts with the evaluation of vital signs and making the decision about whether the patient has any life-threatening hemodynamic instability.

Prevalence of life-threatening situations in older patients is greater than in younger patients. In contrast, a misleading wellness status can be present in the vital signs of older patients despite serious underlying conditions, depending on their decreased physiologic reserves [10]. For example, an older patient with hypertension may have a normal heart rate and normal arterial blood pressure while he/she also has severe hypovolemic shock due to decreased chronotropic response and increased peripheral vascular resistance. Also, in patients using beta-blockers, calcium channel blockers, or digoxin, vital signs may not correlate with the severity of underlying condition or medications such as immunosuppressive drugs, NSAIDs, opioid analgesics, steroids, or chemotherapeutical drugs which can alter the anti-inflammatory response to the disease. Fever response to infections in the older patients can be blunted or delayed during clinical course. In some cases, hypothermia can be observed [5]. In one study, 30% of older patients with AAP did not present with fever and leukocytosis [11].

Muscular defense and rebound signs in the abdominal examination may not be found in the older patients despite serious intra-abdominal diseases because of the thinner abdominal wall, degenerated inflammation process, and abolition of peripheral nerve functions [12]. It was shown that only 17% of older patients presented to the ED with classic symptoms in perforated appendicitis [13]. Negative abdominal examination findings can exist during the course of life-threatening diseases such as mesenteric ischemia or perforation. Pain with specific localization, e.g., pain localized in the lower right quadrant for acute appendicitis, is generally more saddle in older patients than in younger patients or can be seen in atypical localizations [13]. Furthermore, older patients tend to feel the pain specific for renal colic, pancreatitis, myocardial infarction, appendicitis, or peptic ulcer less compared to younger patients. A linear decrease in pain perception is observed with increasing age [14].

Inguinal and umbilical areas must be carefully examined for hernia. Urinary retention can be the cause of a globe in the bladder and responsible for AAP. The bladder globe must therefore always be excluded in older patients with AAP, and digital anal and genital examination must be systematically performed.

15.3.2 Differential Diagnosis

More serious and life-threatening conditions can be detected in older patients as compared to younger patients. While reported with varying frequencies in different series, diseases frequently diagnosed in the older patient group include the following: gallbladder disease, intestinal obstruction, acute appendicitis, diverticulitis, peptic ulcer disease (PUD), mesenteric ischemia, abdominal aortic aneurysm (AAA), pancreatitis, gastroenteritis, and urinary tract infections (UTIs) [7, 15].

The underlying pathology cannot be diagnosed in 20% of older patients who present to the ED with AAP [7]. Those patients were discharged after long periods of observation with the diagnosis of nonspecific abdominal pain (NSAP) [7].

Just like the pediatric patients group, older patients with extra-abdominal diseases can have atypical presentation with AAP as the main symptom. Therefore, life-threatening conditions including myocardial infarction, pneumonia, diabetic ketoacidosis, or intoxications must be systematically considered in the differential diagnosis.

15.3.3 Laboratory Studies

Laboratory test results from blood sampling can help in the differential diagnosis in older patients. Since the findings from history and physical examination are less informative in older patients than in younger patients, the threshold values should be kept at a lower level to order diagnostic tests. The complete blood count (CBC), liver function and renal function tests, pancreatic enzymes, and urinalysis are ordered frequently while planning target-oriented studies in older patients. However, tests including bleeding profile, cardiac enzymes, blood lactate level, C-reactive protein (CRP), and arterial blood gas (ABG) should also be considered in selected cases [16].

Certain characteristics depending on age and comorbidities must be considered when evaluating blood test results in older patients. Although a CBC test is frequently ordered in the management of AAP, it is not generally a diagnostic test. While the finding of leukocytosis indicates the presence of an inflammatory or infectious process, sensitivity and specificity of leukocytosis for the differential diagnosis of AAP are rather low in the older patients as compared to younger patients. Life-threatening conditions may have course with white blood cell (WBC) count that is within normal limits of its range. Therefore, blood tests such as WBC count or CRP should not be accepted as a single parameter that will change the treatment plan in older patients [12]. The other common blood tests performed for evaluation of abdominal pain are:

(1) Renal function tests (urea and creatinine) are needed in older patients to determine the level of age-related renal function loss. Serum electrolyte levels must also be ordered in patients with symptoms including nausea, vomiting, diarrhea, or low oral intake, findings related to dehydration in the physical examination, and previous diuretic use.
(2) Liver function tests and level of pancreatic enzymes (amylase and lipase) guide the diagnosis of biliary and pancreatic diseases common in older patients. However, it must be kept in mind that acute cholecystitis can already have developed despite biochemical tests within normal limits.
(3) Arterial blood gas analysis can be ordered for the evaluation of the acid-base disorders as well as the respiratory status of patients. It is also helpful for the diagnosis of extra-abdominal causes of AAP. ABG analysis is guiding for both diagnosis and treatment of many diseases including diabetic ketoacidosis, renal failure, sepsis, pneumonia, and mesenteric ischemia.
(4) Serum lactate level provides valuable information in the evaluation of both mesenteric ischemia and sepsis in relation with intra-abdominal diseases. Serial measurements of serum lactate levels in patients who are hemodynamically

unstable are important to evaluate the success of the initial resuscitation and to determine the prognosis [17, 18].
(5) Urinalysis must be ordered for the rule out of UTI and hematuria. Tendency for UTI increases in older patients, and such infections can be expressed with nonspecific symptoms including nausea, vomiting, or impairment of oral intake and without symptoms such as fever or dysuria. Urine density can provide information about the hydration status of the patients. Urinary level of ketone can also provide information about the oral intake impairment or the underlying status of ketoacidosis. More of the urinary tract infections in older patients will be discussed in Chap. 16.

15.3.4 Imaging Studies

Management of AAP in older patients has gained a new dimension with the evolution of imaging methods such as ultrasonography (USG) and computerized tomography (CT). EPs have a tendency to perform imaging studies more aggressively in an increasing number of patients in order to decrease diagnostic errors related to unreliable and non-informative findings of the physical examination and indecisive results of laboratory tests [6].

The decision to perform imaging studies in older patients with AAP should be based on the clinical status of the patient, clues obtained from history, and physical examination. The following imagings are classically used in the ED:

(1) Plain abdominal X-rays should not be used systematically in AAP (see review from [19]). Plain films are supplemented by further imaging studies to confirm the diagnosis, to identify the cause and characteristics, or to localize the site of occlusion or of a foreign body [19].

   Plain abdominal radiographs currently have no place in the exploration of abdominal emergencies, due to insufficient diagnostic efficacy, loss of time, additional expense, and unnecessary irradiation [19]. The chest X-ray can diagnose perforation by free air under the diaphragm or pneumonia by infiltrations in the lungs.

(2) Ultrasonography (USG) is becoming the first imaging test used for the differential diagnosis of AAP whatever the age. Despite its advantages, such as quick results, absence of radiation, and that it can be done at the bedside in the ED, it has some disadvantages, including the experience of the technician and quality of the device or the presence of intestinal gas artifacts. USG is the first imaging choice in diseases related to bile ducts as well as in case of abdominal aortic aneurysm (AAA) and aneurysmal rupture. Normal USG findings cannot eliminate serious diseases in older patients.

(3) Computed tomography (CT) is gradually gaining a central position in the management of older patients with AAP. It has been reported that the use of CT in the ED increases diagnostic accuracy from 30–35% to 50–75% in older patients with AAP. The decision to discharge patients or to go for a surgical intervention

has been directly affected in this age group [20, 21]. In a recent study, it has been reported that 55% of CTs performed in older patients with AAP have shown anomalies, including small intestinal obstruction (18%), diverticulitis (9%), non-ischemic vascular diseases (6%), and mesenteric ischemia (4%). Based on the results of this study, 43% of these diagnoses were not suspected before the CT scan. CT scan results have changed the treatment plan and decision for discharge in 65% of older patients [6].

One of the important issues for EPs is the use of contrast products during contrast-enhanced CT scanning when making the decision for advanced imaging studies. While radiation is an important issue in younger patients, nephropathy that can develop in relation with the contrast product becomes a major risk in older patients due to decreased kidney functions. However, the decision for non-contrast or contrast-enhanced CT scanning should be made according to benefit-risk assessment based on the presence of findings in the physical examination suggesting life-threatening conditions and clinical status of the patient. It has been reported that emergent CT scan enhanced with only intravenous (IV) contrast substance does not cause erroneous or delayed diagnoses in patients with AAP [22]. When contrast-enhanced CT scanning indication is obvious, usage of only IV contrast substance appears rational to prevent loss of time and decrease the quantity of contrast substance used in older patients.

15.3.5 Management

The major problem in the management of older patients with AAP in the ED is related to difficulties in establishing a certain diagnosis. Possible reasons include communication problems with older patients, unusual symptoms and clinical findings, and uncertain laboratory presentations. Early use of imaging in appropriate patients may reduce the delay in the diagnosis [23].

Older patients with AAP should be monitored for vital signs, mental status, and respiratory failure. Intravenous fluid management should be started with normal saline or lactated Ringer's solution. The intravascular fluid status should be monitored via blood pressure, heart rate, and urine output. Older patients with AAP should not be fed by mouth until surgical pathology is excluded [24]. Figure 15.1 shows an algorithm of management of older patients with AAP.

A recent study showed that emergent gastrointestinal surgical procedures in older patients did not differ from those in younger patients. However, the morbidity and mortality rates were higher in older patients. Assessing comorbidities, frailty, the diagnosis, and the patient's wishes and status should help in the decision-making for emergency surgical management [23]. Overall mortality approaches 20–25% in older patients who underwent emergent abdominal surgery. The American Society of Anesthesiologists (ASA) grading, interval from onset of symptoms to admission, presence of mesenteric infarction, palliative bypass, and nontherapeutic laparotomy

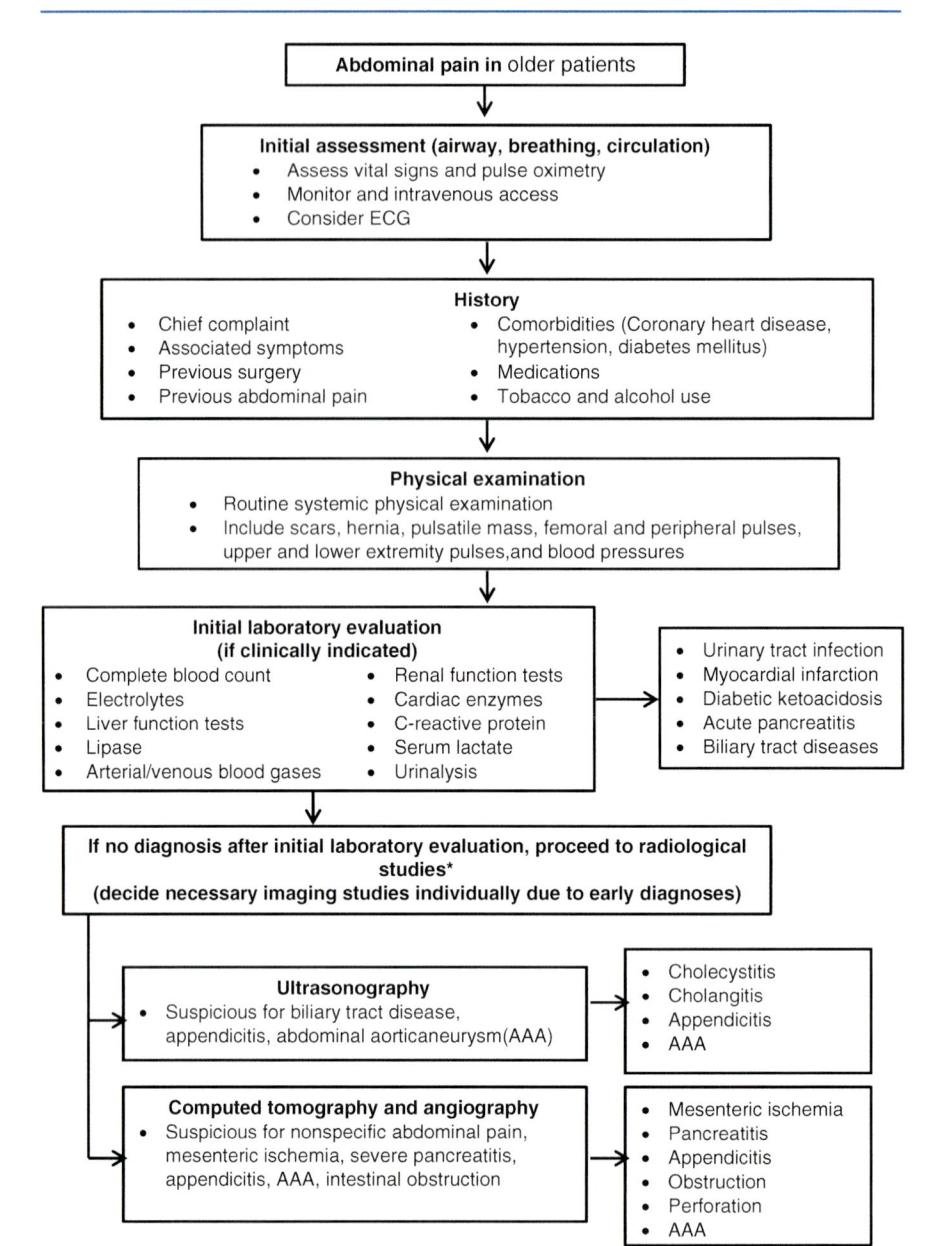

```
┌─────────────────────────────────────────┐
│      Abdominal pain in older patients   │
└─────────────────────────────────────────┘
                    ↓
┌─────────────────────────────────────────┐
│  Initial assessment (airway, breathing, circulation)
│  • Assess vital signs and pulse oximetry
│  • Monitor and intravenous access
│  • Consider ECG
└─────────────────────────────────────────┘
                    ↓
┌─────────────────────────────────────────┐
│                 History                 │
│  • Chief complaint      • Comorbidities (Coronary heart disease,
│  • Associated symptoms    hypertension, diabetes mellitus)
│  • Previous surgery     • Medications
│  • Previous abdominal pain • Tobacco and alcohol use
└─────────────────────────────────────────┘
                    ↓
┌─────────────────────────────────────────┐
│          Physical examination           │
│  • Routine systemic physical examination
│  • Include scars, hernia, pulsatile mass, femoral and peripheral pulses,
│    upper and lower extremity pulses, and blood pressures
└─────────────────────────────────────────┘
                    ↓
┌───────────────────────────────────┐    ┌──────────────────────────┐
│  Initial laboratory evaluation    │    │ • Urinary tract infection│
│       (if clinically indicated)   │    │ • Myocardial infarction  │
│  • Complete blood count           │ →  │ • Diabetic ketoacidosis  │
│  • Electrolytes                   │    │ • Acute pancreatitis     │
│  • Liver function tests           │    │ • Biliary tract diseases │
│  • Lipase                         │    └──────────────────────────┘
│  • Arterial/venous blood gases    │
│  • Renal function tests           │
│  • Cardiac enzymes                │
│  • C-reactive protein             │
│  • Serum lactate                  │
│  • Urinalysis                     │
└───────────────────────────────────┘
                    ↓
┌─────────────────────────────────────────┐
│  If no diagnosis after initial laboratory evaluation, proceed to radiological
│                        studies*
│  (decide necessary imaging studies individually due to early diagnoses)
└─────────────────────────────────────────┘
                    ↓
┌───────────────────────────────────┐    ┌──────────────────────────┐
│         Ultrasonography           │    │ • Cholecystitis          │
│  • Suspicious for biliary tract disease,│ • Cholangitis            │
│    appendicitis, abdominal aorticaneurysm(AAA)│• Appendicitis      │
│                                   │ →  │ • AAA                    │
└───────────────────────────────────┘    └──────────────────────────┘

┌───────────────────────────────────┐    ┌──────────────────────────┐
│  Computed tomography and angiography│  │ • Mesenteric ischemia    │
│  • Suspicious for nonspecific abdominal pain, │ • Pancreatitis    │
│    mesenteric ischemia, severe pancreatitis,  │ • Appendicitis    │
│    appendicitis, AAA, intestinal obstruction  │ • Obstruction     │
│                                   │ →  │ • Perforation            │
│                                   │    │ • AAA                    │
└───────────────────────────────────┘    └──────────────────────────┘
```

*Recent publications recommend not using plain abdominal radiographs in the management of AAP (see review from Dubuisson et al 2015).

Fig. 15.1 Algorithm for acute abdominal pain management in older patients (Adapted from [16])

are predictors of mortality [25]. Twenty-five percent of older patients who have undergone emergency abdominal surgery are faced with local morbidity, and 30% of them are faced with systemic morbidity. The leading local morbidity is wound infection, whereas the leading systemic morbidity is respiratory failure [25].

Another important point is to manage older patients with AAP in a multidisciplinary approach. Recent data have confirmed that multidisciplinary care improves outcomes for older surgical patients [23, 26]. Diagnostic and therapeutic decisions should involve EPs, surgeons, anesthesiologists, and geriatricians. It is recommended that protocol-driven integrating pathways can guide care of older patients effectively, but the critical decisions should be individualized for each patient [23, 26].

15.4 Specific Causes

15.4.1 Acute Mesenteric Ischemia

Acute mesenteric ischemia (AMI) is a disease of older patients with a rate of 0.1–2/1000 acute hospital admissions [27]. It is mostly seen in patients over 70 years old and is more common than abdominal aneurysm in patients older than 75 years of age [28]. Arterial embolism and thrombus are the two most common causes of AMI. Women are affected slightly more frequently, but exact gender ratio differs according to the etiology of AMI (Table 15.1) [29]. Despite many advances in the diagnosis and treatment of AMI in the last 3–4 decades, prognosis is still poor. In-hospital mortality rate ranges from 59 to 93% [29, 30].

AMI can be classified into two main groups: thrombotic and non-thrombotic. Thrombotic AMI can be a result of arterial embolism, thrombosis, and mesenteric venous thrombosis (MVT). Non-thrombotic AMI, mainly named as non-occlusive mesenteric ischemia (NOMI) and secondary to low flow states such as cardiogenic shock, sepsis, and hypovolemia, is primarily seen in patients hospitalized in intensive care units [29–32]. Decreased cardiac output causes diffuse mesenteric vasoconstriction leading to ischemia and necrosis.

Arterial embolism is the most common cause of AMI. Onset is usually rapid. Since superior mesenteric artery (SMA) emerges from the aorta with an acute angle, emboli have an affinity for SMA. Most emboli arise from cardiac origin. Arterial thrombosis has the worst prognosis because it involves the origin of the SMA, and the onset is more insidious. MVT accounts for 10% of AAP. Ninety percent of MVTs have an identifiable cause (Table 15.2) and may be acute or chronic.

Table 15.1 Incidence, mortality, and demographics of patients according to the cause of acute mesenteric ischemia [29]

Etiology	Incidence (%)	Mean mortality (%)	Mean age	Female/male ratio
Arterial embolism	34	66–71	69	1.23
Arterial thrombus	34	70–87	71	1.46
Mesenteric venous thrombosis	13	44	70	0.78
Non-occlusive mesenteric ischemia	19	70–80	69	1.17
Overall		64–74		

Table 15.2 Conditions that predispose to mesenteric venous thrombosis

- Hypercoagulable states (antithrombin III deficiency, protein C/S deficiency, factor V Leiden, PCV, etc.)
- Direct injury or inflammation (surgery, trauma, pancreatitis, cholecystitis, etc.)
- Venous stasis (Budd-Chiari, cirrhosis, postsplenectomy, etc.)

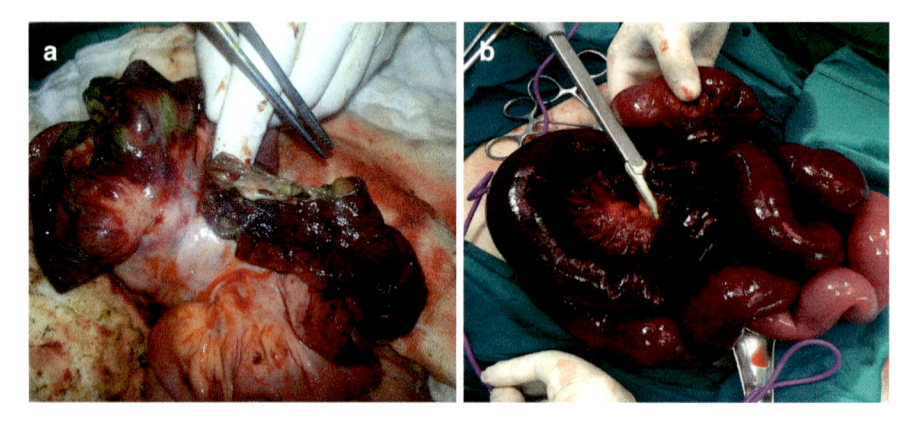

Fig. 15.2 (**a**) Acute mesenteric ischemia resulted in diffuse necrosis and perforation in jejunal segments. (**b**) Mesenteric venous thrombosis causing necrosis, which required surgical treatment

Whatever the cause, the result is a breakdown of mucosal barrier, bacterial translocation, migration of polymorphonuclear leukocytes, and activation of inflammatory pathways. Reperfusion can cause ischemia perfusion injury and worsen the condition. Systemic inflammatory response syndrome, disseminated intravascular coagulation, sepsis, and multiorgan failure are the final expression in these patients.

The most important step in the diagnosis of AMI is clinical suspicion in older patients with chief complaint of AAP. Some risk factors must be recorded such as atrial fibrillation, history of coronary artery disease and myocardial infarction, recent cardiac or vascular surgery, prior embolism, chronic mesenteric ischemia symptoms, history of prior deep venous thrombosis, hypercoagulable states, etc. Only 33% of patients had been suspected of AMI before they died of mesenteric ischemia [29–32].

AAP is the most common symptom of AMI. At the beginning, ischemia causes cramping abdominal pain, but tenderness is minimal. When intestinal necrosis develops, diffuse peritonitis appears with a rigid abdomen and sepsis (Fig. 15.2a). Bowel sounds are usually absent but may be present at the beginning. Depending on the cause, other symptoms such as vomiting, diarrhea, distention, and blood in stool may be present. Older patients may have less frequent abdominal pain and more often symptoms such as tachypnea and mental status changes [29–31].

Laboratory findings are increased WBC (usually > 15,000/mm^3), D-dimer, lactate levels, and metabolic acidosis is observed. Metabolic alkalosis may also be seen because of vomiting. However, sensitivity and specificity of those markers range from 38–96% to 40–84%, respectively. Intestinal fatty acid binding protein has promising results with 90% sensitivity and 89% specificity. Patients may have elevated amylase levels, abnormal liver enzymes, and hyperphosphatemia. Electrocardiography may reveal arrhythmia [29–32].

Pneumatosis intestinalis, free air, air-fluid levels, portal venous gas, thumb printing, or thickening of the bowel wall may be seen on abdominal X-ray, but 25% of patients with AMI have normal findings. Although in classical textbooks, conventional angiography is still accepted as the gold standard for diagnosing AMI, CT angiography has replaced it with a sensitivity and specificity of 94 and 95%. In patients with peritoneal signs, early surgery is indicated because these signs reflect presence of infarction [30, 31]. However, conventional mesenteric angiography may still be the first choice in NOMI [27].

Aggressive volume resuscitation, urinary catheterization, nasogastric decompression, blood sampling for CBC, renal function test, liver function tests, arterial blood gas analysis, and crossmatch should be done. The patient must be stabilized as much as possible before the transfer to the operating room. EPs should consider broad spectrum antibiotic treatment and first dose of anticoagulation therapy in the ED.

Revascularization, assessment of intestinal viability, and resection of necrotic bowel are the main principles of the surgical treatment. The first 6 h of management is critical to decrease the mortality. MVT and NOMI are usually treated nonsurgically. Surgical treatment is indicated in patients with bowel necrosis occurring in 20% of MVT (Fig. 15.2b). Treatment of underlying cause is the mainstay therapy of NOMI. Papaverine infusion via the intra-arterial catheter may be beneficial in resolving vasoconstriction without the need for surgery.

15.4.2 Abdominal Aortic Aneurysm

Abdominal aortic aneurysm is defined by an aortic diameter greater than 3 cm. Prevalence of AAA varies between 4 and 9% in males and 0.2 and 2% in females [33]. Risk factors include old age, male gender, smoking, positive family history, high height, coronary artery disease, hypercholesterolemia, hypertension, and atherosclerosis [33].

AAA is usually asymptomatic. It is frequently found in imaging studies in the ED or in outpatient clinics. However, sometimes patients go to the ED with AAP related to life-threatening rupture. About one half of the patients with aneurysm rupture cannot reach the ED following the rupture. Hypertension, smoking, female gender, larger diameter of the aneurysm, growth rate of the aneurysm, and wall tension of the aneurysm are risk factors for AAA rupture [33, 34].

Older patients with AAA can present with sudden, severe, and unchanging back or abdominal pain depending on the growth rate of the aneurysm. Abdominal pain can be unclear in such patients, and nonspecific symptoms such as syncope, paralysis in the lower extremities, and sensation of fullness in flanks can be the presenting symptoms. Patients who have atypical clinical expression can be misdiagnosed as renal colic, constipation, gas distension, diverticulitis, or NSAP.

Ultrasonography is the first choice imaging study for AAA. Sensitivity of USG approaches 95% and its specificity is 100% for the diagnosis of AAA. Detection of the intra-abdominal free fluid and hemorrhage at bedside are additional advantages in older patients with suspicion of rupture [35].

The second imaging study to be preferred for the diagnosis of AAA or its rupture is CT scan with a sensitivity of approximately 100%. Furthermore, CT scan provides valuable information about the diameter of the aorta, aortic area affected from the aneurism, visceral artery involvement, retroperitoneal bleeding, and renal abnormalities [33]. Detailed information about the aorta and its branches can be obtained with CT angiography, which can provide all information required for the treatment plan of AAA [36].

15.4.3 Intestinal Obstruction

Intestinal obstruction may affect the bowel or the colon. Adhesions as a result of previous surgery and hernias are the most common cause of intestinal obstruction, whereas malignancy is most common in colonic obstruction. Other causes include gallstone ileus, sigmoid volvulus, and diverticulitis. The gallstone ileus is unique to the older population and can cause intestinal obstruction in 20% of patients older than 65 years with a high rate of mortality [16]. Patients usually present with classical findings of intestinal obstruction, air in the biliary tree, and calculus on plain abdominal radiographs [32].

The other signs are colicky abdominal pain with nausea and vomiting. Colonic obstructions may be more insidious in onset [16]. Obstruction in any localization may be complete or incomplete depending on the degree of obstruction. Physical examination usually reveals altered bowel sounds, signs of hypovolemia, distention, and tenderness. Peritoneal signs may be present if necrosis or perforation has developed.

Imaging which shows distended small bowel loops, air-fluid levels, and absence of air in the large bowel should indicate intestinal obstruction. The dilated large bowel with haustral markings is the classical finding of colonic obstruction [16, 32].

The first step in the management of obstruction is the evaluation of vital signs and hydration status. Intravenous hydration, nasogastric decompression, correction of any electrolyte abnormality, urinary catheterization, and diagnostic work-up must be done quickly in the ED. Definitive treatment depends on clinical presentation. If peritoneal findings are present, urgent laparotomy may be necessary. Otherwise, patients may be treated conservatively, and the decision will be made depending on the findings in the follow-up period.

15.4.4 Acute Diverticulitis

Diverticulosis is seen in 10% of the population younger than 40 years of age. Incidence increases with age; 70% of patients older than 80 years have a diverticulosis. The most commonly affected side of the colon is the sigmoid region. About 10–30% of the patients with diverticulosis may have painful diverticular disease or diverticulitis [16, 37].

Painful diverticular disease is characterized by attacks of abdominal pain without inflammatory findings. When fever, leukocytosis, and peritoneal irritation signs are present, it is called diverticulitis, which is associated with microperforation in one of the diverticula. Beyond microperforation, patients may have diverticular perforation causing localized or generalized peritonitis, or abscess [32].

Depending on the extension of the inflammation, clinical signs and management may differ from oral antibiotics in outpatient clinics to urgent laparotomy and supportive care in the intensive care unit. Diagnosis can be made by history and clinical findings. A CT scan may be necessary to make diagnosis and determine the extension of the inflammation. Colonoscopy and barium enema should be avoided in the acute phase of the disease [32].

15.4.5 Acute Appendicitis

Older patients with acute appendicitis (AA) present frequently to the ED with generalized pain, rigidity, hypoactive bowel sounds, longer period of complaints, and a mass. However, it has been shown that this difference is not due to a difference in process of AA in older patients but rather to the late presentation to the ED [16].

Although anorexia, nausea, vomiting, and pain in the right lower quadrant are the main symptoms of patients with AA, clinical findings depend on the stage of the disease at the admission. Findings may not be specific at the beginning, whereas other signs include tachycardia, tachypnea, hypotension, oliguria, and acute abdomen such as rigidity and rebound tenderness (localized or generalized). Fever may not be present.

Ultrasonography is the first choice for the diagnosis of AA. However, since it is operative dependent, it may not always be accurate nor decrease rate of negative appendectomies. In patients with suspected diagnosis or in conditions needed to eliminate other causes of abdominal pain, CT scan with contrast enhanced may be the choice (sensitivity 91–98.5% and specificity 90–98%) [16, 38, 39]. A recent meta-analysis demonstrated that magnetic resonance imaging (MRI) for the diagnosis of AA has a sensitivity and specificity of 96% and 96%, respectively, for the general population and 94 and 97% for pregnant patients [39]. The use of MRI for diagnosis of AA can be used in older patients, but the availability 24 h a day could be a major limitation. Further investigations are needed in older patients.

Appendectomy is the treatment of choice for AA. However, in a report analyzing five randomized control studies, appendectomy versus antibiotic treatment was compared in cases of uncomplicated AA. This meta-analysis demonstrated that antibiotic treatment could be a choice for treatment of uncomplicated AA. But only two studies included patients older than 65 years of age in their analysis [40]. Further investigations are needed in older patients.

15.4.6 Bile Tract Diseases

Disease related to bile ducts is frequently diagnosed in older patients with AAP in the ED. Physiological changes related to bile ducts and bile production appear in relation to advancing age. Lithogenicity of the bile, diameter of common bile duct, and formation of pigmented bile stone increase with advanced age [41]. The frequency of bile stone secondary to these physiological changes increases, and about 30–40% of patients aged 65 years or older have cholelithiasis [5]. In addition, pathologies including choledocholithiasis, gallbladder perforation, gangrenous cholecystitis, bile stone ileus, or pancreatitis related to bile stones are more frequent in older patients compared to younger patients.

The diagnosis of cholecystitis in older patients can be more difficult than in young patients. Systemic symptoms including nausea, vomiting, or fever could be missing in older patients despite the pain or sensation of fullness in the upper right quadrant. Laboratory tests may not be helpful for the diagnosis. WBC count can be in the normal range. Therefore, the threshold for imaging studies must be kept lower for older patients when diseases related to bile ducts are suspected.

The risk of developing gangrenous cholecystitis is greater in older patients. Gangrenous cholecystitis is more frequent, particularly in male patients with comorbidities including coronary artery disease or diabetes mellitus. Clinical status of the patient can be unaltered, even in the presence of gangrene in the gallbladder. Surgery should be planned in the early phase of cholecystitis in older patients [42, 43].

15.4.7 Acute Pancreatitis

The causes of acute pancreatitis (AP) in older patients differ from younger patients. AP related to bile stones and idiopathic etiology is more frequent in older patients. Since gallbladder stones increase with age, cases are related to bile stones in almost half of the patients. Biliary and idiopathic etiologies are the first two causes accounting for over 90% of severe AP in older patients [44].

Serum lipase level is the ancillary tests for the diagnosis of AP because of its high specificity as compared to amylase [15]. It is recommended that if the diagnosis of AP is established by abdominal pain and increases in the serum lipase, a CT scan is not usually required for the diagnosis in the ED or on admission to the hospital [45]. A CT scan should be performed in patients with an uncertain diagnosis, severe clinical pancreatitis, a Ranson score greater than 3 or APACHE II score greater than 8, no improvement within 72 h, and acute deterioration.

AP generally has a benign course in younger patients, whereas major organ failures develop more frequently in older patients. While the rate of local complications of AP is the same in older patients, they should be monitored carefully to detect organ failure. The overall mortality of severe AP in older patients is approximately 15% versus 5% in younger patients [44]. The most frequent complications of severe AP in older patients are acute lung injury and acute respiratory distress syndrome (30.9%), followed by multiple organ dysfunction syndrome (26.6%), electrolyte disturbances (21.3%), renal failure (18.1%), pancreatic encephalopathy (17.1%), and cardiovascular insufficiency (17.0%). The management strategy of severe AP in older patients should be based on these possible complications [44].

Determining the optimum timing for cholecystectomy and endoscopic sphincterotomy in patients with AP secondary to bile duct stones will improve prognosis in older patients and prevent relapses [46].

15.4.8 Peptic Ulcer Disease

Incidence of PUD in older patients is higher as compared to younger patients. The use of NSAIDs and infection due to *Helicobacter pylori* (*H. pylori*) in older patients are factors that increase the frequency of PUD development and secondary gastrointestinal bleeding [47].

In a study involving older patients for whom endoscopy has been carried out for any reason, endoscopy found esophagitis (15.5%), erosive gastritis (24.8%), PUD (26.2%), and nonorganic lesions (31.0%) [48].

Prevalence of *H. pylori* infection is about 70–80% in older patients; however, it falls significantly after 85 years of age. *H. pylori* infection plays a role in the development of gastritis and PUD, and it is also involved in the pathophysiology of lymphoma related to the gastric mucosa and gastric cancer [47].

Symptoms and signs of PUD in older patients can be limited, like in other abdominal diseases. About 30% of patients older than 65 years with confirmed PUD do not have abdominal pain [16]. The most frequently encountered complications include perforation and gastrointestinal bleeding with a high rate of mortality.

15.4.9 Nonspecific Abdominal Pain

Although the ratio varies, 15% of older patients visiting the ED are discharged from the ED with the diagnosis of NSAP [7]. It does not mean the absence of any pathology. In patients discharged from the ED with a diagnosis of NSAP, 2.2% of patients were diagnosed with malignancies within a period of 12 months [49]. EPs should be careful during the management of patients with nonspecific gastrointestinal signs and symptoms and should make recommendations for further studies after the ED care.

15.4.10 Extra-abdominal Causes of Abdominal Pain

Extra-abdominal diseases can be revealed with abdominal pain and other gastrointestinal complaints in older patients as in general population. EPs should not miss cases with acute myocardial infarction (MI). In a study including 65 years of age and older patients with acute MI, 1.3% of patients were discharged without any diagnosis in the ED [50]. The rate of acute MI who had not been diagnosed in the

ED is 0.52% [50]. Symptoms can be abdominal pain, shortness of breath, or weakness, atypical presentation of MI in older patients. Electrocardiogram with 12 leads should be ordered systematically in older patients with abdominal pain.

Conclusion

The management of abdominal pain in older patients is a unique challenge for the EPs. Taking a reliable history from older patients or their relatives, normal or near normal findings in physical examination, and results of laboratory tests within normal ranges contribute to make difficult the differential diagnosis of AAP in older patients in the ED. EPs should use a systematic approach with a more systematic realization of the CT scan in older patients. Most of the older patients with AAP will require surgery, but the mortality is ten times higher than the mortality observed in younger patients.

AAP in older patients may be due to vascular etiology, e.g., mesenteric ischemia and rupture of abdominal aortic aneurysm. Acute appendicitis, pancreatitis, and diverticulitis are uncommon in older patients and usually become apparent lately in their courses. Biliary tract diseases, bowel obstruction, and PUD are more frequent diseases and should be considered in the differential diagnosis. The motto of the classical approach of emergency medicine, "ABC priority," should be always applied in older patients, and extra-abdominal causes like myocardial infarction must be systematically eliminated during the differential diagnosis process in the ED.

References

1. Ergin M, Karamercan MA, Ayranci M et al (2015) Epidemiological characteristics of geriatric patients in emergency departments: results of a multicenter study. Turk J Geriatr 18(4):259–265
2. Bhutto A, Morley JE (2008) The clinical significance of gastrointestinal changes with aging. Curr Opin Clin Nutr Metab Care 11(5):651–660
3. Cotreau MM, von Moltke LL, Greenblatt DJ (2005) The influence of age and sex on the clearance of cytochrome P450 3A substrates. Clin Pharmacokinet 44(1):33–60
4. Radley S, Keighley MR, Radley SC et al (1999) Bowel dysfunction following hysterectomy. Br J Obstet Gynaecol 106(11):1120–1125
5. Leuthauser A, Mc Vane B (2016) Abdominal pain in the geriatric patient. Emerg Med Clin North Am 34(2):363–375
6. Gardner CS, Jaffe TA, Nelson RC (2015) Impact of CT in elderly patients presenting to the emergency department with acute abdominal pain. Abdom Imaging 40(7):2877–2882
7. Lewis LM, Banet GA, Blanda M et al (2005) Etiology and clinical course of abdominal pain in senior patients: a prospective, multicenter study. J Gerontol A Biol Sci Med Sci 60(8):1071–1076
8. van Geloven AA, Biesheuvel TH, Luitse JS et al (2000) Hospital admissions of patients aged over 80 with acute abdominal complaints. Eur J Surg 166(11):866–871
9. Acierno R, Hernandez MA, Amstadter AB et al (2010) Prevalence and correlates of emotional, physical, sexual, and financial abuse and potential neglect in the United States: the National Elder Mistreatment Study. Am J Public Health 100(2):292–297

10. Birnbaumer DM (2014) The elder patient. In: Marx JA (ed) Rosen's emergency medicine: concepts and clinical practice, 8th edn. Saunders, Elsevier, Philadelphia, pp 2351–2355
11. Potts FE, Vukov LF (1999) Utility of fever and leukocytosis in acute surgical abdomens in octogenarians and beyond. J Gerontol A Biol Sci Med Sci 54(2):M55–M58
12. Laurell H, Hansson LE, Gunnarsson U (2006) Acute abdominal pain among elderly patients. Gerontology 52(6):339–344
13. Paranjape C, Dalia S, Pan J et al (2007) Appendicitis in the elderly: a change in the laparoscopic era. Surg Endosc 21(5):777–781
14. Daoust R, Paquet J, Piette E et al (2016) Impact of age on pain perception for typical painful diagnoses in the emergency department. J Emerg Med 50(1):14–20
15. Hendrickson M, Naparst TR (2003) Abdominal surgical emergencies in the elderly. Emerg Med Clin North Am 21(4):937–969
16. Lyon C, Clark DC (2006) Diagnosis of acute abdominal pain in older patients. Am Fam Physician 74(9):1537–1544
17. di Grezia F, di Panzillo EA, Russo S et al (2016) Prognostic role of lactate on mortality in younger and older patients with cardiorespiratory failure admitted to an acute intensive care unit. Aging Clin Exp Res 28(3):40712
18. Haas SA, Lange T, Saugel B et al (2016) Severe hyperlactatemia, lactate clearance and mortality in unselected critically ill patients. Intensive Care Med 42(2):202–210
19. Dubuisson V, Voïglio EJ, Grenier N et al (2015) Imaging of non-traumatic abdominal emergencies in adults. J Visc Surg 152:S57–S64
20. Esses D, Birnbaum A, Bijur P et al (2004) Ability of CT to alter decision making in elderly patients with acute abdominal pain. Am J Emerg Med 22(4):270–272
21. Lewis LM, Klippel AP, Bavolek RA et al (2007) Quantifying the usefulness of CT in evaluating seniors with abdominal pain. Eur J Radiol 61(2):290–296
22. Alabousi A, Patlas MN, Sne N et al (2015) Is oral contrast necessary for multi detector computed tomography imaging of patients with acute abdominal pain? Can Assoc Radiol J 66(4):318–322
23. Launay-Savary MV, Rainfray M, Dubuisson V (2015) Emergency gastrointestinal surgery in the elderly. J Visc Surg 152(6 Suppl):S73–S79
24. Chang C, Wang S (2007) Acute abdominal pain in the elderly. Int J Gerontol 1(2):77–82
25. Arenal JJ, Bengoechea-Beeby M (2003) Mortality associated with emergency abdominal surgery in the elderly. Can J Surg 46(2):111–116
26. Griffiths R, Beech F, Brown A et al (2014) Peri-operative care of the elderly 2014: Association of Anaesthetists of Great Britain and Ireland. Anaesthesia 69(Suppl 1):81–98
27. Tilsed JV, Casamassima A, Kurihara H et al (2016) ESTES guidelines: acute mesenteric ischaemia. Eur J Trauma Emerg Surg 42(2):253–270
28. Kärkkäinen JM, Lehtimäki TT, Manninen H et al (2015) Acute mesenteric ischemia is a more common cause than expected of acute abdomen in the elderly. J Gastrointest Surg 19(8):1407–1414
29. Schoots IG, Koffeman GI, Legemate DA et al (2004) Systematic review of survival after acute mesenteric ischaemia according to disease aetiology. Br J Surg 91(1):17–27
30. Carver TW, Vora RS, Taneja A (2016) Mesenteric ischemia. Crit Care Clin 32(2):155–171
31. Cangemi JR, Picco MF (2009) Intestinal ischemia in the elderly. Gastroenterol Clin N Am 38(3):527–540
32. Spangler R, Van Pham T, Khoujah D et al (2014) Abdominal emergencies in the geriatric patient. Int J Emerg Med 7:43
33. Moll FL, Powell JT, Fraedrich G et al (2011) Management of abdominal aortic aneurysms clinical practice guidelines of the European society for vascular surgery. Eur J Vasc Endovasc Surg 41(Suppl 1):S1–S58
34. Brown PM, Zelt DT, Sobolev B (2003) The risk of rupture in untreated aneurysms: the impact of size, gender, and expansion rate. J Vasc Surg 37(2):280–284

35. Guirguis-Blake JM, Beil TL, Sun X et al (2014) Primary care screening for abdominal aortic aneurysm: a systematic evidence review for the U.S. Preventive Services Task Force. Agency for Healthcare Research and Quality (US) Report No:14-05202-EF-1
36. Qanadli SD, Mesurolle B, Coggia M et al (2000) Abdominal aortic aneurysm: pretherapy assessment with dual-slice helical CT angiography. AJR Am J Roentgenol 174(1):181–187
37. Jacobs DO (2007) Clinical practice. Diverticulitis. N Engl J Med 357(20):2057–2066
38. Akkapulu N, Kıymazaslan B, Düzkalır HG et al (2013) The efficacy of abdominal ultrasonographic examination in preventing negative appendectomies. J Acad Emerg Med 12(3):118–121
39. Duke E, Kalb B, Arif-Tiwari H et al (2016) A systematic review and meta-analysis of diagnostic performance of MRI for evaluation of acute appendicitis. AJR Am J Roentgenol 206(3):508–517
40. Sallinen V, Akl EA, You JJ et al (2016) Meta-analysis of antibiotics versus appendectomy for non-perforated acute appendicitis. Br J Surg 103(6):656–667. (Epub - ahead of print)
41. Ross SO, Forsmark CE (2001) Pancreatic and biliary disorders in the elderly. Gastroenterol Clin N Am 30(2):531–545
42. Ambe PC, Weber SA, Christ H et al (2015) Primary cholecystectomy is feasible in elderly patients with acute cholecystitis. Aging Clin Exp Res 27(6):921–926
43. Bourikian S, Anand RJ, Aboutanos M et al (2015) Risk factors for acute gangrenous cholecystitis in emergency general surgery patients. Am J Surg 210(4):730–733
44. Xin MJ, Chen H, Luo H et al (2008) Severe acute pancreatitis in the elderly: etiology and clinical characteristics. World J Gastroenterol 14(16):2517–2521
45. Banks PA, Bollen TL, Dervenis C et al (2013) Classification of acute pancreatitis—2012: revision of the Atlanta classification and definitions by international consensus. Gut 62(1):102–111
46. Sandblom G, Bergman T, Rasmussen I (2008) Acute pancreatitis in patients 70 years of age or older clinical medicine. Geriatrics 1:27–32
47. Pilotto A, Franceschi M (2014) Helicobacter pylori infection in older people. World J Gastroenterol 20(21):6364–6373
48. Pilotto A, Maggi S, Noale M et al (2010) Development and validation of a new questionnaire for the evaluation of upper gastrointestinal symptoms in the elderly population: a multicenter study. J Gerontol A Biol Sci Med Sci 65(2):174–178
49. Ferlander P, Elfström C, Göransson K et al (2016) Nonspecific abdominal pain in the emergency department: malignancy incidence in a nationwide Swedish cohort study. Eur J Emerg Med Epub ahead of print
50. Wilson M, Welch J, Schuur J et al (2014) Hospital and emergency department factors associated with variations in missed diagnosis and costs for patients age 65 years and older with acute myocardial infarction who present to emergency departments. Acad Emerg Med 21(10):1101–1108

Urinary Tract Infections in Older Patients

16

Roberta Petrino, Aldo Tua, and Fabio Salvi

16.1 Introduction

Urinary tract infection (UTI) is one of the most common infections in both community-dwelling and long-term care resident, as well as hospitalised older adults. The prevalence of UTI increases with age in both sexes, being higher for women than men at all ages [1].

Case definitions are central to any discussion about epidemiology of UTI. The spectrum of urinary conditions ranges from asymptomatic bacteriuria, to symptomatic (uncomplicated/complicated) UTI, to UTI-associated sepsis requiring hospitalisation (Table 16.1) [2].

ASB is very common in older people: 10.6–16% in older women and 3.6–19% in older men living in the community and up to 50% in older women and up to 40% in older men living in long-term care facilities [3]. Its presence does not necessarily indicate acute illness and is not, on its own, an indication for treatment [4]. Symptomatic UTI requires the presence of new urinary tract symptoms (such as frequency, urgency, dysuria, new incontinence, haematuria, or costovertebral or suprapubic tenderness) together with a urine culture with an identified urinary pathogen (Fig. 16.1) [3]. It represents 5% of all ED visits made annually by older adults in the United States, with a prevalence of 16.5% in a cohort of community-dwelling older women [6]. However, diagnosis becomes problematic when a patient, usually a frail older adult, is unable to provide a clear history of acute urinary

R. Petrino (✉) • A. Tua
Emergency Medicine Unit, S. Andrea Hospital, Vercelli, Italy
e-mail: ropetrino@gmail.com

F. Salvi
Department of Geriatrics and Geriatric Emergency Care, INRCA-IRCCS, Ancona, Italy
e-mail: F.SALVI@inrca.it

© Springer International Publishing Switzerland 2018
C. Nickel et al. (eds.), *Geriatric Emergency Medicine*,
https://doi.org/10.1007/978-3-319-19318-2_16

Table 16.1 Classification of UTI (modified from Mody and Juthani-Metha [2])

Anatomical level of infection	Cystitis, urethritis, pyelonephritis, prostatitis
Grade of severity of infection	Uncomplicated and complicated UTIs, urinary tract-driven sepsis, septic shock
Underlying risk factors	Prostatic hypertrophy, permanent catheterisation, incontinence, high motor dependency
Microbiological findings	Recurrent infections, multiresistant bacteria, antibiotic abuse

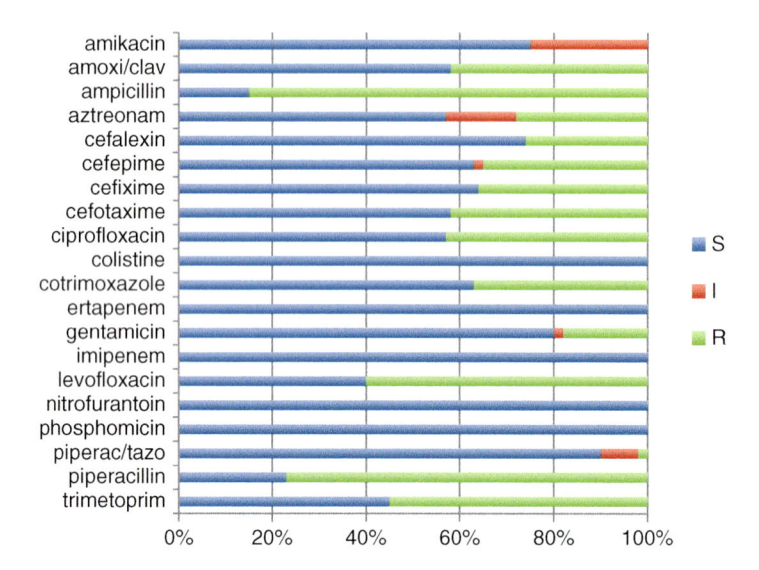

Fig. 16.1 Resistance to antibiotics in a sample of 350 *E. coli*-positive urine cultures in a North Italian series [5]

symptoms and/or present with nonspecific symptoms such as acute functional decline, confusion (delirium), or generalised weakness.

16.2 Symptoms of UTI

In adult patients, symptoms, signs, and laboratory findings focus on the anatomical level and the degree of severity of the infection (Table 16.2). The risk factor analysis contributes to define any additional therapeutic measure required (i.e. drainage).

Older people with UTI can present with these classical symptoms, but often, particularly when they have communication barriers, typical symptoms may be absent, masked, or impossible to ascertain. In this case, the predominant clinical expression could be lethargy or agitation (i.e. hypoactive or hyperactive delirium), fever or hypothermia (sepsis), hypotension and tachycardia (septic shock), acute functional decline (or fall), generalised weakness, and so on [7].

In older adults, the diagnosis of UTI should be always based on a full clinical assessment. The very high prevalence of asymptomatic bacteriuria (with positive

16 Urinary Tract Infections in Older Patients

Table 16.2 Anatomical localisations of UTI and classical related symptoms

Urethra and bladder: lower urinary tract infection (LUTI)	• Dysuria or frequency with or without fever and chills • Tenderness over the bladder • Lower back pain • Urgency, spasm after voiding • Cloudy urines, haematuria • Generally acute onset
Kidney: upper urinary tract infection (UUTI) or pyelonephritis	• Loin pain, flank tenderness • Fever > 38°C • Rigours or other manifestations of infection
Prostate: prostatitis	• Pain in the lower back, perirectal area, and testicles • High fever and chills • Swelling of the prostate with possible obstruction • Urinary retention, which can cause abscesses or seminal vesiculitis
Bloodstream: urosepsis	• Symptoms of UTI and systemic symptoms • Presence of bacteria in the blood diagnosed by blood culture

dipstick test) together with the high prevalence of atypical presentations or inability to provide a clear history of acute urinary symptoms in older patients (especially in the presence of indwelling catheter holders) risks overdiagnosis and consequent overtreatment. Potentially unnecessary use of antibiotics leads to increased resistance of the common uropathogens, specifically the emergence of multidrug-resistant ESBL-producing *Escherichia coli* and *Klebsiella* species. Additionally, overuse of antibiotics increases the risk of antibiotic-related complications such as increasing number of MRSA infections and clostridial diarrhoea, as well as unnecessary costs. There is also an opportunity cost in terms of missed diagnoses—incorrect interpretation of urine dipstick testing can lead to the true diagnoses being missed and delays in treatment.

16.2.1 Asymptomatic Bacteriuria

ASB is defined as the presence of bacteria in the urine in quantities of 10^5 colony-forming units per millilitre (cfu/mL) or more in two consecutive urine specimens in women or one urine specimen in men, in the absence of clinical signs or symptoms suggestive of a UTI [8]. It is more common in diabetic older patients, while it is constant in indwelling catheter holders and very frequent in incontinent women. The prevalence of ASB is estimated to be between 6 and 10% in women older than 60 years and approximately 5% in men older than 65 [9]. In institutionalised adults the incidence of bacteriuria is even higher, with estimates ranging from 25 to 50% for women and 15 to 35% for men. Table 16.3 shows the prevalence of bacteriuria in different countries and ages. Although ASB increases the risk of symptomatic

Table 16.3 Prevalence of asymptomatic bacteriuria according to age in different countries [10]

Country	Age (years)	Men (%)	Women (%)
Japan	50–59	0.6	2.8
	60–69	1.5	7.4
	>70	3.6	10.8
Sweden	62	6	16
	79	6	14
Scotland	65–74	6	16
	>75	7	17

UTI, it should not be treated except in those patients undergoing invasive genitourinary procedures [3].

A common clinical scenario is an older patient, maybe living in a residential home, who is referred to the ED with a history of increasing confusion, being unable to provide clear associated symptoms. The patient could have dark and offensive smelling urine; the dipstick test is positive for leucocyte esterase and nitrites. A urine culture is sent (and will be positive), UTI is diagnosed, and antibiotic treatment is started. However, fever or other indices of systemic inflammation (hypothermia, CRP, raised white cell count) or genitourinary tract infection are lacking; other sources of infection (pneumonia, diverticulitis, endocarditis, etc.) have not been ruled out; and alternative diagnoses of acute confusion have not been adequately taken into account. For example, the patient could have recently started codeine for knee pain, and this could be the cause of increasing confusion, constipation, reduced fluid intake with consequent dehydration, and change in the character of urine that is chronically bacteriuric. An apparently simple and well-managed clinical case becomes a misdiagnosis and a missed diagnosis of the true cause of delirium [4]. Moreover, unnecessary antibiotic treatment may frequently cause harm (rash, drug interactions, development of antibiotic resistance, and disruption of intestinal microbiome) [11].

16.2.2 Symptomatic Urinary Tract Infection

In older patients the symptoms and signs of UTI may be atypical and difficult to distinguish from other urinary diseases. Older adults with UTI are more likely to present to the ED with altered mental status rather than fever or classic urinary symptoms; however, when present, acute dysuria is more specific for UTI than urinary frequency or urgency [6]. Atypical presentations also abound in older patients with pyelonephritis, but fever and chills are more consistently present [6]. Another important symptom of UTI could be the pain in the suprapubic area, the flank, or the back, which in the non-cooperative patient could be suggested by agitation, irritability, and increased confusion (delirium) with increased incidence of falls. Even if incontinence could be a risk factor for UTI, it may also represent a symptom of the disease. When UTI evolves into sepsis or septic shock, typical symptoms—like hypotension, tachycardia, tachypnoea, anorexia, respiratory distress, and abdominal tenderness—may occur but can be delayed or onset abrupt.

As mentioned above, the simple evidence of cloudy or malodorous urine is not sufficient to start an antimicrobial treatment, as it could be due to epithelial cells or mucus, dehydration, or poor hygiene, while the evidence of haematuria could be due to different causes, such as cancer or medication. In older patients also fever may be absent or late in onset, or they could be hypothermic with sepsis. When present, fever is the most important sign, but it is important to exclude other sources of infection.

16.3 Microbiology

The vast majority of UTI are due to infection by *Escherichia coli*, *Proteus mirabilis*, *Klebsiella pneumoniae*, *Enterococcus*, *Pseudomonas*, and *Staphylococcus* spp. [12, 13]. Older patients have a lower incidence of *Escherichia coli* and a higher incidence of polymicrobial infections [12, 13]. In community-living postmenopausal women, *E. coli* is the most common urinary isolate, accounting for 75–82% of UTIs [12, 13]. Gram-positive organisms including *Enterococcus* and *Staphylococcus* accounted for 4.5% and 4.1% of cases, respectively [12, 13]. *Klebsiella* sp. was the second most common (12%) followed by *Enterococcus faecalis* (8%) [12, 13]. It is postulated that the postmenopausal state changes the vaginal microbial environment of older women, which together with worsening of incontinence and disability, and greater exposure to antibiotics, leads to change the profile of uropathogens causing UTI in community-dwelling and institutionalised women [12, 13]. In nursing homes the microbiology of UTI changes according to the presence of a long-term catheter [12, 13].

16.3.1 Antimicrobial Resistance

Multidrug-resistant organisms (MDROs) are increasing over time, due to the widespread and frequently inappropriate use of antibiotics for UTI [14]. Although MDROs are more common in healthcare settings, the prevalence of resistant urinary pathogens in community populations is also growing [5]. Figure 16.1 shows the antimicrobial resistance in *E. coli*-positive urinary cultures in a North Italian environment, with a high prevalence of older people [5]. These data suggest that it is important to know the epidemiology and antibiotic sensibility in each environment, setting, and geographical location, to be able to conduct a correct education of doctors to use antibiotics that are effective and that are not increasing resistances, which vary widely among Europe.

16.4 Risk Factors for UTI

A variety of factors predispose older adults to infections. Immunity is modified by age or by chronic diseases and can increase likelihood to contract infection. Also the need for invasive procedures, prosthetic devices, urinary catheterisation, and long-term care facilities is all increasing the risk of UTI and of acquired MDROs [15].

In community-dwelling older adults, one of the strongest predictors for developing UTI is having a history of UTI. Other risk factors associated with developing UTI in older women include a history of urinary incontinence, the presence of a cystocele, and a history of diabetes mellitus. A change in vaginal flora as a result of declining oestrogen levels is thought to predispose postmenopausal women to UTI, which is not decreased by oestrogen replacement therapy. In men the most important predisposing factors for UTI are prostatic hypertrophy causing urinary retention and high post-void residuals.

Residents in long-term care facilities are more likely to suffer from significant functional and cognitive impairment, both of which have been shown to increase the risk of developing UTI. Disorders such as dementia, Parkinson's disease, and stroke often lead to voiding abnormalities, impede adequate self-hygiene, and increase the need for urinary catheterisation.

The major age-related risk factors for UTI are:

- Faecal incontinence (and constipation)
- Incomplete bladder empting
- Vaginal atrophy, oestrogen deficiency
- Urinary incontinence, cystocele/prolapse
- Dehydration, impaired fluid intake
- Long-term indwelling urinary catheter
- Diabetes or immunosuppression
- Prostatic hypertrophy
- Bladder or prostate cancer

16.5 Diagnosis of UTI

16.5.1 Diagnosis of UTI in Community-Dwelling Older Adults

The diagnosis of symptomatic UTI in community-dwelling older adults who are cognitively intact requires the presence of genitourinary symptoms in the setting of urinary tract inflammation demonstrated by pyuria (Fig. 16.2) and a documented microbiologic pathogen. Although urinary symptoms are common in community-dwelling older adults, not all patients who present with urinary symptoms have symptomatic UTI, and overuse of antibiotics for the treatment of UTI in this population remains a significant problem [16]. It is important to interpret correctly also the other signs and symptoms described above and evaluate if they are really related to urinary infection.

A screening for ASB is recommended only for patients about to undergo invasive urological procedures (prostatic transurethral resection, procedures that may cause haematuria), while it should not be routinely undertaken in other groups (people with diabetes, long-term care residents, or patients undergoing urinary catheter insertion).

Fig. 16.2 Pyuria sample

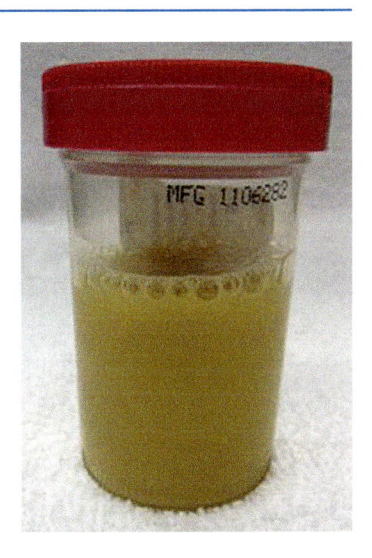

16.5.2 Diagnostic Criteria of UTI in Community-Dwelling Older Adults

In older adults who are cognitively intact and present with symptoms suggestive of UTI, a urinary dipstick (Fig. 16.3) can be helpful to exclude UTI if there are no nitrates or leucocytes (high negative predictive value), but in other scenarios it is reasonable to treat based on local antimicrobial guidance and send a midstream sample for subsequent review.

16.5.3 Diagnosis of UTI in Patients with Communication Barriers

The diagnosis of symptomatic UTI in older people with communication barriers is more challenging, as according to definitions of there should be localised genitourinary symptoms, the incidence of which will be low. Institutionalised older adults, indeed, often have significant underlying medical comorbidities such as dementia and stroke, which impair their ability to communicate, and are more likely to present with atypical or nonspecific symptoms when infected. The high prevalence of bacteriuria in long-term care facility patients makes it difficult for providers to distinguish symptomatic UTI from ASB, risks overtreatment, and selection of MDROs.

To improve infection control practices and prevent the negative effects of overuse of antibiotics, several consensus guidelines have been developed to assist providers in the diagnosis and treatment of UTI in long-term care residents [17]. Importantly, healthcare professionals should not use dipstick testing to diagnose UTI in adults with urinary catheters. Dipstick testing is not an effective method for detecting urinary tract infections in catheterised adults. This is because there is no

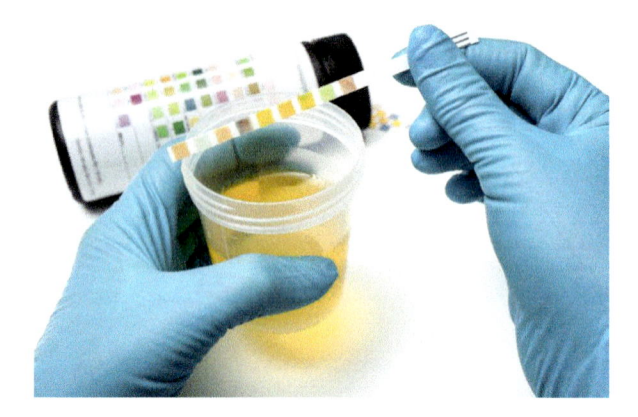

Fig. 16.3 Dipstick urine analysis: in 60 s the doctor and the nurse may have information on the presence of blood, nitrates, proteins, pH, and specific gravity in the urine sample

Table 16.4 Minimum criteria for initiating antibiotics for UTI in long-term care residents

1. At least one of the following subcriteria of signs or symptoms
    - Acute dysuria or acute pain, swelling, or tenderness of the testes, epididymis, or prostate
    - Fever or leucocytosis and at least one of the following localising urinary tract subcriteria:
        – Acute costovertebral angle pain or tenderness
        – Suprapubic pain
        – Gross haematuria
        – New or marked increase in incontinence
        – New or marked increase in urgency
        – New or marked increase in frequency
    - In the absence of fever or leucocytosis, two or more of the following localising urinary tract subcriteria:
        – Suprapubic pain
        – Gross haematuria
        – New or marked increase in incontinence
        – New or marked increase in urgency
        – New or marked increase in frequency
2. One of the following microbiological subcriteria
    - At least 10^5 cfu/mL of no more than two species of microorganisms in a voided urine sample
    - At least 10^2 of any number of organisms in a specimen collected by in-and-out catheter

Adapted from [17]

relationship between the level of pyuria and infection in people with indwelling catheters (the presence of the catheter invariably induces pyuria without the presence of infection). A negative dipstick test can be a useful method to rule out UTI in these patients [11].

For residents without an indwelling urinary catheter, the diagnosis of UTI in the revised McGeer criteria is illustrated in Table 16.4 [17].

16.5.4 Diagnostic Algorithm for UTI in Older Adults in Long-Term Care Facilities

The minimum laboratory evaluation for suspected UTI should include urinalysis to evaluate for pyuria and urinary dipstick to evaluate for evidence of leucocyte esterase and nitrates. If pyuria is present or the urinary dipstick is positive for leucocyte esterase or nitrate test, a urine culture should be obtained to search the presence of bacteriuria and to document antimicrobial susceptibility testing [18]. The absence of both leucocyte esterase and nitrite has been shown to have 98% negative predictive value for the diagnosis of UTI. When an older person is unable to provide a definitive history of acute urinary symptoms, a UTI should be diagnosed only when evidence exists of bacteriuria (base on urine culture) and systemic inflammation (fever/hypothermia, raised white cell count, or CRP), and, importantly, no other more likely cause of acute illness exists, after a careful/full clinical assessment [11]. Older patients with acute mental status changes accompanied by bacteriuria and pyuria, without clinical instability or other signs or symptoms of UTI, can reasonably be observed for resolution of confusion for 24–48 h without antibiotics, while searching for other causes of confusion (i.e. dehydration, hypoxia, polypharmacy adverse reactions) [19].

16.5.5 UTI in Older Patients with Long-Term Indwelling Urinary Catheter

Bacteriuria is constant in patients with catheter, because the device provides a focus for bacterial biofilm formation (Fig. 16.4). So the first preventive action for the older patient is to minimise the use of indwelling catheters, which will be colonised, even with a close drainage system. So it is important to address all the reasons for catheterisation, such as prostatic hypertrophy or other obstruction, or in cooperative patients, for example, with neurological bladder, consider intermittent self-catheterisation. In any case, the antibiotic prophylaxis in patients with long-term indwelling catheter is not indicated [3].

16.6 Treatment of UTI

In older patients who have nonspecific symptoms, the decision to start a specific antibiotic may be challenging. In this setting it is widely spread the use of empiric antimicrobial therapy, even without a clear evidence of infection, and this has often led to antibiotic overuse and increase in resistance.

A full diagnostic workup should be always performed, urine microscopy and ideally with culture, and the treatment started, trying to target the causative organism only following indications reported above. It is important to use an antibiotic

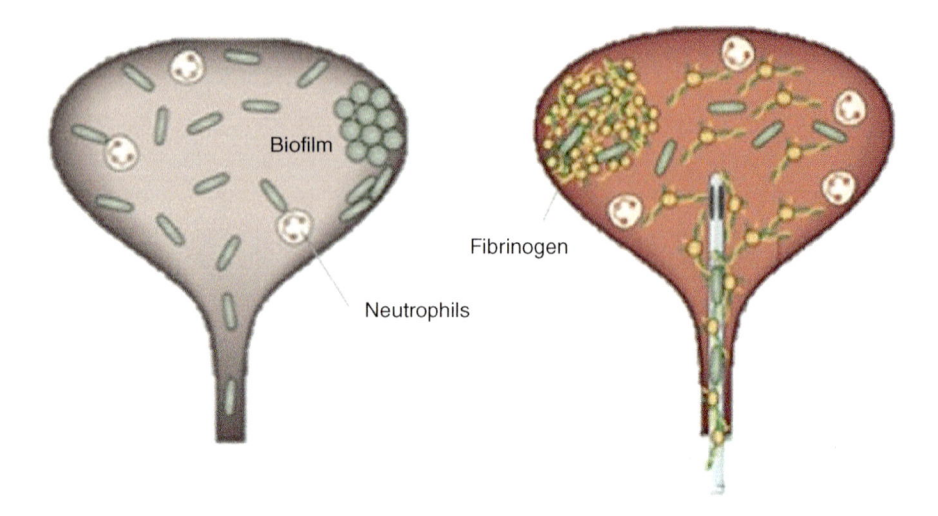

Fig. 16.4 The bladder without catheter on the *left* and with catheter on the *right*. Fibrinogen bridges maintain the biofilm in catheter holder, and inflammation of the bladder is increased and developed

with a narrow spectrum of action, to avoid the onset of *Clostridium difficile* enteritis that may increase morbidity and mortality. It is also important to consider dose-adjusting needs, due to the frequent presence of chronic renal failure [20].

As already explained above, one of the most important issues a doctor faces with treating UTIs is to know the microbiology of the region where he or she is operating and the specific resistance of bacteria to the available and commonly used antibiotics. So when possible, a urine culture should be performed. For an uncomplicated UTI, 3 days of treatment will usually suffice, whereas for complicated UTI (signs of systemic inflammation or altered anatomy), up to 14 days may be required, possibly intravenously if the patient's illness severity or inability to comply with oral medication dictates that is necessary. The choice of antibiotic will depend on a knowledge of local resistance patterns. Prostatitis occurs not infrequently in older men and, when present, requires at least 4 weeks of an antibiotic that has good tissue penetration, such as ciprofloxacin or cotrimoxazole.

16.7 Prevention of UTIs

Several strategies can be taken to try to prevent UTIs in older patients:

1. Avoid long-term catheterisation when possible. It is necessary to reassess the reason for catheter insertion and try to remove it, monitoring the new onset of obstruction.
2. Look for clinical predisposing factors to UTI, such as diabetes or urological disease (stones or tumours). Similarly, search for constipation (and tendency to

faecal impaction), chronic urinary retention (post-void residual scan), and other anatomical abnormalities.
3. Increase mobility of patients. Several studies demonstrated a reduced rate of UTIs up to 60% in older patients that were mobilised.
4. Use of cranberry juice or capsules is no longer recommended [21]).

Conclusion

In this chapter we have highlighted the key issues of diagnosing and managing UTI in older people. The take-home messages can be encapsulated in these points:

1. UTI is a very common disease in older patients and can be present in very atypical, often neuropsychiatric ways, such as delirium [22].
2. Asymptomatic bacteriuria is common but should not be treated.
3. When a treatment is necessary, it should be targeted on epidemiological and microbiological findings to limit antibiotic resistance as much as possible [23].
4. Treatment should be short for uncomplicated UTI.
5. Prevention measures such as avoiding catheter when not necessary and improving mobility of the patients should be fostered.

References

1. Foxman B (2003) Epidemiology of urinary tract infections. Dis Mon 49(2):53–70
2. Mody L, Juthani-Metha M (2014) Urinary tract infections in older woman. A clinical review. JAMA 311(8):844–854
3. Nicolle LE, Bradley S, Colgan R et al (2005) Infectious diseases society of America guidelines for the diagnosis and treatment of asymptomatic bacteriuria in adults. Clin Infect Dis 40(5):643–654
4. Ninan S, Walton C, Barlow G (2014) Investigation of suspected urinary tract infection in older people. BMJ 348:g4070
5. Das R, Perrelli E, Towle V et al (2009) Antimicrobial susceptibility of bacteria isolated from urine samples obtained from nursing home residents. Infect Control Hosp Epidemiol 30(11):1116–1119
6. Liang SY (2016) Sepsis and other infectious disease emergencies in the elderly. Emerg Med Clin N Am 34:501–522
7. Limpawattana P, Phungoen P, Mitsungnern T et al (2016) Atypical presentations of older adults at the emergency department and associated factors. Arch Gerontol Geriatr 62:97–102
8. Adedipe A, Lowenstein R (2006) Infectious emergencies in the elderly. Emerg Med Clin N Am 24(2):433–448
9. Grabe M, Bartoletti R, Bjerklund-Johansen TE, Çek HM, Pickard RS, Tenke P, Wagenlehner F, Wullt B (2014) Guidelines on urological infections. European Association of Urology
10. Nicolle LE (1997) Asymptomatic bacteriuria in the elderly. Infect Dis Clin N Am 11(3):647–662
11. Scottish Intercollegiate Guidelines Network (2012) SIGN guideline 88. Management of suspected bacterial urinary tract infection in adults. www.sign.ac.uk/guidelines/fulltext/88/index.html
12. Caljouw MA, Den Elzen WP, Cools HJ et al (2011) Predictive factors of urinary tract infections among the oldest old in the general population. A population-based prospective follow-up study. BMC Med 9:57

13. Hu KK, Boyko EJ, Scholes D et al (2004) Risk factors for urinary tract infections in postmenopausal women. Arch Intern Med 164(9):989–993
14. Rao GG, Patel M (2009) Urinary tract infection in hospitalized elderly patients in the United Kingdom: the importance of making an accurate diagnosis in the post broad-spectrum antibiotic era. J Antimicrob Chemother 63:5–6
15. Swami SK, Liesinger JT, Shah N et al (2012) Incidence of antibiotic-resistant *Adv PSA337* bacteriuria according to age and location of onset: a population-based study from Olmsted County, Minnesota. Mayo Clin Proc 87(8):753–759
16. Juthani-Mehta M, Quagliarello VJ (2010) Infectious diseases in the nursing home setting: challenges and opportunities for clinical investigation. Clin Infect Dis 51(8):931–936
17. Loeb M, Bentley DW, Bradley S et al (2001) Infect Control Hosp Epidemiol 22:120–124
18. Stone ND, Ashraf MS, Calder J et al (2012) Surveillance definitions of infections in long-term care facilities: revisiting the McGeer criteria. Infect Control Hosp Epidemiol 33(10):965–977
19. Schulz L, Hoffman RJ, Pothof J, Fox B (2016) Top ten myths regarding the diagnosis and treatment of urinary tract infections. J Emerg Med 51:25–30
20. Hooton TM (2012) Clinical practice. Uncomplicated urinary tract infection. N Engl J Med 366(11):1028–1037
21. Jepson RG, Craig JC (2009) Cranberries for preventing urinary tract infections. Cochrane Database Syst Rev 1:CD001321
22. Cove-Smith A, Almond M (2007) Management of urinary tract infections in the elderly. Trends Urol Gynaecol Sexual Health:30–35
23. Mckinnell JA, Stollenwerk NS, Jung CW et al (2011) Nitrofurantoin compares favourably to recommended agents as empirical treatment of uncomplicated urinary tract infections in a decision and cost analysis. Mayo Clin Proc 86(6):480–488

Management of Acute Chest Pain in Older Patients

17

Tim Arnold, Ursula Müller-Werdan, and Martin Möckel

17.1 Introduction

Chest pain is the most frequent leading symptom in the emergency department (ED) and challenges the team, because it has many differential diagnoses but also because some of them are serious life-threatening diseases and others only cause discomfort. In addition, many patients with chest pain are 75 years and older. In the ED, chest pain is the most frequent leading symptom, but only 10% of all ED visitors will be diagnosed with acute myocardial infarction (AMI) [1], and 36% of chest pain are related to musculoskeletal conditions, 19% to gastrointestinal and 5% to respiratory conditions, 10% account for stable angina, and 1.5% percent for acute cardiac ischemia [2]. They often do not present with a typical set of symptoms and many of them suffer from multimorbidity.

The challenge in frail older people (many of whom will have impaired communication) is to identify the leading cause of chest pain. Furthermore, in the frailest, the focus of management may shift from preventing mortality to dignity, autonomy, and comfort.

T. Arnold
Division of Emergency and Acute Medicine, Campus Virchow-Klinikum and Campus Mitte; Charité – Universitätsmedizin Berlin, Berlin, Germany

U. Müller-Werdan
Department of Geriatric Medicine, Campus Benjamin Franklin, Charité – Universitätsmedizin Berlin, Berlin, Germany

M. Möckel (✉)
Division of Emergency and Acute Medicine, Campus Virchow-Klinikum and Campus Mitte; Charité – Universitätsmedizin Berlin, Berlin, Germany

Department of Cardiology, Campus Virchow-Klinikum and Campus Mitte; Charité – Universitätsmedizin Berlin, Berlin, Germany
e-mail: martin.moeckel@charite.de

17.2 Differential Diagnosis

It is crucial to distinguish rapidly between life-threatening and benign causes of chest pain, whereas the "big five of chest pain" (AMI, pulmonary arterial embolism, aortic dissection, tension pneumothorax, and—very rare—the Boerhaave's syndrome) are the most relevant pathologies that must be ruled out. Aortic dissection type A and Boerhaave's syndrome will require immediate surgical intervention independent of age. Pulmonary embolism (PE) is primarily treated by anticoagulation also in older patients, and fibrinolysis is limited to a small group of patients in shock. Therefore, the most challenging differential diagnosis with respect to an age-related management is the AMI.

It has to be taken into account that the top ten diagnoses among patients presenting with chest pain contain also cardiomyopathy, atrial fibrillation, heart failure, and arterial hypertension [1]. These patients may not profit from coronary angiography as they often are at high risk for renal failure and other complications without having a culprit coronary artery lesion. It is to emphasize that age, multimorbidity, and frailty should not promote therapeutic nihilism in consideration of chest pain, but it is crucial that risks and benefits not only of the diagnostic but also possible therapeutic approaches are discussed in a patient-centered conversation.

17.2.1 Pulmonary Embolism

Aging is a major risk factor for vein thrombosis and thus for PE, too. Vein thrombosis is very rare in young individuals (<1 per 10,000 per year) but increases to ~1% per year in older patients [3]. This emphasizes that aging is one of the strongest and most prevalent risk factor for venous thrombosis [3].

Typical symptoms for PE are less likely to occur in older patients. According to a study published in 2014, only 64% of all patients with PE and older than 60 years suffered from unexplained dyspnea, pain on inspiration was found in 49%, and only 37% suffered from acute chest pain. Hemoptysis was only found in 3% [4]. Older patients are more likely to present with syncope.

The main diagnostic steps in suspected PE are to calculate the pretest probability using the Wells score followed by further diagnostic tests, whether it is D-dimer testing or a computed tomography of the chest—at least depending on the pretest probability. Not only the Wells score but also D-dimer cutoff values are barely evaluated in older patients, so it is not surprising that only 5% of patients older than 80 years have a negative D-dimers (compared with 50% of patients less than 50 years) [5].

Thus the failure rate of Wells score combined with a qualitative point of care D-dimer test to exclude PE was shown to be 6% in older patients, whereas in younger patients several studies found a failure rate below 1% [6].

Age-adjusted D-dimer levels are beginning to be implemented into decision scores, like in the revised Geneva score of "not high" or Wells score of "low."

PE can be diagnosed by computed tomography pulmonary angiography (CTPA) or lung ventilation-perfusion scan, whereas the CT scan remains the gold standard.

As the radiation exposure especially in younger individuals needs to be taken into account, it is more the contrast-induced kidney injury in older patients that is to be weighed up. After all, literature tells that patients aged 64 years or older show a prevalence of chronic kidney disease from 23.4 to 35.8% [7].

Although older patients are more likely to experience adverse effects of systemic anticoagulation, the therapeutic approach is not different than in younger individuals.

17.2.2 Type A Aortic Dissection

Type A aortic dissection is an uncommon disease with an incidence ranging from 5 to 30 cases per million people per year, but because of the frequently fatal outcome, finding the right diagnosis fast could save the patient's life. Nevertheless, many patients with aortic dissection die before presentation to the hospital or prior to diagnosis [8].

Several studies found that up to 32% of all patients with type A dissection are 70 years or older. In younger individuals the underlying disease usually is Marfan syndrome; in older patients, hypertension, atherosclerosis, and iatrogenic dissection are in the foreground [9].

Like in other acute diseases, older patients with type A aortic dissection are less likely to present with typical symptoms like acute chest or back pain (76.5% in >70 years vs. 88.5% in <70 years); in older patients fewer show murmur of aortic regurgitation (28% in >70 years vs. 47.1% in <70 years) [9].

Still, an abrupt onset of chest pain (leading symptom in up to 76% >70 years and 88% in <70 years) in combination with a low blood pressure is the most common symptom for a type A dissection, if it is in the young or the old [9].

Older patients are less likely to undergo surgical treatment and more likely to be treated conservatively, which means by medical treatment. It was significantly shown that only 64% in the >70 years older patients are treated by surgery compared to 86% in the <70 years older patients; medical approach represents 36% vs. 14% [9].

The overall mortality for patients treated surgically is around 27%, where there is a significant difference for the younger ones (23%) and those >70 years age (38%) [9]. The most common in-hospital complications are myocardial, mesenteric and limb ischemia, renal failure, cardiac tamponade, and coma or altered consciousness. In relation to those complications, there are no significant differences between younger or older patients [9].

17.2.3 (Tension) Pneumothorax

Primary spontaneous pneumothorax usually occurs in tall, lean, and young men aged between 20 and 25—but the spontaneous pneumothorax has two age peaks with the second peak and mostly secondary spontaneous pneumothorax in older patients aged 80 years and older due to changes in the chest wall as well as underlying lung diseases like emphysema or chronic obstructive lung disease [10]. At least, old patients are at a higher risk of fractures not only because potential medical side effects compromising walking stability and therefore a higher risk of falls but also because of osteoporosis. There is only limited data on pneumothorax in older patients, but so far, it seems like older patients compared to younger ones present less often with a typical sudden onset of pleuritic pain or even don't have any pain, so the major symptom is unspecific dyspnea [11]. Thus, the diagnosis of pneumothorax is significantly less often made in older patients; the mean delay to presentation as well as the duration of hospitalization is much longer. In contrast to the mostly benign clinical course of a primary spontaneous pneumothorax, due to underlying lung disease and limited pulmonary reserve, the secondary spontaneous often is a life-threatening event [10].

The therapeutic approach does not differ between younger or older patients, at least in both the first step is a chest drainage.

17.2.4 Other Differential Diagnoses Leading to Chest Pain

One-third of all patients >65 years suffer from a fall once a year; in the older individuals literature even tells us that in those aged >80 years even 50% suffer from a fall per year. Two-thirds of those who fall will fall again within 6 months [12], who falls once will fall twice. Roughly estimated, every tenth fall causes any fracture and, in the same frequency, mild injuries like hematoma, cuts, or grazes [13]. It is crucial to ask for falls and injuries, while taking the patients' history in those who present with chest pain, the clinical examination must address signs of a trauma like hematoma, bone bruise, and pneumothorax. In the differential diagnostic workup, chest X-ray with focus on rip fractures as well as pneumothorax should be performed; sometimes only a CT scan of the chest reveals injuries.

If patients suffer from fever, (productive) coughing, and reduced general condition, pneumonia or other pulmonary infections need to be taken into account in those presenting with chest pain. Within the older population, those with more advanced age are more susceptible to pneumonia with incidence rates of 52.3 cases per 1000 persons in those aged at least 85 years [14]. It remains a big challenge to diagnose "pneumonia" in older patients, as they complain significantly fewer symptoms than younger patients do. Often delirium, worsening of chronic confusion or falls may be the only manifestation [15].

Other conditions causing chest pain like the very rare Boerhaave's syndrome or herpes zoster and postherpetic neuralgia or even just a trivial muscle pain should be considered. Boerhaave's syndrome is more common in patients aged 50–70 years; herpes zoster often has a typical set of symptoms (though the variety of symptoms in older patients can be widely spread from constant to intermittent, from burning to itching pain) often followed or combined with a typical rash, whereas in the majority of cases the rash follows the pain. Postherpetic neuralgia is the most menacing complication of herpes zoster in older patients. The occurrence of postherpetic neuralgia, defined as a pain 1 month after rash onset, is estimated up to 68% in patients older than 60 years [16].

17.3 Acute Coronary Syndromes

17.3.1 General Aspects

Twenty to twenty-five percent of patients presenting in the ED with chest pain suffer from acute coronary syndrome (ACS). According to the AHA and ESC guidelines, an ECG must be obtained within 10 min after initial presentation to the ED in patients with chest discomfort or other symptoms or other symptoms consistent with ACS.

17.3.2 Definitions

ACS is an umbrella term including acute myocardial infarction (NSTEMI and STEMI) and unstable angina.

17.3.2.1 STEMI

According to the universal definition, a STEMI is a syndrome out of symptoms of a myocardial ischemia combined with persistent characteristic ECG changes [17]. Those are new ST-elevations at the J-point in at least two adjacent leads at a minimum of 0.1 mV except of the leads V2-3. Here, a ST-segment elevation of minimum 0.25 mV in men younger than 40 years as well as at minimum 0.2 mV in men older than 40 years needs to be found. In women, the lower limit for a ST-segment elevation in lead V2-3 is 0.15 mV. The appearance of a new left bundle branch block accompanied by typical symptoms for ACS is a STEMI equivalent. It remains a big challenge to put the left bundle branch block in the right context. It is well known that the prevalence of left bundle branch block and other cardiac conduction abnormalities increases with age, so it might be difficult to find out whether it is old or new. In addition, left bundle branch block is a marker both of age and severe heart disease but not exclusively coronary disease [18]. At least, when left bundle branch block is present, the suspicion of acute myocardial infarction should be increased, efforts should be made to obtain previous ECGs, and more definitive tests like point of care troponin test should be performed.

17.3.2.2 NSTE-ACS

In contrast to the STEMI, there are no mandatory ECG changes in NSTEMI. Thus, the measurement of the biomarker troponin is the most important diagnostic approach after a thorough clinical assessment of the patient. In contrast to unstable angina, troponin is elevated in NSTEMI; a typical dynamic over the 99th percentile of the reference value is required [1].

17.3.3 Symptoms

Typical symptoms for an ACS are tightness in the chest, chest pain, and radiation in the left arm and the chaws, often accompanied by dyspnea and vegetative symptoms like diaphoresis and nausea/vomiting.

Atypical symptoms (defined as absence of chest pain) occur more often among older patients with ACS in up to 40% [19]. Literature shows that the average age of patients presenting with atypical symptoms was 73 years, whereas the average age of patients presenting with typical symptoms was 66 years [20]. Because of delays in finding the diagnosis and initiating treatment, atypical presentation of ACS is shown to be a negative predictor for death with a threefold higher in-hospital death rate than in typical ACS. Canto et al. found that in 434,877 patients diagnosed with myocardial infarction, up to 33% did not present with typical chest pain [3].

Although chest pain remains a common presentation of ACS regardless of age, older patients were more likely to present with dyspnea (49%), diaphoresis (26%), nausea and vomiting (24%), and syncope (19%) as a primary complaint [20].

Especially in older patients who already suffer from another acute illness (infections or worsening of a comorbid condition), the risk for development of an ACS increases.

17.3.4 Diagnosis

Initial steps in the workup are a focused patient's history (history of coronary heart disease, comorbidities, and prior medication) as well as a physical examination (heart murmurs, tachycardia or arrhythmia, crackling noises in lung auscultation, blood pressure). An assessment of the patients general appearance is crucial (are they cold sweated, pale, restless and anxious?). These initial steps are challenging in older patients because due to limitations of memory, polypharmacy, and multimorbidity. Necessary information can often not obtained from the patient but from relatives and records.

Further key components in diagnosing ACS are ECG findings and biomarkers (specifically cardiac troponin), while other reasons for an elevated troponin should be considered. In fact studies could show that the workup progress in older patients takes much longer than in younger ones, for instance, the average time between presentation and first ECG is 40 min, where it takes 7 min longer in patients >75 years [20].

The performance of a global assessment whether if it is in the emergency setting or completed when the patient's condition has stabilized is considered best practice (see Chap. 6). It should assess medical and psychosocial items and use simple tests for the rapid detection of concomitant diseases, an evaluation of the patient's autonomy and his/her social conditions. Main items to be assessed are the evaluation of cognition and dependence (daily living) as well as a somatic geriatric (minimal nutrition assessment) and a psychological (simplified geriatric depression score) evaluation [21].

17.3.5 Specific Differential Diagnosis

There are several other reasons for an elevation of troponin than myocardial ischemia, especially in older patients and multimorbid patients (Table 17.1).

17.3.6 Treatment

In general, older patients have a high risk of complications during antithrombotic therapy and revascularization. The ACC/AHA guidelines thus recommend for older patients [22, 23]:

(a) Decisions on management should reflect considerations of general health, comorbidities, cognitive status, and life expectancy (Ic)
(b) Attention should be paid to altered pharmacokinetics and sensitivity to hypotensive drugs (Ib)
(c) Intensive medical and interventional management of ACS may be undertaken but with close observation for adverse effects of these therapies (Ib)

Furthermore, the 2015 ESC guidelines for the management of acute coronary syndromes in patients presenting without persistent ST-segment elevation emphasize that despite the lower rate of revascularization in older patients, its benefit appears to be maintained at older age. According to paying attention to altered pharmacokinetics and possible adverse effects of therapies, 10–15% of patients were deemed to have contraindications for aspirin, beta-blockers, and statins. Nevertheless, it has to be suggested—based on registry data—that even in the very old patient, adherence to recommended therapies within 24 h of admission reduces in-hospital mortality [23]. This benefit was observed despite the increased risk of side effects

Table 17.1 Reasons for the elevation of cTn other than myocardial ischemia

Chronic or acute kidney failure
Heart failure—acute or chronic
Hypertensive crisis
Tachy- or bradyarrhythmias
Lung arterial embolism, pulmonary hypertension
Critical ill patients with respiratory insufficiency and septic condition
Acute neurological disease, i.e. stroke or subarachnoid bleeding
Aortic dissection, aortic valve diseases or hypertrophic cardiomyopathy
Contusion of the heart, ablation therapy, pacemaker stimulation, cardioversion or endomyocardial biopsy
Hypothyroidism
Takotsubo cardiomyopathy
Rhabdomyolysis
Myocarditis
Infiltrative myocardial disease like amyloidosis, hemochromatosis, sarcoidosis and sclerodermia
Drugs toxicity, i.e. adriamycine, 5-fluorouracile, herceptine, snake venoms

from pharmacological treatment and, specifically, the increased risk of bleeding events associated with antithrombotic therapy in older patients [23]. However, the management strategy must take into account possible end-stage diseases like cancer or dementia and the hereby-accompanied quality of life into account and weigh up costs and benefits of diagnostic and therapeutic interventions.

17.3.6.1 Cardiac Catheterization

More than half of all ACS trials in the last decade did not enroll patients >75 years. This subgroup only accounted for 9% of all patients enrolled in trials [20]. Among patients >75 years of age, the likelihood of catheterization decreased by 15% each year of advancing age [24]. Due to the exclusion of patients based on age, there is only limited evidence for the use of cardiac catheterization in older patients with ACS. For the same reason, there still is uncertainty about the benefits and risks in the use of newer medication in ACS. Comorbidities do not simplify the decision-making either, and older populations are heterogeneous in ways not captured by standard assessments.

Older patients >75 years undergo less cardiac catheterization than younger ones. In the USA, about 77% of older patients undergo cardiac catheterization, compared to 91% in younger patients [24].

The 2015 ESC guidelines for the management of acute coronary syndromes in patients presenting without persistent ST-segment elevation recommend an early invasive strategy with PCI within 48 h after initial presentation for all high-risk NSTE-ACS patients, whereas high risk implies indicators such as recurrent angina, elevated cardiac markers, ST-segment depression, heart failure, arrhythmias, prior coronary bypass or PCI. It was shown that the older population has a greater benefit in terms of absolute and relative risk reduction in reducing death with early invasive strategy, but these benefits coexist with an increase in major bleeding events [23].

17.3.6.2 Pharmacological Treatment

It has been shown that in-hospital administration of antiplatelet therapy decreases by age, while this is more pronounced for clopidogrel than for aspirin.

According to the ESC guidelines for the management of acute coronary syndromes in patients presenting without persistent ST-segment elevation guidelines, dual antiplatelet therapy and therefore the use of aspirin and one of the two more potent P2Y12 inhibitors ticagrelor or prasugrel in suspected ACS are highly recommended. The benefit of aspirin does not seem to be affected by age, and its benefit is greatest in highest-risk populations such as older patients [20]. As adjunct to the use of aspirin, the guidelines give a class Ia recommendation for a dual antiplatelet therapy without modification based on age, but there is still a lack of age subgroup data on efficacy and safety of this therapy from randomized trials. In contrast, the 2014 ACC/AHA guidelines for the management of patients with non-ST elevation acute coronary syndromes recommend that either clopidogrel or ticagrelor should be administered in addition to aspirin for up to 12 months to all patients with NSTE-ACS without contraindications who are treated with either an early invasive or ischemia-guided strategy [23].

17.3.6.3 Ticagrelor

A substudy of the Platelet Inhibition and Patient Outcomes (PLATO) trial published in 2012 could show that the clinical benefit of ticagrelor over clopidogrel in patients with acute coronary syndrome with respect to the composite of cardiovascular death, myocardial infarction, and stroke or all-cause mortality, was not significantly different between patients aged ≥75 and those aged <75 years [25]. The authors observed no increased risk of major bleeding complications with ticagrelor versus clopidogrel in patients aged ≥75 years or patients aged <75 years. Side effects like dyspnea and ventricular pauses were more common during treatment with ticagrelor than clopidogrel, with no evidence of an age-by-treatment interaction and no effect on mortality [25].

17.3.6.4 Prasugrel

Prasugrel has several limitations especially in older patients. It should not be given in those with a history of stroke or TIA or patients older 75 years as well as patients with a body weight less than 60 kg.

However, because it still remains unclear whether ticagrelor or prasugrel has a better net clinical benefit in older patients with NSTE-ACS when compared with clopidogrel, the 2015 enrolled "POPular AGE trial (Ticagrelor or Prasugrel Versus Clopidogrel in older Patients With an Acute Coronary Syndrome and a High Bleeding Risk: Optimization of Antiplatelet Treatment in High-risk Older)" is designed to address the optimal antiplatelet strategy in older patients NSTE-ACS patients [26].

In this randomized, controlled, open label, multicenter trial with an estimated enrollment of 1000 patients aged 70 years and older, presenting with non-ST elevation acute coronary syndrome, patients will be randomized to either clopidogrel or one of the P2Y12 inhibitors ticagrelor or prasugrel. Patients will be followed for 1 year for outcomes such as bleeding episodes requiring medical intervention and net clinical benefit, defined as all-cause mortality, nonfatal myocardial infarction, nonfatal stroke, and PLATO major and minor bleeding [27].

17.3.7 Prognosis and Outcomes

In-hospital death rate in patients <65 and NSTE-ACS is 1 in 100, whereas this risk increases dramatically to one in ten in patients >85 years. The 1-year mortality rate for NSTE-ACS patients >75 years is one in five increasing to one in four in patients >85 years [20].

The trends to higher mortality among those not undergoing catheterization were no longer significant after adjustment for predictors of mortality and propensity for cardiac catheterization in the overall population [24]. This supports the need for further studies in higher age populations, as it is suspected that effective therapies are withhold from old people due to the lack of data and higher absolute complication rates.

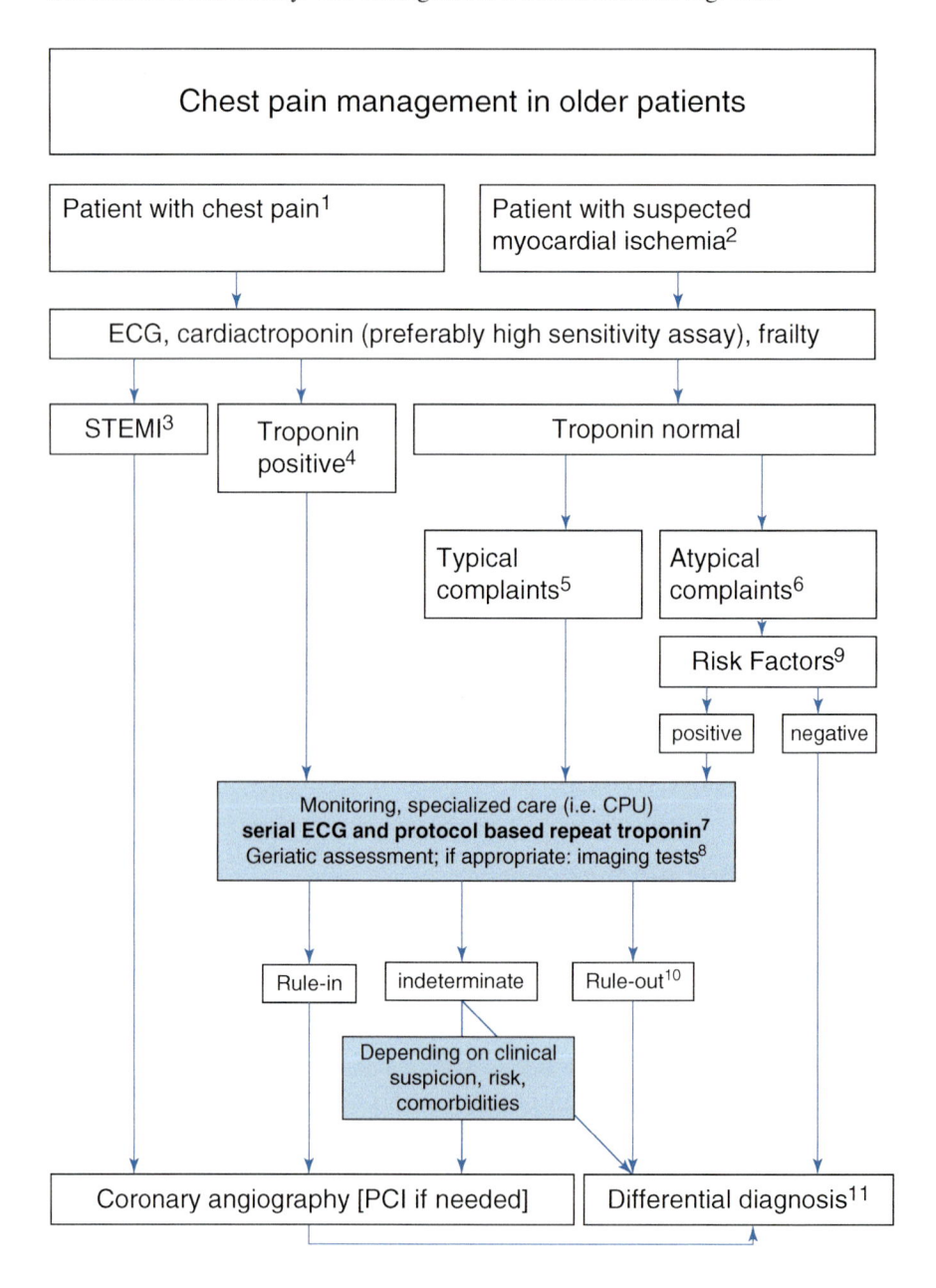

17.4 General Management of Chest Pain in Older Patients

The general management of acute chest pain should be basically the same as in the general population [28], but frailty needs to be recognized early, and a holistic assessment is mandatory. The management is summarized in Fig. 17.1.

```
Chest pain management in older patients

Patient with chest pain[1]          Patient with suspected myocardial ischemia[2]

        ECG, cardiactroponin (preferably high sensitivity assay), frailty

STEMI[3]   Troponin positive[4]                Troponin normal

                                    Typical complaints[5]    Atypical complaints[6]

                                                             Risk Factors[9]
                                                             positive    negative

            Monitoring, specialized care (i.e. CPU)
            serial ECG and protocol based repeat troponin[7]
            Geriatic assessment; if appropriate: imaging tests[8]

            Rule-in   indeterminate   Rule-out[10]

                      Depending on clinical
                      suspicion, risk,
                      comorbidities

        Coronary angiography [PCI if needed]     Differential diagnosis[11]
```

Fig. 17.1 Management of chest pain in older patients. (*1*) Nontraumatic chest pain without evident extracardiac source; (*2*) other symptoms include dyspnea and vegetative symptoms like sweating, nausea, vomiting, and shock; (*3*) STEMI patients are directly ruled in for acute coronary angiography and PCI; (*4*) troponin positive means above the 99%tile in high-sensitive (HS) assays and above assay-dependent cutoffs in conventional sensitive assays (only if the CV does not allow to use the 99%tile cutoff); (*5*) typical complaints denote chest pain with radiation in the jaw, back, and both arms, which is not released by the use of nitroglycerin; (*6*) atypical complaints are punctual, "stabbing" chest pain or episodes which have released already spontaneously or during exertion; specific rule-out strategies are discussed elsewhere; (*7*) HS troponin every 3 h or in shorter intervals if implemented as protocol, conventional troponin every 6 h; repeat ECG at every clinical event (arrhythmias, significant change of symptoms) and when troponin is repeated; (*8*) geriatric assessment and comorbidities influencing cardiac troponin levels are crucial; early echocardiography is used in unclear cases to diagnose important differential diagnoses like pulmonary embolism, aortic dissection, or severe heart failure but also to detect regional wall motion abnormalities which support the suspicion of AMI; (*9*) for risk stratification established scores like TIMI, GRACE, or the HEART score should be used; (*10*) in case of a negative initial evaluation, an early stress test should be applied within 3 days; (*11*) differential diagnoses include the important entities mentioned under (*8*) but also benign disorders like musculoskeletal caused pain, which can be diagnosed on an outpatient basis. Abbreviation: CPU, chest pain unit

In older patients with acute coronary syndrome, the diagnosis is frequently hampered by nonspecific symptoms, and these patients often seek medical help later than they often seek younger individuals. Older patients with acute coronary syndrome are still less frequently being referred to percutaneous coronary intervention (PCI) than younger patients, although statistically even octogenarians profit from PCI more than from thrombolysis or purely drug therapy. Radial access may be of special benefit in older patients, allowing for an early mobilization of frail individuals and reducing bleeding complications in patients with per se high risk due to age. The presence of comorbidities in geriatric individuals dictates the necessity of implementing a comprehensive geriatric assessment [6].

Conclusions

The management of chest pain in older patients is a major challenge due to the lack of data from clinical studies. In general, the same principles as for other patients apply, but frailty should be assessed early, and multimorbidity and polypharmacy need to be taken into account. Compared to younger patients, atypical symptoms are more common, and the index chest pain event may be "hidden." In addition, confusional states are often exacerbated by hospitalization and may be a symptom of myocardial infarction due to hypotension and pre-shock.

References

1. Mockel M, Searle J, Muller R, Slagman A, Storchmann H, Oestereich P, Wyrwich W, Ale-Abaei A, Vollert JO, Koch M, Somasundaram R (2013) Chief complaints in medical emergencies: do they relate to underlying disease and outcome? The charite emergency medicine study (Charitem). Eur J Emerg Med 20:103–108
2. Ebell MH (2011) Evaluation of chest pain in primary care patients. Am Fam Physician 83:603–605
3. Engbers MJ, Van Hylckama Vlieg A, Rosendaal FR (2010) Venous thrombosis in the elderly: incidence, risk factors and risk groups. J Thromb Haemost 8:2105–2112
4. Schouten HJ, Geersing GJ, Oudega R, Van Delden JJ, Moons KG, Koek HL (2014) Accuracy of the wells clinical prediction rule for pulmonary embolism in older ambulatory adults. J Am Geriatr Soc 62:2136–2141
5. Righini M, Le Gal G, Bounameaux H (2015) Venous thromboembolism diagnosis: unresolved issues. Thromb Haemost 113:1184–1192
6. Lucassen W, Geersing GJ, Erkens PM, Reitsma JB, Moons KG, Buller H, Van Weert HC (2011) Clinical decision rules for excluding pulmonary embolism: a meta-analysis. Ann Intern Med 155:448–460
7. Zhang QL, Rothenbacher D (2008) Prevalence of chronic kidney disease in population-based studies: systematic review. BMC Public Health 8:117
8. Khan IA, Nair CK (2002) Clinical, diagnostic, and management perspectives of aortic dissection. Chest 122:311–328
9. Mehta RH, O'gara PT, Bossone E, Nienaber CA, Myrmel T, Cooper JV, Smith DE, Armstrong WF, Isselbacher EM, Pape LA, Eagle KA, Gilon D, International Registry of Acute Aortic Dissection Investigation (2002) Acute type A aortic dissection in the elderly: clinical characteristics, management, and outcomes in the current era. J Am Coll Cardiol 40:685–692
10. Sahn SA, Heffner JE (2000) Spontaneous pneumothorax. N Engl J Med 342:868–874
11. Liston R, Mcloughlin R, Clinch D (1994) Acute pneumothorax: a comparison of elderly with younger patients. Age Ageing 23:393–395
12. Chang JT, Morton SC, Rubenstein LZ, Mojica WA, Maglione M, Suttorp MJ, Roth EA, Shekelle PG (2004) Interventions for the prevention of falls in older adults: systematic review and meta-analysis of randomised clinical trials. BMJ 328:680
13. Büscher A (2006) Expertenstandard Sturzprophylaxe In Der Pflege. Deutsches Netzwerk Für Qualitätsentwicklung In Der Pflege, 1. Is it a book, please edit according to Springer
14. Stupka JE, Mortensen EM, Anzueto A, Restrepo MI (2009) Community-acquired pneumonia in elderly patients. Aging Health 5:763–774
15. Marrie TJ (2000) Community-acquired pneumonia in the elderly. Clin Infect Dis 31:1066–1078
16. Schmader K (1998) Postherpetic neuralgia in immunocompetent elderly people. Vaccine 16:1768–1770
17. Thygesen K, Alpert JS, Jaffe AS, Simoons ML, Chaitman BR, White HD, Joint ESC/ACCF/AHA/WHF Task Force for the Universal Definition of Myocardial Infarction; Authors/Task Force Members Chairpersons, Thygesen K, Alpert JS, White HD, Biomarker Subcommittee, Jaffe AS, Katus HA, Apple FS, Lindahl B, Morrow DA, ECG Subcommittee, Chaitman BR, Clemmensen PM, Johanson P, Hod H, Imaging Subcommittee, Underwood R, Bax JJ, Bonow JJ, Pinto F, Gibbons RJ, Classification Subcommittee, Fox KA, Atar D, Newby LK, Galvani M, Hamm CW, Intervention Subcommittee, Uretsky BF, Steg PG, Wijns W, Bassand JP, Menasche P, Ravkilde J, Trials & Registries Subcommittee, Ohman EM, Antman EM, Wallentin LC, Armstrong PW, Simoons ML, Trials & Registries Subcommittee, Januzzi JL, Nieminen MS, Gheorghiade M, Filippatos G, Luepker RV, Fortmann SP, Rosamond WD, Levy D, Wood D, Trials & Registries Subcommittee, Smith SC, Hu D, Lopez-Sendon JL, Robertson RM, Weaver D, Tendera M, Bove AA, Parkhomenko AN, Vasilieva EJ, Mendis S, ESC Committee for Practice Guidelines (CPG), Bax JJ, Baumgartner H, Ceconi C, Dean V, Deaton C, Fagard R, Funck-Brentano C, Hasdai D, Hoes A, Kirchhof P, Knuuti J, Kolh P,

Mcdonagh T, Moulin C, Popescu BA, Reiner Z, Sechtem U, Sirnes PA, Tendera M, Torbicki A, Vahanian A, Windecker S, Document Reviewers, Morais J, Aguiar C, Almahmeed W et al (2012) Third universal definition of myocardial infarction. J Am Coll Cardiol 60:1581–1598
18. Friesinger GC, Smith RF (2000) Old age, left bundle branch block and acute myocardial infarction: a vexing and lethal combination. J Am Coll Cardiol 36:713–716
19. Canto JG, Shlipak MG, Rogers WJ, Malmgren JA, Frederick PD, Lambrew CT, Ornato JP, Barron HV, Kiefe CI (2000) Prevalence, clinical characteristics, and mortality among patients with myocardial infarction presenting without chest pain. JAMA 283:3223–3229
20. Alexander KP, Newby LK, Cannon CP, Armstrong PW, Gibler WB, Rich MW, Van De Werf F, White HD, Weaver WD, Naylor MD, Gore JM, Krumholz HM, Ohman EM, American Heart Association Council on Clinical Cardiology; Society of Geriatric Cardiology (2007) Acute coronary care in the elderly, part I: non-St-segment-elevation acute coronary syndromes: a scientific statement for healthcare professionals from the American Heart Association Council on clinical cardiology: in collaboration with the society of geriatric cardiology. Circulation 115:2549–2569
21. Hanon O, Baixas C, Friocourt P, Carrie D, Emeriau JP, Galinier M, Belmin J, De Groote P, Benetos A, Jourdain P, Berrut G, Aupetit JF, Jondeau G, Danchin N, Forette F, Komajda M, French Society of Gerontology and Geriatrics; French Society of Cardiology (2009) Consensus of the French society of gerontology and geriatrics and the French society of cardiology for the management of coronary artery disease in older adults. Arch Cardiovasc Dis 102:829–845
22. Alexander KP, Newby LK, Armstrong PW, Cannon CP, Gibler WB, Rich MW, Van De Werf F, White HD, Weaver WD, Naylor MD, Gore JM, Krumholz HM, Ohman EM, American Heart Association Council on Clinical Cardiology; Society of Geriatric Cardiology (2007) Acute coronary care in the elderly, part ii: St-segment-elevation myocardial infarction: a scientific statement for healthcare professionals from the American Heart Association Council on clinical cardiology: in collaboration with the society of geriatric cardiology. Circulation 115:2570–2589
23. Amsterdam EA, Wenger NK, Brindis RG, Casey DE Jr, Ganiats TG, Holmes DR Jr, Jaffe AS, Jneid H, Kelly RF, Kontos MC, Levine GN, Liebson PR, Mukherjee D, Peterson ED, Sabatine MS, Smalling RW, Zieman SJ, ACC/AHA Task Force Members (2014) 2014 aha/Acc guideline for the management of patients with non-St-elevation acute coronary syndromes: a report of the American college of cardiology/American Heart Association task force on practice guidelines. Circulation 130:E344–E426
24. Alexander KP, Newby LK, Bhapkar MV, White HD, Hochman JS, Pfisterer ME, Moliterno DJ, Peterson ED, Van De Werf F, Armstrong PW, Califf RM, Symphony and 2nd Symphony Investigators (2006) International variation in invasive care of the elderly with acute coronary syndromes. Eur Heart J 27:1558–1564
25. Husted S, James S, Becker RC, Horrow J, Katus H, Storey RF, Cannon CP, Heras M, Lopes RD, Morais J, Mahaffey KW, Bach RG, Wojdyla D, Wallentin L, PLATO study group (2012) Ticagrelor versus clopidogrel in elderly patients with acute coronary syndromes: a substudy from the prospective randomized platelet inhibition and patient outcomes (Plato) trial. Circ Cardiovasc Qual Outcomes 5:680–688
26. Berg JMT (2014) Ticagrelor or prasugrel versus clopidogrel in elderly patients with an acute coronary syndrome and a high bleeding risk: optimization of antiplatelet treatment in high-risk elderly (popular age). Am Heart J 170(5):981–985.e1
27. Qaderdan K, Ishak M, Heestermans AA, De Vrey E, Jukema JW, Voskuil M, De Boer MJ, Van't Hof AW, Groenemeijer BE, Vos GJ, Janssen PW, Bergmeijer TO, Kelder JC, Deneer VH, Ten Berg JM (2015) Ticagrelor or prasugrel versus clopidogrel in elderly patients with an acute coronary syndrome: optimization of antiplatelet treatment in patients 70 years and older--rationale and design of the popular age study. Am Heart J 170:981–985 e1
28. Mockel M, Giannitsis E, Mueller C, Huber K, Jaffe AS, Mair J, Plebani M, Thygesen K, Lindahl B (2016) Rule-in of acute myocardial infarction: focus on troponin. Eur Heart J Acute Cardiovasc Care 6(3):212–217

Dyspnoea in Older People in the Emergency Department

18

F. Javier Martín-Sánchez and Juan González del Castillo

18.1 Introduction

Breathlessness is one of the most common complaints and is the main cause for the admission of older patients presenting to the ED. Dyspnoea is a potentially serious syndrome and can represent life-threatening emergencies [1]. In fact, dyspnoea is one of the highest mortality of all non-trauma complaints [2].

18.2 Definition

Dyspnoea is a difficult symptom to assess and is often caused by life-threatening conditions [3]. Dyspnoea is a subjective symptom of breathlessness (air hunger). Acute respiratory failure (ARF) is a condition in which the cardiorespiratory system fails in one or both of its gas exchange functions, i.e. oxygenation ($PaO_2 < 60$ mmHg) and/or elimination of carbon dioxide (arterial carbon dioxide pressure ($PaCO_2$) >45 mmHg). ARF can also be suspected by the presence of dyspnoea or other 'simple' clinical features such as polypnoea >30 per min, contraction of the accessory inspiratory muscles, abdominal respiration, cyanosis, asterixis, decreased level of consciousness and symptoms and signs of heart failure [4, 5] (Fig. 18.1).

Age-related changes of the cardiorespiratory system should be taken into account in the assessment and management of dyspnoea. Figure 18.2 shows the main changes secondary to ageing in the pulmonary, cardiovascular and central nervous systems. Changes due to ageing in both the pulmonary and cardiovascular systems make older people more vulnerable to significant acute injury and less likely to

---

F.J. Martín-Sánchez, MD, PhD (✉) • J.G. del Castillo, MD, PhD
Emergency Department, Hospital Clínico San Carlos,
C/ Profesor Martín-Lagos s/n, 28040 Madrid, Spain
e-mail: fjjms@hotmail.com

© Springer International Publishing Switzerland 2018
C. Nickel et al. (eds.), *Geriatric Emergency Medicine*,
https://doi.org/10.1007/978-3-319-19318-2_18

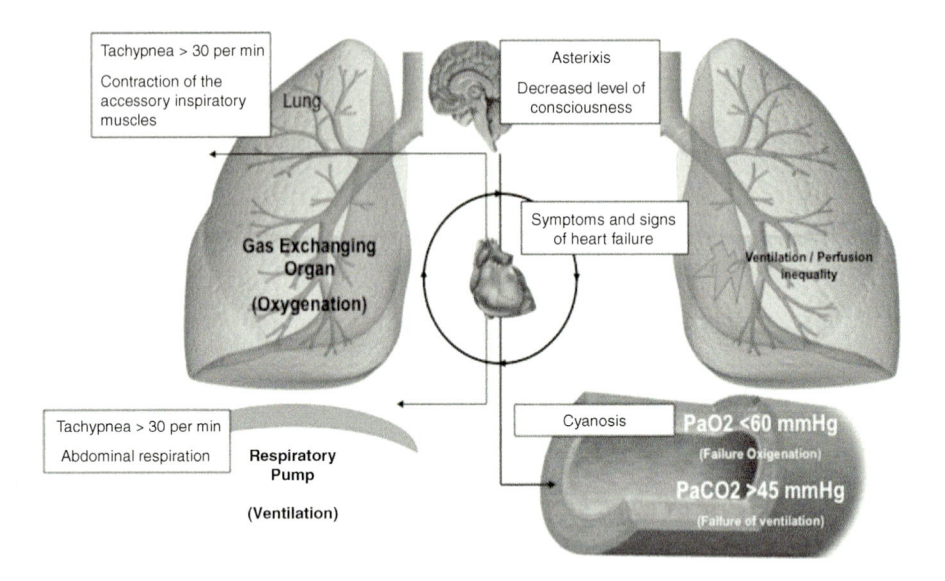

Fig. 18.1 Symptoms and signs of acute respiratory failure

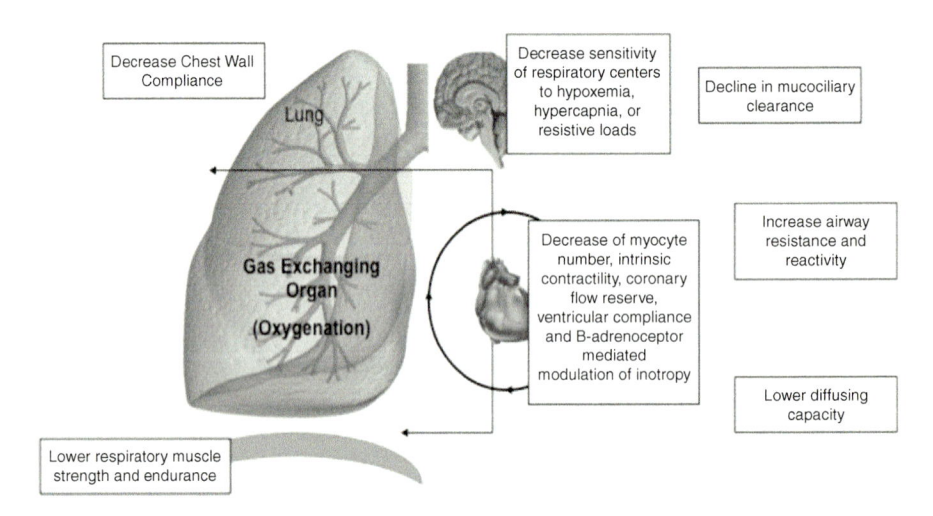

Fig. 18.2 Age-related changes of the cardiorespiratory system

present with the classical symptoms and signs of dyspnoea, which are associated with a worse prognosis.

18.3 Aetiology

Dyspnoea is the main clinical presentation of cardiac and respiratory disorders, although many other potential aetiologies may also be present [4, 5]. Dyspnoea is caused by chest wall and pleural abnormalities, lung and airway disease, acute heart failure (AHF) or central and peripheral nervous system condition alterations. In the EPIDASA study, AHF (43%), pneumonia (35%), COPD exacerbations (32%) and pulmonary embolism (PE) (18%) were the main causes of dyspnoea in older patients, being associated with a high mortality [3]. Acute dyspnoea in the older is more likely to be due to multiple causes (50% had more than two diagnoses), including non-cardiopulmonary factors (i.e. metabolic acidosis, acute intra-abdominal or renal pathology and sepsis) and therefore require a more extensive work-up [3].

18.4 Diagnosis

Dyspnoea is due to multiple causes and the diagnostic work-up of emergency physicians involves wide differential diagnoses (Table 18.1). Diagnosis by emergency physicians is even more complex and less accurate in older patients [3]. The appropriate initial diagnosis and treatment of patients attended for dyspnoea in the ED are associated with shorter hospital and intensive care unit (ICU) stay and a better short-term prognosis [3].

Table 18.1 Aetiology of dyspnoea in older patients in the emergency department[a]

Lung and airway disease
- Acute exacerbation of COPD
- Pneumonia
- Acute asthma
- Upper airway obstruction
- Lung cancer
- Pulmonary fibrosis
- Bronchiectasis
- Tuberculosis

Acute heart failure
- Ischaemic disease
- Heart valve disease
- Arrhythmia

Vessels
- Hypertension
- Pulmonary embolism

Chest wall and pleural abnormalities
- Kyphoscoliosis
- Chest wall trauma
- Pleural effusion
- Pneumothorax
- Muscle abnormalities

Central and peripheral nervous system
- Drugs: Sedatives
- CNS: Stroke, trauma, etc.
- PNS: Guillain-Barre syndrome, myelitis, tetanus, spinal cord trauma, amyotrophic lateral sclerosis, myasthenia, botulism, etc.

Other
- Shock
- Anaemia

[a]50% of older patients have two aetiologies [3]

The differential diagnosis of dyspnoea in older patients attended in the ED is usually achieved according to the clinical history, physical examination, 12-lead electrocardiogram, chest X-ray and laboratory tests. Further tests such as determination of biomarkers, arterial or venous blood gas, ultrasound, computed tomography, ventilation/perfusion scan or other tests should be performed taking into account previous findings. The diagnosis of pneumonia is based on chest X-rays [6], while the diagnosis of heart failure is based on electrocardiogram, chest radiographs and natriuretic peptide type B values [7], and the diagnosis of pulmonary embolism is based on prediction rules (Wells rule and revised Geneva score), D-dimer (age-adjusted cut-offs) and computerized tomography [8]. There are no definitive diagnostic or imaging tests to diagnose an exacerbation of COPD or asthma. Moreover, asthma present in the most advanced ages is often diagnosed as COPD, thereby leading to under or inappropriate treatment [9].

18.4.1 Symptoms and Signs

Regarding dyspnoea, it is important to ascertain the time of presentation, precipitating factors and additional treatment given, the baseline functional status and exercise tolerance, the clinical history (comorbidities, tobacco consumption, use of home oxygen, number of previous hospital admissions or ED visits, and ventilation in an ICU) as well as the usual medical treatment.

Questions about associated symptoms such as chest pain, palpitations, diaphoresis, paroxysmal nocturnal dyspnoea, orthopnoea, leg swelling, fever, cough and changes in sputum or haemoptysis should also be considered. The older tends to present more atypical (i.e. confusion, fall, functional impairment or decompensation of chronic disease) and fewer typical symptoms (i.e. paroxysmal nocturnal dyspnoea in heart failure, chest pain in myocardial infarction (MI), fever, cough, sputum or dyspnoea in pneumonia) compared to younger adults.

Physical examination has a twofold objective. The first is to identify high-risk patients in the initial assessment even before obtaining the clinical history. Severe respiratory distress includes the inability to complete sentences in one breath or lie supine, the use of accessory muscles, agitation or other altered mental status, diaphoresis, hypotension, tachypnoea, tachycardia and silent chest. Signs of imminent respiratory failure include confusion or coma, cyanosis and feeble respiratory effort. The level of consciousness or vital signs in older people may be altered by age-related changes, comorbidities or medications. Elevated jugular venous pressure and pulsus paradoxus can occur in some conditions that compromise right heart filling. The second objective of the physical examination is to provide essential elements for differential diagnosis, although no finding on physical examination can rule out a significant condition. Cardiac and pulmonary auscultation may reveal abnormal (inspiratory or expiratory stridor, wheezing or rales) or diminished breath or heart sounds and murmurs. On physical examination of older patients, there is a greater probability of detecting less specific (i.e. rales, oedema) and reproducible (i.e. elevated jugular venous pressure) signs and a lesser probability of identifying specific (i.e. third heart sound) signs [10–12].

18 Dyspnoea in Older People in the Emergency Department

The presence of breathlessness, fatigue or tiredness increased time to recover after exercise or confusion, and a past history of chronic heart failure or coronary disease suggest an episode of acute heart failure. Silent acute MI is well recognized in older people, especially in those over 85 years old. Acute presentation of dyspnoea, especially if accompanied by tachypnoea, tachycardia, pleuritic chest pain, haemoptysis or syncope, with recent immobilization (i.e. bed rest, recent trauma or surgery or recent hospitalization) or hypercoagulability (i.e. cancer), indicates the possible presence of a pulmonary embolism. Asthma and COPD exacerbations are frequently accompanied by cough, tachypnoea, intermittent chest pain, sputum production, wheezing and decreased or absent breath sounds. The most complex task is to distinguish between asthma and COPD [9]. The presentation of pneumonia is usually more subtle. It is important to consider spontaneous pneumothorax or pulmonary embolism in patients showing a sudden deterioration in the ED, especially in those with underlying asthma and COPD.

18.4.2 Electrocardiogram

The electrocardiogram may show new features suggestive of acute cardiac ischaemia (ST segment or T wave), pulmonary embolism (S1Q3T3 and right ventricle overload) as well as other conditions.

18.4.3 Chest Radiography

A chest X-ray is usually diagnostic of pneumonia (infiltrate), pneumothorax (air in pleural space) and AHF (cardiomegaly, redistribution of pulmonary vessels, Kerley lines, peribronchial cuffing, consolidation, cotton wool appearance, pleural effusion). Chest X-ray has showed a low sensitivity and negative predictive value in identifying pulmonary opacities. A chest X-ray may be unremarkable in many patients with mildly or moderately severe COPD, in most patients with asthma, in almost 20% patients with heart failure and in 30% of patients with pneumonia, being more frequent in the early phase or when accompanied by dehydration or neutropenia. Thus, on suspicion of pneumonia the radiography should be repeated at 24–48 h, or a computerized tomography should be performed. Rib fractures may be found in older patients with an altered mental status or a history of falls.

18.4.4 Laboratory Tests

In reference to routine laboratory test immediately performed in ED, it is recommended to request a blood count and biochemistry including electrolytes, renal and liver function tests and thyroid hormones. Inadequate inflammatory response as a consequence of immunosenescence may condition C-reactive protein (CRP) and leukocyte results, underestimating the severity of the infectious process.

18.4.5 Biomarkers

Troponin, natriuretic peptides, procalcitonin and D-dimer are markers, which can significantly contribute to the aetiologic diagnosis of an acute dyspnoea. Troponin, natriuretic peptides and procalcitonin (PCT) in conjunction with lactate are also prognostic markers, and these parameters are valuable for stratifying disease severity according to initial values and plasma kinetics during the clinical course of the disease.

Troponin is a marker of myocardial damage and may be useful for the aetiologic diagnosis of an acute coronary event but also in the short-term prognostic stratification of AHF and PE [13]. Serial measurements of cardiac biomarkers are necessary to rule out an acute coronary syndrome. Nonetheless, troponin has limited specificity and may be elevated in other conditions (i.e. sepsis).

D-dimer values may be obtained in cases with a low to intermediate risk of PE (i.e. Wells or Geneva criteria) since a negative D-Dimer value allows PE to be ruled out. D-dimer values are more likely to be falsely increased in older patients (sensitivity of ELISA D-dimer tests is around 100% irrespective of age; however the specificity is lower than 15% in older people with frailty because of multiple underlying comorbidities). Recent evidence suggests using age-adjusted cut-offs to improve the performance of D-dimer testing in older people [8, 14].

The addition of a single natriuretic peptide type B measurement improves the diagnostic accuracy and prognosis of AHF in the ED compared to standard clinical judgement in ED patients with dyspnoea [15]. BNP and NT-proBNP are both accurate in the diagnosis of AHF and are recommended to exclude cardiac causes of dyspnoea [15]. It is known that these values rise with age, sex, renal function, nutritional state and in other associated acute conditions (atrial fibrillation, pulmonary thromboembolism, sepsis, anaemia, ischaemic heart disease, myocardiopathies, etc.) [16]. In general, it is considered that BNP < 100 pg/mL and NT-proBNP < 300 pg/mL almost certainly rule out the diagnosis of AHF. To the contrary, from a diagnostic point of view, different cut-offs of NT-proBNP have been described based on the age group (<50 years, 450 pg/mL; 50–75 years, 900 pg/mL; >75 years, 1.800 pg/mL) [15]. With regard to the prognostic value of NT-proBNP, it is known that a cut-off of ≥5.180 pg/mL is associated with 30-day mortality in the older population attended for AHF in a hospital ED, regardless of the presence of other factors which may influence interpretation such as the severity of the acute episode or a reduction in glomerular filtration (Martin-Sanchez et al. 2012).

PCT is the prehormone of calcitonin, which is normally secreted by the thyroid gland in response to hypercalcemia and is induced by bacterial infection. Elevated PCT concentrations (higher than 0.25 ng/mL) may indicate an infectious aetiology of dyspnoea [17]. In suspected lower respiratory tract infections (CAP or COPD exacerbation), determination of PCT concentrations was useful as a guide to reduce the total antibiotic exposure and antibiotic prescriptions on admission [4, 5]. The BACH trial showed that patients with a diagnosis of AHF and elevated PCT concentrations had a worse outcome if not treated with antibiotics. PCT may aid in the decision to administer antibiotics to patients presenting for AHF and in whom there is clinical uncertainty regarding the involvement of a superimposed bacterial infection [18].

The panel of markers (troponin I, myoglobin, creatinine kinase-myocardial band isoenzyme, D-dimer, and B-type natriuretic peptide) did not improve the area under the ROC curve for diagnosing the combined set of clinical conditions (AHF, PE, MI) [19].

18.4.6 Arterial Blood Gas

Oxygenation can usually be measured using transcutaneous pulse oximetry, but in some cases (delirium, hypothermia, hypoperfusion or carbon monoxide poisoning) it can be more difficult. Arterial blood gas allows the assessment of oxygen saturation and CO2 retention. Only PaO2 and SaO2 changed clinically significantly with increasing age, whereas the other analyses were virtually independent of age [20].

18.4.7 Bedside Ultrasound

The integrated use of bedside ultrasound (lung-cardiac-inferior vena cava) may help to diagnosis some life-threatening causes of dyspnoea, including pericardial tamponade, pneumothorax, pleural effusion, MI and PE [21]. This technique allows assessment of lung sliding and quantification of pulmonary lines, the degree of vena cava collapse, the qualitative assessment of the left ventricular ejection fraction, the presence of pericardial effusion, dilatation of the right ventricle, cardiac wall motion abnormalities and deep venous thrombosis.

Regarding lung ultrasound, predominant A lines plus lung sliding indicated asthma or COPD. Multiple anterior diffuse B lines with lung sliding indicate pulmonary oedema. A normal anterior profile plus deep venous thrombosis indicate PE. Anterior absent lung sliding plus A lines plus lung point indicate pneumothorax. Anterior alveolar consolidations, anterior diffuse B lines with abolished lung sliding, anterior asymmetric interstitial patterns, posterior consolidations or effusions without anterior diffuse B lines indicate pneumonia. A previous study, which included 260 patients with mean age 68 (SD 16) years, showed correct diagnoses in 90.5% of cases with the use of these profiles [22].

Some authors have proposed new alternative algorithms for the diagnostic approach to dyspnoea, especially in cases in which biomarkers induce diagnostic uncertainty and differential diagnosis with pulmonary disease is difficult [4, 5, 21, 23].

18.4.8 Chest Computed Tomography

Chest computed tomography (CT) is the most sensitive test to diagnose lung pathologies (i.e. cancer, pneumonia, interstitial lung disease, pulmonary oedema) and may be used when diagnosis cannot be definitively made by other modalities. A CT angiogram is the test of choice for diagnosing PE and aortic syndrome. The triple rule out protocol (coronary acute syndrome, pulmonary embolism, aortic syndrome) may be helpful in the evaluation of selected patients, but it should not be routinely used [24].

18.5 Treatment

The initial evaluation of dyspnoea includes the identification of high-risk patients, respiratory and haemodynamic stabilization, diagnosis and treatment of rapidly reversible causes that require immediate intervention and evaluation of the need for admission to the intensive care unit. This decision should not be based on age alone but also on factors such as the patient's baseline functional level and comorbidities, severity of illness and preferences for life support.

Potential high-risk patients are older patients with a history of trauma, severe underlying lung or heart disease, abnormal vital or hypoperfusion signs, accessory muscles used, cyanosis, decreased level of consciousness or agitation and rapid clinical deterioration. In these patients, hypoxaemia should be treated with oxygen therapy, airway management, and ventilation support should be considered. Bedside ultrasound and an electrocardiogram should be performed to rule out life-threatening causes (upper airway foreign body or anaphylaxia, pneumothorax tension, pericardial tamponade, acute coronary syndrome with ST-segment elevation and arrhythmia). Polymedication may affect the respiratory and cardiac systems.

Secondarily, after ruling out life-threatening conditions or stabilizing high-risk patients, hypoxaemia should be treated with oxygen therapy and complementary tests requested. The initial treatment must be guided by the suspected aetiology of dyspnoea. Thirdly, the patient should be monitored non-invasively and treatment started according to aetiology identified. Fourthly, the clinical situation and response to initial treatment should be reevaluated. Fifthly, patient risk should be stratified, and lastly, the decision-making process and design of an individualized care plan should be undertaken. Indeed, the outcome of the patient depends on the appropriate initial treatment administered in the ED (Fig. 18.3).

18.5.1 Oxygen and Non-invasive Ventilation (NIV)

Oxygen supplementation is only needed in patients with hypoxaemia. The target of oxygen saturation is greater than or equal to 92% (90% in COPD). Incorrect use of oxygen therapy is associated with an increase of hypercapnia and acidosis in COPD patients. In a recent meta-analysis, NIV was recommended as first-line treatment in cases of acute cardiogenic pulmonary oedema and COPD, especially with moderate-severe acute respiratory failure [25, 26]. NIV has been associated with reduced mortality, avoidance of endotracheal intubation and a reduction in treatment failure [25, 26].

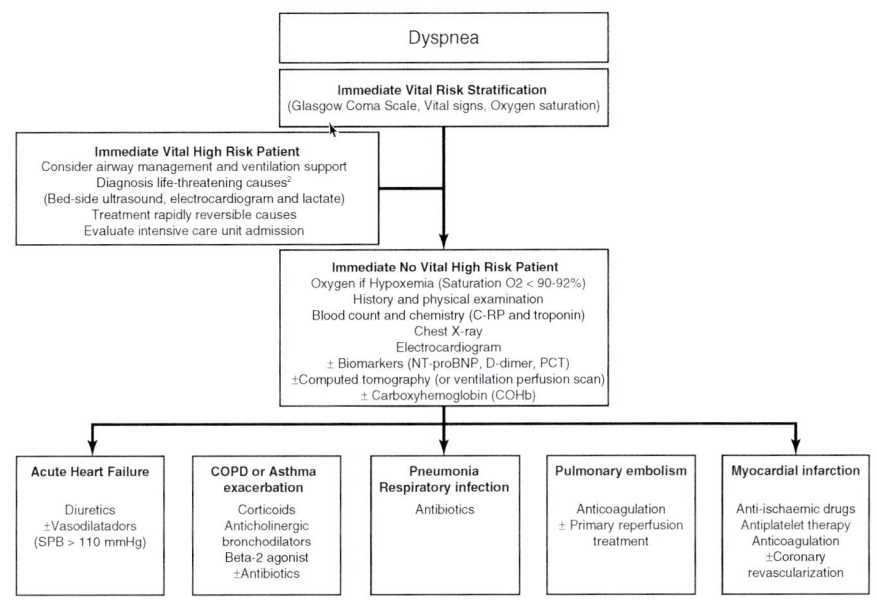

18 Dyspnoea in Older People in the Emergency Department

Fig. 18.3 Treatment algorithm for dyspnoea in the older

18.5.2 Diuretics

Intravenous diuretics are the treatment of choice in pulmonary congestion. In older people, AHF with preserved systolic function is frequent, and therefore an appropriate relation between diuretics (cardiac failure) and vasodilators (vascular failure) is needed [27].

18.5.3 Bronchodilators

Short-acting beta 2 agonists and anticholinergic bronchodilators (nebulized or inhaled) plus corticosteroids (oral or intravenous) are mainstays of therapy for acute exacerbations of asthma and COPD [28]. Theophylline is not recommended in older people because of its limited benefits, narrow therapeutic window and risk of cardiovascular events.

Side effects of beta-2 agonist are more frequent in older people and include tachycardia, tremors, QT prolongations and decreased serum potassium levels. The coexistence of cardiovascular disorders increases the frequency and severity of side effects. Beta-2 agonist use was associated with increased all-cause mortality, cardiovascular death, heart failure hospitalization and major adverse cardiovascular events in patients with chronic heart failure [29]. Currently, there is insufficient evidence to suggest that acute treatment with inhaled beta-2 agonists should be avoided in patients with dyspnoea caused by heart failure [30].

Doses of oral prednisone higher than 60 or 125 mg of intravenous methylprednisolone have not proven to be more effective. Local (hoarseness, cough, candidiasis) and systemic (cataracts and osteoporosis) adverse effects can be more frequent in older patients and are associated with the route and time of corticosteroid administration.

18.5.4 Antibiotics

Antibiotics are currently recommended for pneumonia, respiratory infection and COPD exacerbations when bacterial infection is suspected or when a severe situation such as when ventilatory support is needed. The most predictive factor associated with bacterial infection is an increase in sputum volume and purulence [31].

With respect to the timing of the antibiotic treatment, patients with pneumonia should start appropriate antibiotic treatment early, especially those with severe sepsis and septic shock. Although current guidelines for treating CAP without severe sepsis and septic shock do not recommend administering antibiotics within a certain time limit, the recommendation is to start antibiotics as soon as the diagnosis of CAP is established and while the patient is still in the ED [6]. Stable patients with an atypical presentation, however, should not be prioritized over other patients in the ED and should not receive antibiotics unless the diagnosis of pneumonia is established [32].

Regarding empirical antibiotic treatment, the recommendations depend on the specific organism suspected and guidelines in conjunction with the severity of the clinical situation and local microbial resistance [6].

18.5.5 Anticoagulation

Anticoagulation is the treatment of choice in PE. Older people are at increased risk of bleeding when under anticoagulation therapy compared with younger patients. Acute-phase treatment consists of administering parenteral anticoagulation (unfractionated heparin, low-molecular-weight heparin or fondaparinux) over the first 5–10 days. Parenteral heparin should overlap with the initiation of a vitamin K antagonist; alternatively, it can be followed by the administration of one of the new oral anticoagulants which may be started directly or after 1–2 days of administration of parenteral anticoagulation [8].

In older patients admitted to hospital, thromboprophylaxis with low-molecular-weight heparin (LMWH), low-dose unfractionated heparin (LDUH) or fondaparinux is recommended [33].

The use LMWH often requires adjustment according to creatinine clearance. Long-term use of heparin has been associated with increased osteopenia in older people.

18.5.6 Management of Comorbidities

The clinician must also take into account the comorbidities of the patient (i.e. malnutrition, diabetes mellitus, anaemia, renal failure) as well as the functional and mental status in order to provide the most appropriate care.

Geriatric assessment adapted to the ED that includes brief scales related to clinical, mental, functional and social aspects has been proposed to help in decision-making and in the design of care planning [10–12]. Comprehensive rehabilitation including exercise, nutritional support and education is a first therapeutic option of choice in the care of these individuals [28].

18.6 Risk Stratification

Ray et al. described several variables associated with in-hospital death in patients attended in the ED for dyspnoea including inappropriate treatment in ED, clinical signs of acute ventilatory failure or PaCO2 > 45 mmHg, elevated BNP or NT-proBNP levels and renal failure [3]. Several models of 30-day mortality risk stratification have been developed to help in the decision-making process for the admission and placement of patients. These models include the Pulmonary Embolism Severity Index (PESI)for PE, the Pneumonia Severity Index (PSI)or CURB-65 for pneumonia and the CHR risk model (EFFECT heart failure mortality prediction for heart failure). However, these scores have not been validated in very old patients.

Observation or short-stay units play a fundamental role since they allow several hours to evaluate response to treatment, which helps decision-making as well as patient education and the establishment of a continuity of care plan at discharge. The final decision should always be individualized taking into account functional, mental and social aspects that allow patient adherence to therapy and outpatient monitoring.

Conclusions
- Dyspnoea is one of the most common and dangerous complaints and the main cause of hospital admission among older people presenting to the ED.
- Dyspnoea is a symptom which is difficult to assess and is often caused by life-threatening conditions.
- Missed diagnosis or delayed treatment in older people with dyspnoea attending the ED is associated with a worse prognosis.
- Biomarkers, bedside ultrasound and triple-rule-out CT may play a role in the differential diagnosis between cardiac and noncardiac dyspnoea in older patients attended in the ED.
- Treatment should be guided by the underlying cause of dyspnoea.

Further studies are needed to define the correct treatment when two or more diagnoses coexist and/or comorbidities are present in older patients with dyspnoea in the ED.

References

1. Pines JM et al (2013) National trends in emergency department use, care patterns, and quality of care of older adults in the United States. J Am Geriatr Soc 61:12–17
2. Safwenberg U, Terént A, Lind L (2007) The emergency department presenting complaint as predictor of in-hospital fatality. Eur J Emerg Med 14:324–331
3. Ray P et al (2006) Acute respiratory failure in the elderly: etiology, emergency diagnosis and prognosis. Crit Care 10:R82
4. Delerme S et al (2008) Acute respiratory failure in the elderly: diagnosis and prognosis. Age Ageing 37:251–257
5. Delerme S et al (2008) Usefulness of B natriuretic peptides and procalcitonin in emergency medicine. Biomark Insights 3:203–217
6. González Del Castillo J et al (2014) Consensus guidelines for the management of community acquired pneumonia in the elderly patient. Rev Esp Geriatr Gerontol 49:279–291
7. McMurray JJ et al (2012) ESC guidelines for the diagnosis and treatment of acute and chronic heart failure 2012: the task force for the diagnosis and treatment of acute and chronic heart failure 2012 of the European Society of Cardiology. Developed in collaboration with the Heart Failure Association (HFA) of the ESC. Eur J Heart Fail 14:803–869
8. Konstantinides SV et al (2014) 2014 ESC guidelines on the diagnosis and management of acute pulmonary embolism. Eur Heart J 35:3033–3069
9. Scichilone N et al (2014) Diagnosis and management of asthma in the elderly. Eur J Intern Med 25:336–342
10. Martín-Sánchez FJ et al (2013) Management of acute heart failure in Spanish emergency departments based on age. Rev Esp Cardiol 66:715–720
11. Martín Sánchez FJ et al (2013) Prognostic role of NT-proBNP in emergency department in the elderly with acute heart failure. Rev Esp Geriatr Gerontol 48:155–160
12. Martín-Sánchez FJ et al (2013) Key points in healthcare of frail elders in the emergency department. Med Clin (Barc) 140:24–29
13. Jacob J et al (2013) Prognostic value of troponin in patients with acute heart failure attended in Spanish emergency departments: TROPICA study (TROPonin in acute heart failure). Med Clin (Barc) 140:145–151
14. Righini M et al (2014) Age-adjusted D-dimer cutoff levels to rule out pulmonary embolism: the ADJUST-PE study. JAMA 311:1117–1124
15. Januzzi J et al (2008) Amino-terminal pro–B-type natriuretic peptide testing for the diagnosis or exclusion of heart failure in patients with acute symptoms. Am J Cardiol 101:29–38
16. Gaggin HK et al (2013) Biomarkers and diagnostics in heart failure. Biochim Biophys Acta 1832:2442–2450
17. Cinar O et al (2012) Evaluation of mid-regional pro-atrial natriuretic peptide, procalcitonin, and mid-regional pro-adrenomedullin for the diagnosis and risk stratification of dyspneic ED patients. Am J Emerg Med 30:1915–1920
18. Maisel A et al (2012) Use of procalcitonin for the diagnosis of pneumonia in patients presenting with a chief complaint of dyspnoea: results from the BACH (biomarkers in acute heart failure) trial. Eur J Heart Fail 14:278–286
19. Singer AJ et al (2009) The incremental benefit of a shortness of-breath biomarker panel in emergency department patients with dyspnoea. Acad Emerg Med 16:488–494
20. Klæstrup E et al (2011) Reference intervals and age and gender dependency for arterial blood gases and electrolytes in adults. Clin Chem Lab Med 49:1495–1500
21. Prosen G et al (2011) Combination of lung ultrasound (a comet-tail sign) and N-terminal pro-brain natriuretic peptide in differentiating acute heart failure from chronic obstructive pulmonary disease and asthma as cause of acute dyspnoea in prehospital emergency setting. Crit Care 15:450
22. Lichtenstein DA et al (2008) Relevance of lung ultrasound in the diagnosis of acute respiratory failure: the BLUE protocol. Chest 134:117–125

23. Kajimoto K et al (2012) Rapid evaluation by lung-cardiac-inferior vena cava (LCI) integrated ultrasound for differentiating heart failure from pulmonary disease as the cause of acute dyspnoea in the emergency setting. Cardiovasc Ultrasound 10:49
24. Rogers IS et al (2011) Usefulness of comprehensive cardiothoracic computed tomography in the evaluation of acute undifferentiated chest discomfort in the emergency department (CAPTURE). Am J Cardiol 107:643–650
25. Mariani J et al (2011) Noninvasive ventilation in acute cardiogenic pulmonary edema: a meta-analysis of randomized controlled trials. J Card Fail 17:850–859
26. Lightowler JV et al (2003) Noninvasive positive pressure ventilation to treat respiratory failure resulting from exacerbations of chronic obstructive pulmonary disease: Cochrane systematic review and metaanalysis. BMJ 326:185
27. Holzer-Richling N et al (2011) Randomized placebo controlled trial of furosemide on subjective perception of dyspnoea in patients with pulmonary oedema because of hypertensive crisis. Eur J Clin Investig 41:627–634
28. Incalzi RA et al (2014) Chronic obstructive pulmonary disease in the elderly. Eur J Intern Med 25:320–328
29. Hawkins NM et al (2010) Baseline characteristics and outcomes of patients with heart failure receiving bronchodilators in the CHARM programme. Eur J Heart Fail 12:557–565
30. Maak CA et al (2011) Should acute treatment with inhaled Beta agonists be withheld from patients with Dyspnoea who may have heart failure? J Emerg Med 40:135–145
31. Miravitlles M et al (2014) Spanish guideline for COPD (GesEPOC). Update 2014. Arch Bronconeumol 50(Suppl 1):1–16
32. Yahav D et al (2013) Time to first antibiotic dose for patients hospitalised with community-acquired pneumonia. Int J Antimicrob Agents 41:410–413
33. Geerts WH et al (2008) Prevention of venous thromboembolism: American College of chest physicians evidence-based clinical practice guidelines (8th edition). Chest 133(6 Suppl):381S–453S

Management of Back Pain in Older Patients

19

Jennifer Truchot and Jean Laganier

19.1 Introduction

Chronic low back pain (CLBP) in older adults is very common, disabling, and remains poorly understood [1]. Osteoarticular pain represents more than half of the sources of pain in older patients [2, 3]. CLBP in older patient is associated with a high morbidity, because of the polypathologic characteristic, which requires a more specific management [4]. Recent studies revealed that the prevalence of pain declines with age; however, the degree of pain interference with quality of life increases with age [5].

One of the missions of the ED physician's evaluation is to diagnose the potential life-threatening condition, which manifest as LBP.

As with most emergency presentations, the patient arrives with an undefined complaint requiring diagnosis. Lower back pain can be benign in most cases, but can also be the symptom of a more serious illness.

LBP is classified into organic pain associated with organic disorders (such as spondylolisthesis, spinal stenosis, osteoporotic vertebral fracture) and functional pain associated with only physiological age-related lesions. Both should be treated with the right intervention after accurate diagnosis. The functional pain requires therapeutic exercise and life guidance. It remains important to systematically search for a systemic disease causing the pain, for a neurologic compromise that might require an urgent surgical evaluation and for a social or psychological distress that might amplify the pain and complicate management [6, 7].

J. Truchot (✉)
Emergency Department, Hôpital Lariboisière, APHP, Paris, France
e-mail: Jennifer.truchot@aphp.fr

J. Laganier
Geriatrics Department, Hôpital Lariboisière, APHP, Paris, France
e-mail: Jean.laganier@aphp.fr

Many patients stay quite functional; however, LBP remains one of the most disabling and therapeutically challenging pain conditions afflicting older adults [8]. In the ED, managing CLPB in older patients can be difficult, due to diagnosis issues, accurate evaluation of pain, and the iatrogenic risk.

Chronic pain has been showed to be associated with depression [9, 10], decreased appetite [11], impaired sleep [12], and decreased quality of life [13] in the general population.

However, studies examining the consequences of LBP on the quality of life of older patients are still too rare, in contrast to the extensive research on working-aged adults with LBP. The generalizability and the relevance of these results to the older population are unknown.

19.2 Epidemiology

LBP is the third most frequent cause of physician visits in patients over the age of 65 [14]. However, little research has been done in the area of LBP in older people; the prevalence of LBP is therefore uncertain. Many factors influence the evaluation of prevalence such as cognitive impairment, a difficulty expressing pain complaints, co-morbidities, and resignation to perceived effects of aging. The development of this symptom is associated with postural load conditions reflecting the patient's lifestyle and the age-related changes in lumbar spine structures.

An American study with the use of the National Electronic Injury Surveillance System evaluated all cases of LBP presenting to emergency departments between 2004 and 2008. Incidence rate ratios were calculated according to age, sex, and race. LBP demonstrates a bimodal distribution with peaks between 25 and 29 years of age (2.58/1000 person-years) and 95–99 years of age (1.47/1000) without differentiation by underlying etiology. Older patients were found to be at a greater risk of hospital admission for low back pain [15].

A Japanese study even showed a prevalence of LBP of 54% among 745 randomly selected older patients living in an urban area (the percentage with low back pain during the preceding month) [16]. The prevalence of LBP exceeded 70% among 703 older persons working in rural/mountainous areas. The prevalence was lower with 42% patients staying in an urban health institution. These results confirm that LBP seems to be associated with the patient's lifestyle [16].

19.3 Pathophysiology

Aging is associated with decreased muscle strength and mass (sarcopenia). It may be due to a decrease in number of muscle fibers and of the size of individual fibers. Type II (fast-twitch) fiber atrophy is associated with aging, resulting in slower muscle contractile properties. This phenomenon can however be avoided with training. Decreased muscle quality (due to increased intramuscular fat infiltration) is associated with aging muscle. Facet joint degeneration is associated with the aging spine.

Desiccation of the disc occurs with time. The changes in the disc height affect the amount of loading on the facet joints.

Bad posture, irregular movement of the lower back, and reduced muscle strength can increase the nociceptive stimuli. As a consequence to this pain, motion restriction may lead to the contracture of the intervertebral joints and atrophy of the other lumbar spine structures, resulting in a vicious circle of pain.

Among all the previously cited changes in lumbar spine structures, age-related degeneration of intervertebral disk cartilages and of intervertebral joints is a common cause of LBP. Kirkaldy-Willis classified the development of LBP into the following three stages [17]:

Dysfunction Rupture occurs in the intervertebral cartilages. Lesions such as damage to the intervertebral joints and mechanical inflammation develop.

Instability The function of the intervertebral disks is disrupted; the degenerative processes progress in the intervertebral joints, while instability develops in the motor functional unit. Symptoms such as LBP and lower limb neurological symptoms become more severe.

Restabilization Movement is restricted due to spur formation on the vertebral bodies, thickening, and deformation of intervertebral joints. The severity of pain can decrease.

Assessing trunk muscle composition and core muscle integrity could be an essential approach to manage LBP, maintain functional mobility, and reduce the risk of falls in older adults.

19.4 Clinical Presentation

The diagnosis of LBP in older patients in the ED should be based on careful history taking and physical findings. Osteoarthritis is the first cause of CLBP in older patients, before inflammatory rheumatism. It can be a challenge to identify inflammatory pain in older patients, especially in the ED, with specific issues such as overcrowding and lack of time. Movement can aggravate LBP, as it would be for mechanical pains. Inflammatory clinical signs are not always present. It is particularly important to confirm the kind of activities of daily living inducing the clinical symptoms. Many different clinical presentations of CLBP exist; among those are some diagnosis pitfalls. Comprehensive assessment should therefore include an exhaustive investigation of the patient's pain and medical history and a complete physical examination.

19.4.1 History

Older patients are more likely to be admitted to the hospital [15] and to have a serious cause of LBP, such as a fracture, a tumor, an infection, or intra-abdominal process [7,

18]. A systematic approach for all patients helps avoiding missing those etiologies associated with high morbidity and mortality. The duration of symptoms is an important element of history taking. Back pain is considered acute if it has been present for 0–6 weeks, subacute if it has been present for 6–12 weeks, and chronic if it has been present for longer than 12 weeks. A back pain of more than 6 weeks should be considered particularly concerning [19]. Trauma history is fundamental, even a minor trauma can cause fractures in older patients. Back pain that is sudden and severe may be indicative of an acute abdominal process such as a ruptured abdominal aortic aneurysm. Back pain due to mechanical cause is often intermittent, positional, and pain is maximal at onset. Historical features that should be searched for also include systemic symptoms such as fever, chills, night sweats, or weight loss.

19.4.2 Physical Examination

The physical examination of patients with LBP can be accomplished quickly in the ED and should be very rigorous. It is first necessary to examine if there is a deformity of the lumbar spine, the range of motion, and the presence of neurological symptoms of the lower limb.

The back evaluation should begin with an inspection of the skin looking for signs of infection or trauma. Patients who present very severe and acute pain can present more serious causes of back pain such as aortic aneurysm, spinal infection, or nephrolithiasis (Corwell 2010). The physical exam should include the evaluation for intrathoracic or intra-abdominal causes for pain. When the patient is able, four ranges of motion with the back should be performed. These motions will provide important information about the range of motion, symmetry, and reproduction of pain [20]. Hip joints must be carefully examined as hip pathology can mimic LBP [21]. Straight-leg and crossed straight-leg tests are also important tests to perform in the evaluation of LBP.

The most important aspect of a complete back pain physical exam remains the neurologic evaluation. It is important to assess each of the spinal nerve roots. Sensation, motor function, and plantar and Achilles deep tendon reflexes should all be assessed.

The final aspect of a complete physical evaluation in older patients with back pain is the rectal exam to evaluate rectal tone and sensation, for prostatic and rectal masses, and for perirectal abscesses.

The following physical examination findings must be considered as red flags for serious causes of back pain: pulsatile abdominal mass, fever, hypotension and hypertension, pale appearance, focal neurologic signs, saddle anesthesia with decreased anal sphincter tone, and acute urinary retention [18, 22].

19.4.3 Inflammatory Lower Back Pain

The most frequent causes of inflammatory LBP are microcrystalline rheumatism in the ED as well as in general medicine. Among those, the prevalence of chondrocalcinosis increases with age. It is most frequently manifested by acute pain but also sometimes by a more chronic or continuous pain.

Spondylodiscitis should always be considered in case of LBP associated with fever. Some inflammatory diseases can also manifest themselves at an older age. For instance, rheumatoid polyarthritis can be seen, in a less aggressive and destructive presentation than in younger patients [23]. Horton's disease prevalence increases with age but is rarely associated with LBP. Lupus, connectivitis, and systemic diseases are rarely described in older patients but should be still considered as a possible diagnosis.

Multiple myeloma can lead to LBP in older patients. Metastasis can also be revealed by a pain complaint. These two diagnoses must be evoked when facing an inflammatory LBP. Osteoarticular paraneoplastic syndromes can also be frequent at this age, and LBP can be a revealing mode.

Therefore, when an inflammatory origin is suspected in the ED, hospitalization will be required for further examination and complementary exams.

19.4.4 Osteoporotic Fracture

Reduced bone mass in older patients may result in the development of osteoporosis and leads to an increased risk of traumatic and nontraumatic osteoporotic fracture. The pain from osteoporotic fracture can be severe and abrupt. Imaging must be performed in the ED whenever a fracture is suspected. The fracture usually heals, and the pain decreases within 2 or 3 months. If the pain continues for more than 2 or 3 months, pseudoarthrosis of the vertebral body has to be suspected. This hypothesis is evaluated by examination of whether or not there is a difference in the anterior height of the injured vertebral body on radiographs (between standing lateral and supine lateral plain).

The elements in favor of an osteoporotic fracture include a LBP associated with a kyphotic and scoliotic spine deformity, neurological symptoms of the lower limb, and the notion of a recent fall. Often no specific trauma history can be identified.

19.4.5 Lumbar Spinal Canal Stenosis

Lumbar spinal canal stenosis involves age-related degeneration of the vertebral bodies, vertebral arches, and intervertebral disks, including the spinal canal. This degeneration causes deformation of the vertebrae, resulting in the narrowing of the space, which contains the cauda equina and nerve roots. This can cause LBP and neurological symptoms of the lower limb. Claudication is a characteristic symptom of lumbar spinal canal stenosis. Prolonged effort, continuous walking, or standing can cause excessive dynamic loading on the spinal canal. The factors leading to lumbar spinal canal stenosis are age-related changes in lumbar spine structures (loss in intervertebral disc height, reduction in the length of the vertebral column, etc.) and postural factors (weakening of trunk muscles and increased load on spinal canal). Segmental instability starting in the middle age (degenerative spondylolisthesis) and spondylolytic spondylolisthesis, previous lumbar surgery, also lead to spinal canal stenosis. While the primary factor of LBP in older patients is age-related changes in the lumbar spine structures, posture should be evaluated with attention. Backward bending of the lumbar spine due to weakening of trunk muscles may cause narrowing of the spinal canal and deformation of the posterior structures.

19.4.6 Lower Back Pain: Pitfalls in Older Patients

Diagnosis pitfalls among older patients are frequent and should always be evoked in the ED. Any acute behavior change in older patients must arise the suspicion of acute pain. Indeed, this specific population often suffers from many different pathologies, and history taking can be difficult because of frequent cognitive function alterations. LBP can be the symptom revealing severe acute conditions such as myocardial infarction, gastric ulcer, or sigmoiditis. Acute renal lithiasis and pyelonephritis can be responsible for LBP; therefore, a urine analysis test must be performed in the ED in every case of LBP in the older patients. An older patient who presents with back pain, abdominal pain, and hypotension should be considered to have an aortic dissection or ruptured abdominal aortic aneurysm (AAA) until proven otherwise. The prevalence of AAA increases with age, and approximately 4–8% of individuals over the age of 65 will have an AAA [22].

19.4.7 Osteoarthritis

Osteoarthritis is a disease of the cartilage and the bone. It is not only a simple deterioration related to aging. This pain is frequent and manifests itself like a mechanical pain, leading to difficulty to walk. This handicap can be severe. The physician should keep in mind there is no correlation between the severity of the lesions and the intensity of the pain. It is therefore important to dissociate the deterioration of the bone structure, the intensity of pain, and the handicap.

19.4.8 The Challenge of Evaluating Pain in Older Patients

There are several challenges to measuring pain in older patients. First since pain is a subjective phenomenon, it is difficult to measure. The different tools available in the ED for the specific geriatric population will however be described. The present pain complaint should always be described in terms of intensity, quality, location(s) (as radiation), pattern (onset, duration, and frequency), and aggravating and relieving factors [24, 25]. Nonverbal cues (e.g., guarding, grimacing, and restricted movement) should be noted, even more if the patient is unable to provide a precise description of the pain. In circumstances where self-report is impossible to obtain, information and history must be gathered from other sources, such as the primary caregiver. This can be difficult in the ED since the patients are sometimes brought alone, without any family or without their complete medical files.

Weiner et al. studied the validity of pain measurement in older patients with CLBP and found a "modest correlation between self-reported pain and disability and pain behaviors observed during the performance of axial specific ADL tasks" [26]. Another more recent study of community dwellers showed that "back pain was most often associated with difficulty in standing in one place, pushing or pulling a large object, and walking a half-mile" [27]. Low back pain in older women has also been associated to difficulty, but not an inability to perform basic and instrumental ADLs [28]. Weiner et al. [29] revealed that LBP was linked to lower extremity pain and self-reported difficulty in performing functional tasks, but not with observed function.

In all cases, it is fundamental to obtain and evaluate detailed information on the nature of the pain in the lower back and lower limbs, and on how the pain influences the activities of daily living. The treatment must be decided in order to improve the patient's quality of life.

19.5 Investigations

The confirmation of an accurate diagnosis of LBP in emergency is possible with only the use of a complete clinical examination and rigorous history taking. It is recommended to perform X-ray or at best and if possible an MRI only if there are any concerning features in the history or physical exam, or if the pain persists after 4–6 weeks of conservative management.

Even though X-rays are not recommended for the management of simple nude back pain (Corwell 2010) [30] in older patients, X-rays can be helpful as they can show some of the pathology frequently associated in older patients (vertebral fractures, malignancy or infection, spondylolisthesis) [20, 31]. MRI is the gold standard for evaluating the cause of acute back pain [32]. MRI can not only identify lesions within the bone marrow but also explore the state of the spinal canal, the spinal cord, the disk space, and vertebral bodies. In the case of osteoporotic fracture, a low-intensity area on a T1-enhanced image indicates a new fracture. This is particularly important in older patients, for which MRI and other imaging methods may show false-positive findings and should always be considered with caution in the ED.

In the ED, in most cases, uncomplicated acute LBP, with or without radiculopathy, is a benign condition that can be managed without imaging. Even though recommendations for the use of imaging exist, a recent American study on a large cohort of 14,838 patients shows that more than half of patients presenting to the ED with LBP did not have a valid indication to receive imaging. They presented uncomplicated LBP and could have avoided a visit to the ED [33]. An important proportion (30.1%) of patients received non-indicated imaging; 26.2% event received advanced imaging (MRI or CT) [33]. These results confirm the need for improvement in the quality of care by reducing unnecessary imaging and the radiation exposure for patients presenting LBP.

The ED physicians must always keep in mind that imaging diagnosis in older patients may provide objective evidence; it can also reveal frequent false-positive findings. Therefore, it should not be concluded that the clinical findings are attributable to abnormalities on imaging findings without rigorous previous clinical examination.

19.6 Treatment

In older patients, musculoskeletal pain remains underdiagnosed and undertreated [34]. Some patients will never express this pain and consequently will receive no treatment [35]. In the specific context of management in emergency of the older population, often suffering from many disorders including cognitive disorder, pain management will be complex. It will be a real challenge to evaluate and consider the patient in its globality and complexity [25] [36]. The goal remains in all time to maintain the patient's autonomy and his functional performance.

In all cases, it is recommended according to the AGS 2002:

- To use the minimal dosage for pain medication
- To adapt supplementary dose to pain reevaluation
- To increase progressively dosage
- To use medication with a short elimination half-life
- To encourage oral medication

19.6.1 The Basics of Treatment of Lower Back Pain in Older Patients

Even though adverse drug reactions in older patients are a significant increased risk, pharmacologic treatment remains the main modality. Considering age-associated changes of pharmacokinetics and pharmacodynamics, the risk of interactions must be evaluated. Despite these challenges, pain in older patients must be controlled and requires trials of different agents with cautious titration of medication. Once treatment is initiated, the physician must regularly and carefully monitor for drug side effects and adverse events [37, 38]. The ED setting allows the initiation and the monitoring of the treatment efficacy and adverse events.

The first choice of treatment for older patients with lumbar spine disorder will be medication (oral, transdermal, suppository, or intravenous).

19.6.1.1 Nonopioid Analgesics

Most mild or moderate LBP in older patients responds well to acetaminophen. This medication is well tolerated, provided that renal and hepatic functions are normal [39].

Long-term use of non-steroidal anti-inflammatory drugs (NSAIDs), because of the association with gastrointestinal bleeding and renal dysfunction, is risky in older patients. The risk of bleeding can be lowered with the prescription of proton pump inhibitors [40, 41]. Therefore, prolonged use of NSAIDs in older patients should be avoided whenever possible. This specific older population already has a higher risk of bleeding as they often use medication such as anticoagulants or antiaggregants. The risk of aggravating a preexisting renal failure is also important. Therefore, since NSAIDs have shown no superiority in pain relief, they should be avoided and should be considered only in patients younger than 75 years old.

Bed rest and corsets can be prescribed to stabilize the lumbar region and relieve pain. However, caution should be taken, because prolonged bed rest and corset use can weaken the trunk muscles of the patients with degenerative disease in the lumbar region. Pressure ulcer has been associated with corset use; therefore, close monitoring and reeducation must be programmed after prescription of a corset.

Patients with lumbar degenerative spondylolisthesis and those with degenerative scoliosis may be prescribed braces for use during effort and for protection against postural loading.

The utmost caution is required for osteoporotic fracture. Resting remains the main treatment.

19.6.1.2 Opioids

Initial doses should be lower, and titration should be slow in older patients. Codeine and tramadol can be used with the same caution as morphine in older patients. Tramadol is used for mild to moderate pain, but always with caution because of the risk of dizziness and seizure (by reducing the seizure threshold). A reevaluation of the pain and the absence of adverse events must be programmed as soon as possible after the initiation of treatment. Laxatives must be prescribed in all cases to prevent iatrogenic constipation. Antiemetics may be needed as well. Falls, dizziness, and gait disturbances can be frequent and monitored carefully.

Morphine is often used in patients older than 85 years old (16%), more frequently than in patients aging from 70 to 85 years (6%) [34]. Morphine prescription in older patients must be developed with caution [42]. Safety has been shown to be superior to NSAIDs [43]. Oral treatment should be preferred with an initial low dosage. Adverse events must be carefully monitored, among those respiratory and neurologic effects especially for patients with altered cognitive functions.

19.6.1.3 Adjuvant Treatments

Bisphosphonates can be of use in the acute phase of an osteoporotic fracture; however, there is no evidence of their efficacy in the management of acute LBP in older patients.

Steroids must be avoided because of the numerous adverse events, especially in older patients. A recent study found that adding a single dose of 8 mg intravenous dexamethasone to current routine care significantly reduced pain at 24 h compared with placebo in ED patients with LBP. Pain scores at 6 weeks were further decreased in both groups, but the effect of dexamethasone over placebo was not sustained. However, there was no difference in functional scores. In this specific population of older patients, steroids are not recommended in usual care [44].

Antidepressants: Although tricyclic antidepressants such as amitriptyline hydrochloride and nortriptyline hydrochloride have been used to treat patients with neuropathic pain, anticonvulsants such as gabapentin and carbamazepine could be more effective [45]. In particular, gabapentin seems to be more effective and better tolerated in older patients.

Finally, other specific treatment for specific diagnosis must always be considered, such as antibiotics for spondylodiscitis or radiotherapy for metastasis.

19.6.2 Surgical Treatment

The surgical and anesthetic risk must always be considered with great caution and with regard to a clear benefit for the relief of pain. Surgical treatment can be required for lumbar spinal canal stenosis in older patients. For patients who develop claudication when moving over a distance of less than 200 m, show rapid progression of symptoms, and do not respond to medical therapy within a month and a half, surgical treatment based on the results of reevaluation should be considered. When surgery is performed too late, recovery may be poor due to progression of more permanent symptoms. Close cooperation between primary care physicians and specialists is therefore required in the evaluation of the symptoms and the surgical risk.

When decompression is performed for lumbar spinal canal stenosis, it is important to avoid unnecessarily extensive decompression. For this, it is necessary to determine responsible spinal levels as closely as possible with the accurate analysis of neurological findings, the possible use of nerve blocks and imaging diagnosis.

Cementoplasty even in fresh cases of osteoporotic spine fracture can be a valid technique. It is also recommended when there is a significant risk of progressive collapse or there is evidence of spinal pseudoarthrosis and persistent pain when making positional changes.

Spine fusion is sometimes performed on patients with spondylolisthesis, only when the lesions are dynamic, the treatment is combined with instrumentation, when the patients present sufficient bone mass and functional activity. However, many patients with lumbar spine slippage do not require spine fusion if the lesions do not involve dynamic factors.

Spinal stenosis with neuropathic pain may be managed conservatively with analgesia and surgically with spinal decompression, and some evidence exists supporting the use of spinal nerve blocks to reduce symptoms on a short-term basis [46]. Recent meta-analyses of pooled data from studies have produced positive results for the technique of spinal nerve block [47, 48].

However, European guidelines for the management of CLBP concluded that the evidence for steroid injections in radicular pain was conflicting. In conclusion, there is not enough evidence to support epidural steroid injections for spinal stenosis and for radicular pain or sciatica in older patients.

Percutaneous epidural adhesiolysis is a technique used to treat patients with refractory pain resulting of either epidural scarring following spinal surgery or spinal stenosis due to compression of intraspinal vascular and neural structures. However, there is limited evidence to support consideration of this technique for spinal stenosis and radicular symptoms in older adults.

19.6.3 Exercise Therapy for Functional Low Back Pain

LBP is considered to be functional in the absence of neurological symptoms in the lower limbs, and if imaging does not reveal evident organic abnormalities besides intervertebral joint deformation and disk degeneration (in accordance to the patient's age). In addition to slight kyphosis and a reduced range of motion, these patients often show weakness of the trunk muscles. Prolonged exertion and an active lifestyle may cause LBP for these patients. A study showed improvement of symptoms after trunk muscle training in older patients, and confirmed that the intensity of the pain improves as the trunk muscles strengthen, more specifically the back muscles [49]. Therapeutic exercise should therefore be prescribed based on the evaluation of a specialist and according to the pain reduction allowed by medication.

Conclusion
The association of a high prevalence of LBP and low care-seeking in older patient suggests that ED physicians should inquire systematically about low back and/or leg pain (Fig. 19.1).

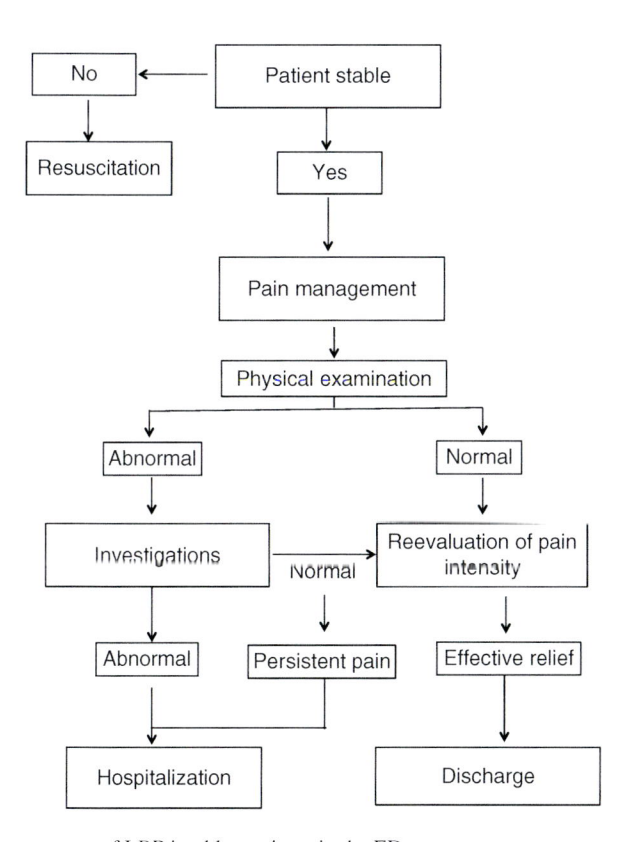

Fig. 19.1 Management of LBP in older patients in the ED

A better understanding of clinical manifestations of pain in the older patients, improved methods of assessment, and the use of both pharmacologic and non-pharmacologic treatments can result to a more favorable outcome in the ED.

The ED physician's role is fundamental to prevent aggravation of the symptoms and physical decline.

More research is needed to explore the consequences of LBP on the quality of life of older patients and to improve the management in the ED.

References

1. Jakobsson U, Klevsgard R, Westergren A, Rahm HI (2003) Old people in pain: a comparative study. J Pain Symptom Manag 26:625–636
2. D'Astolfo CJ, Humphreys BK (2006) A record review of reported musculoskeletal pain in Ontario long-term facility. BMC Geriatr 6(1):5. doi:10.1186/1471-2318-6-5
3. Edmond SL, Felson DT (2000) Prevalence of back symptoms in elders. J Rheumatol 27:220–225
4. Barkin RL, Barkin SJ, Barkin DS (2005) Perception, assessment, treatment, and management of pain in the elderly. Clin Geriatr Med 21:465–490
5. Thomas E, Peat G, Harris L, Wilkie R, Croft PR (2004) The prevalence of pain and pain interference in a general population of older adults: cross-sectional findings from the North Staffordshire Osteoarthritis Project (NorStOP). Pain 110(1–2):361–368
6. Deyo RA, Rainville J, Kent DL (1992) What can the history and physical examination tell us about low back pain? JAMA 268:760–765
7. Deyo RA, Weinstein JN (2001) Low back pain. N Engl J Med 344:363–370
8. Hartvigsen J, Frederiksen H, Christensen K (2006) Back and neck pain in seniors—prevalence and impact. Eur Spine J 15(6):802–806. doi:10.1007/s00586-005-0983-6
9. Bair MJ, Robinson RL, Katon W, Kroenke K (2003) Depression and pain comorbidity: a literature review. Arch Intern Med 163(20):2433–2445
10. Fishbain DA, Cutler R, Rosomoff HL, Rosomoff RS (1997) Chronic pain-associated depression: antecedent or consequence of chronic pain? A review. Clin J Pain 13(2):116–137
11. Bosley BN, Weiner DK, Rudy TE, Granieri E (2004) Is chronic nonmalignant pain associated with decreased appetite in older adults? Preliminary evidence. J Am Geriatr Soc 52(2):247–251
12. Ancoli-Israel S, Soares CN, Gaeta R, Benca RM (2004) Insomnia in special populations: effects of aging, menopause, chronic pain, and depression. Postgrad Med 116:33–47. doi:10.3810/pgm.12.2004.suppl38.260
13. Cooper JK, Kohlmann T (2001) Factors associated with health status of older Americans. Age Ageing 30(6):495–501
14. Bressler HB, Keyes WJ, Rochon PA, Badley E (1999) The prevalence of low back pain in the elderly. A systematic review of the literature. Spine 24(17):1813–1819
15. Waterman BR, Belmont PJ Jr, Schoenfeld AJ (2012) Low back pain in the United States: incidence and risk factors for presentation in the emergency setting. Spine J 12:63–70
16. Ando M, Yamamoto H et al (1986) J West Jpn Res Soc Spine 12(1):172–175
17. Keim HA, Kirkaldy-Willis WH (1980) Low back pain. Clin Symp 32(6):1–35
18. Corwell BN (2010) The emergency department evaluation, management, and treatment of back pain. Emerg Med Clin North Am 28(4):811–39
19. Della-Giustina DA (1999) Emergency department evaluation and treatment of back pain. Emerg Med Clin North Am 17:877–893
20. Hazzard WR, Halter JB (2009) Hazzard's geriatric medicine and gerontology. McGraw-Hill Medical, New York, p 1634

21. Sauter S, Hadler NM (2000) Back pain in elderly people. In: Evans JG, Williams TF, Beattie BL et al (eds) Oxford textbook of geriatric medicine, 2nd edn. University of Oxford Press, Oxford, pp 391–397
22. Winters ME, Kluetz P, Zilberstein J (2006) Back pain emergencies. Med Clin North Am 90:505–523
23. Laiho K, Tuomilehto J, Tilvis R (2001) Prevalence of rheumatoid arthritis and musculoskeletal diseases in the elderly population. Rheumatol Int 20:85–87
24. Hadjistavropoulos T, Herr K, Turk DC, Fine PG, Dworkin RH, Helme R, Jackson K, Parmelee PA, Rudy TE, Lynn Beattie B, Chibnall JT, Craig KD, Ferrell B, Ferrell B, Fillingim RB, Gagliese L, Gallagher R, Gibson SJ, Harrison EL, Katz B, Keefe FJ, Lieber SJ, Lussier D, Schmader KE, Tait RC, Weiner DK, Williams J (2007) An interdisciplinary expert consensus statement on assessment of pain in older persons. Clin J Pain 23:S1–S43
25. Herr K (2005) Pain assessment in the older adult with verbal communication skills. In: Gibson SJ, Weiner DK (eds) Pain in older persons, vol 35. IASP Press, Seattle, pp 111–133
26. Weiner D, Pieper C et al (1996) Pain measurement in elders with chronic low back pain: traditional and alternative approaches. Pain 67:461–467
27. Edmond SL, Felson DT (2003) Function and back symptoms in older adults. J Am Geriatr Soc 51:1702–1709
28. Leveille SG, Guralnik JM, Hochberg M et al (1999) Low back pain and disability in older women: independent association with difficulty but not inability to perform daily activities. J Gerontol 54A:M487–M493
29. Weiner DK, Haggerty CL, Kritchevsky SB et al (2003) How does low back pain impact physical function in independent, well-functioning older adults? Evidence from the health ABC cohort and implications for the future. Pain Med 4:311–320
30. Isaacs DM, Marinac J, Sun C (2004) Radiograph use in low back pain: a United States emergency department database (2014-01-16) analysis. J Emerg Med 26:37–45
31. Weiner AL, MacKenzie RS (1999) Utilization of lumbosacral spine radiographs for the evaluation of low back pain in the emergency department. J Emerg Med 17:229–233
32. Miller JC, Palmer WE, Mansfield FL et al (2006) When is imaging helpful for patients with back pain? J Am Coll Radiol 3:957–960
33. Schlemmer E, Mitchiner JC, Brown M, Wasilevich E (2015) Imaging during low back pain ED visits: a claims-based descriptive analysis. Am J Emerg Med 33(3):414–418. doi:10.1016/j.ajem.2014.12.060. Epub 2014 Dec 31
34. Hartikainen SA, Mantyselka PT, Louhivuori-Laako KA, Sulkava RO (2005) Balancing pain and analgesic treatment in the home-dwelling elderly. Ann Pharmacother 39:11–16
35. McCarberg BH (2007) Rheumatic diseases in the elderly: dealing with rheumatic pain in extended care facilities. Rheum Dis Clin N Am 33:87–108
36. Leland JY (1999) Chronic pain: primary care treatment of the older patient. Geriatrics 54:33–37
37. AGS Panel on Persistent Pain in Older Persons (2002) The management of persistent pain in older persons. J Am Geriatr Soc 50(6 Suppl):S205–S224
38. Cavalieri TA (2002) Pain management in the elderly. J Am Osteopath Assoc 102:481–485
39. Stucki G, Johannesson M, Liang MH (1996) Use of misoprostol in the elderly: is the expense justified? Drugs Aging 8:84–88
40. Greenberger NJ (1997) Update in gastroenterology. Ann Intern Med 127:827–834
41. Topol EJ (2004) Failing the public health—rofecoxib, Merck, and the FDA. N Engl J Med 351(17):1707–1709
42. Pergolizzi J, Böger RH, Budd K et al (2008) Opioids and the management of chronic severe pain in the elderly: consensus statement of an International Expert Panel with focus on the six clinically most often used World Health Organization Step III opioids (buprenorphine, fentanyl, hydromorphone, methadone, morphine, oxycodone). Pain Pract 8:287–313
43. Podichetty VK, Mazaneck D, Biscup RS (2003) Chronic non-malignant musculoskeletal pain in older adults: clinical issues and opioid intervention. Postgrad Med J 79:627–633

44. Balakrishnamoorthy R, Horgan I, Perez S, Steele MC, Keijzers GB (2015) Does a single dose of intravenous dexamethasone reduce Symptoms in Emergency department patients with low Back pain and RAdiculopathy (SEBRA)? A double-blind randomised controlled trial. Emerg Med J 32(7):525–530. doi:10.1136/emermed-2013-203490. Epub 2014 Aug 13
45. Jacox A, Carr DB, Payne R, Berde CB, Breitbart W, Cain JM et al (1994) Management of cancer pain. Clinical practice guideline no. 9. AHCPR publication no. 94-0592. Agency for Health Care Policy and Research, US Department of Health and Human Services, Public Health Service, Rockville
46. Snyder DL, Doggartt D, Turkelson C (2004) Treatment of degenerative lumbar spinal stenosis. Am Fam Physician 70:517–520
47. Abdi S, Datta S, Trescottt A et al (2007) Epidural steroids in the management of chronic spinal pain: a systematic review. Pain Physician 10:185–212
48. Stafford MA, Peng P, Hill DA (2010) Sciatica: a review of history, epidemiology, pathogenesis and the role of epidural steroid injection in management. BJA 99:461–473
49. Handa N, Yamamoto H et al (1997) Exerc Ther Physiother 8(1):63–69

Part III

Special Considerations in Frail Older People

Medicine in Older Patients: Evidence Based?

20

Simon P. Mooijaart

20.1 The Success of Clinical Guidelines

Increasingly, medical doctors are supposed to treat their patients according to clinical guidelines—a synthesis of existing literature, translated into standardized advice with respect to treatment of patients in a given situation. The implementation of such clinical guidelines has had great success: stringent cardiovascular risk management in combination with early revascularization therapies has resulted in a decreased risk of cardiovascular disease and associated complications including death in the last decades. In some Western countries, cardiovascular disease is no longer the number one cause of death, with cancer being the leading cause. However, despite the clinical guidelines, in older patients the risk of cardiovascular has not decreased. Rather, older patients often have multiple diseases, and implementation of all clinical guidelines for these individual diseases in one patient is burdensome, not effective or may even be harmful [1].

20.2 Evidence-Based Medicine

The term 'evidence-based medicine' was coined in 1992 by David Sacket et al. and was defined as 'the conscientious, explicit and judicious use of current best evidence in making decisions about the care of individual patients   [It] means integrating individual clinical expertise with the best available external clinical evidence from systematic research' [2].

S.P. Mooijaart, MD, PhD
Department of Internal Medicine, Section of Gerontology and Geriatrics,
Leiden University Medical Center, PO 9600, 2300 RC Leiden, Netherlands
e-mail: s.p.mooijaart@lumc.nl

In short, when making clinical decisions, three main elements should guide clinical decision making: the individual patient situation and preference, the knowledge and expertise of the physician and the available scientific evidence. The integration of these three elements is what makes medicine evidence based. However, all of these elements may be different for an older patient when compared to a younger patient, raising the questions whether medicine in older patients is actually evidence based [3].

20.3　The Ageing Process

The older patient is different from the younger patients in a large number of aspects. To understand these differences, it is useful to look at what the ageing process is and how it affects an ageing human organism [4]. Although there are many different definitions of ageing, there are also a number of commonalities in their key elements. When combined, a working definition of ageing could be 'an accumulation of damage that results from internal and external stressors, ultimately leading to loss of function and increased risk of disease and mortality'.

The cascade of event starts with 'stressors' from outside and inside the body, which cause damage. Evident stressors from outside the body include, for instance, sunlight: ultraviolet radiation causes DNA damage in the skin. Other external stressors are, for instance, inhaled air, which causes reactive oxygen species in the lungs, or even worse polluted air, which contains toxins that cause DNA damage in lung tissue or are absorbed into the blood stream and cause damage elsewhere in the body. Stressors from inside the body include metabolism, degradation, cell death and cell division. All these processes may lead to an accumulation of damage: toxic by-products, DNA damage or deposits of harmful material.

As a result of the damage inflicted on tissues, there is a loss of integrity and a loss of tissue and organ function. This can be observed on the outside of the body by just looking at the skin: loss of elasticity results in more wrinkles, loss of subcutaneous fat makes the skin thinner and hyperpigmentation leads to spotting. These external manifestations of ageing are accompanied by internal manifestations. Clearance by the kidney gradually declines with age: at the age of 85 years, the average clearance is between 50 and 60 cc/min. Such changes can have significant effects on some medications. Other tissue changes include, for instance, the loss of muscle mass and strength ('sarcopenia') [5].

The ageing process does not affect every individual at the same pace. One patient of 85 years old may be very vital, with few morbidities and functioning independent, whereas another 65-year-old patient has a high burden of comorbidities and problems with mobility and memory. Obviously, the second patient is 20 years younger if we study their passports. The ageing process has however influenced the first patient much less, so that despite the 20 years difference in calendar age, the biological age of the 85-year-old patients may even be lower than those of the 65-year-olds. In all diseases, calendar age is a risk for poor outcome, but an individual patient may have a different risk than somebody of the same calendar age, because their biological age is different. Looking at somebody from the outside will already give away the biological age of hair and skin, which may also reflect the biological age on the inside: organ function. Indeed, facial age is already a better predictor of calendar age of disease and mortality.

A term often used to describe vulnerable older patients is 'frailty'. The term is a reflection of accumulation of deficits [6], decreased resilience and increased risk of adverse outcomes [7]. Although the basic idea is similar, several definitions exist, which overlap but also differ. Likewise, many different measurement instruments exist. All associate with adverse outcome. However, what these measurements have in common is that they are time-consuming and cannot always be administered to patients in the acute setting, such as in the emergency department. Screening instruments that can be administered in limited time also exist, but their performance in predicting adverse outcome is relatively poor.

20.4 The Older Patient

As a result of the ageing process, the older patient that presents to the hospital acutely differs from the younger patient in a number of aspects.

As the definition of ageing already told us, older patients have an increased risk of disease and mortality. Older patients have higher risk than younger patients to get cancer, cardiovascular disease, hypertension, osteoporosis and osteoarthritis. This rising incidence with increasing age has led some disease to be called 'age-related disease'. In the clinic, we observe that compared to younger patients, older patients have more comorbidities and therefore also more polypharmacy. An average individual of 60 years old will already have two or more chronic conditions.

Because of loss of function of tissues and organs, there is loss of resilience to external stressors. Loss of muscle mass, for instance, leads to a decrease in muscle strength, which may then cause functional dependency and risk of falls. And if a patient with low reserve in muscle strength is admitted to the hospital and bedbound for a week, additional muscle loss will occur, frequently leading to even more functional dependence.

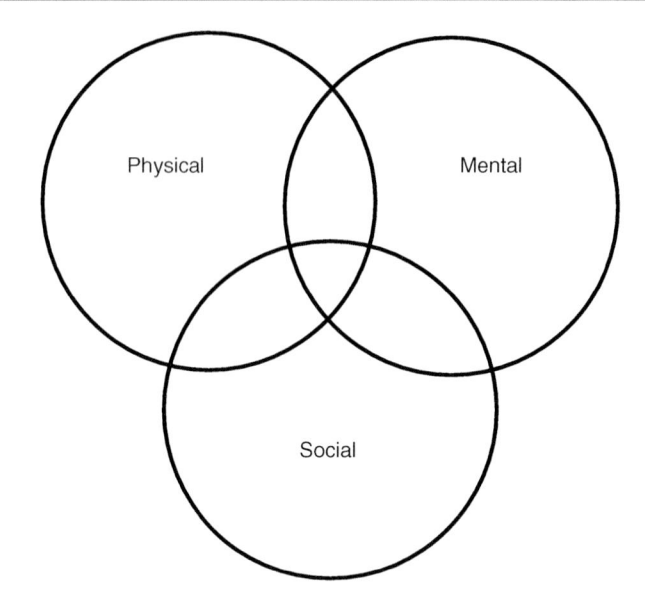

[Venn diagram with three overlapping circles labeled "Physical", "Mental", and "Social"]

The altering of the body as a result of the ageing process also leads to unexpected observations. For instance, whereas in middle age high blood pressure is associated with an increased risk of cardiovascular disease, in a population of 85-year-olds, those with the highest blood pressure have a higher life expectancy compared to those with lower blood pressure. One explanation may be that to maintain adequate perfusion through stiffened arteries by atherosclerosis, a higher blood pressure is needed and that those older patients able to successfully raise their blood pressure apparently are more resilient also to other stressors. For the acute setting, this is also very relevant as it may lead to atypical presentations: an 89-year-old with a systolic blood pressure of 120 mmHg may have a severe sepsis.

In the older patient with a somatic disease, there is an intricate relationship between physical, mental and social function. For instance, an older patient presenting to the emergency department with a severe somatic disease, such as infection or fracture, is at higher risk of getting a delirium. A decrease in physical function may lead to social isolation if mobility of the patient is lost, causing the patient inability to go home after hospitalisation or the other way around: a patient with a depression is at higher risk of social isolation functional decline. As with ageing in general, the same applies to each of these domains: one older patient may be very vulnerable in the physical domain while being mentally very vital, and another patient may be socially isolated and forgetful while being physically vital. These differences are very individual, and therefore, the older patient population is very heterogeneous and the typical older patients do not exist.

Older patients are also different with respect to their treatment preferences. Much more than in younger patients, older patients value the quality of life versus length of life [8]. Whereas a young adult with cancer will typically want the most aggressive treatment to increase the chance of a long life, an older adult may prefer not receiving intensive treatment that reduces the quality of life in what is maybe the last months of their life. Not infrequently older patients choose to not have chemotherapy or an operation but prefer to spend time with their families and make other arrangements regarding the end of their life. However, this also is very individual and may vary between older patients. In similar situations, they may make different choices; decisions should be informed and part of a shared decision-making process.

20.5 Scientific Evidence

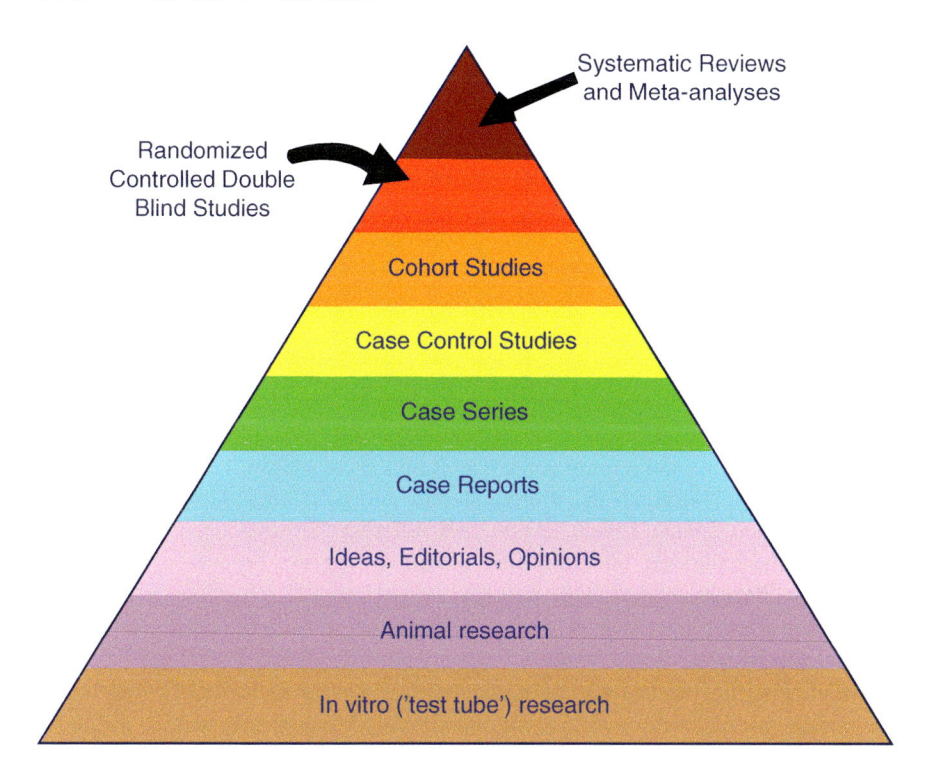

Pyramid of evidence (from top to bottom): Systematic Reviews and Meta-analyses; Randomized Controlled Double Blind Studies; Cohort Studies; Case Control Studies; Case Series; Case Reports; Ideas, Editorials, Opinions; Animal research; In vitro ('test tube') research.

Scientific evidence is generated in different types of studies of which the relevance for clinical patient care varies. The 'pyramid' of 'evidence' has been widely accepted and shows that at the APEX randomised controlled trials (RCTs) and meta-analyses of RCTs are regarded to have the highest level of evidence. In clinical guidelines, such studies (if conducted properly) would lead to clinical recommendations with a 'high level of evidence'. Because of this wording, the term 'evidence-based medicine' has sometimes been confused with 'medicine based on RCTs', disregarding the other two elements of EBM: patient situation and preference and the physicians' knowledge and clinical expertise.

The fundamental problem with scientific evidence is that older patients are systematically excluded from RCTs, and the older patients that do participate in such trial are not representative of the older patient in clinical practice. In a meta-analysis of all RCTs in 2012, only 7% specifically included older patients [9], much less than the typical proportion of older patients in practice. Another study showed that only 14% of participants in trials on acute coronary syndrome are over 75 years of age [10], whereas their proportion is much larger in the emergency department. Generally, older patients who participate in clinical studies are healthier than patients who visit the doctor. Exclusion criteria often include the use of concomitant medication, renal failure of cognitive impairment. Inclusion criteria often include the willingness and capability to (repeatedly) visit a study centre, obviously selecting for fit and mobile older patients.

Furthermore, RCTs do not study end points so relevant for older patients, such as physical function, cognitive function and quality of life. Typical end points studied in RCTs usually include incidence of cardiovascular disease (in cardiovascular research) or 5- or 10-year survival (in oncology research).

As a result of the underrepresentation of representative older patients in RCTs, the validity of published study for the older patient with multimorbidity is limited.

20.6 Physician Knowledge and Experience

The basis of clinical decision making is balancing the 'benefits' and 'harms' of different treatment strategies with respect to a certain end point, like putting blocks on both sides of a scale and seeing which way it tips. Increasingly, these balances have become implicit, informed by clinical studies and guidelines. However, in older patients the benefits and harms may be very different than in younger patients: the blocks on the scale may have different weight. In general, because of the ageing process, the risks are higher: there is also a higher chance of side effects and complications but also a higher risk of long rehabilitation as a result of decreased physical reserve. The benefits of treatments in older people are—again, on average—smaller. There are less life-years to win from treatment, and in the presence of comorbidity, there may also be less to win in symptom control. An older patient with dyspnoea may have a combination of several causes: anaemia, heart failure and chronic obstructive pulmonary disease. Treating only one of these causes may lead to some symptom improvement but no complete disappearance.

When making the balance of benefits and harms in older patients, we even might want to consider using another scale: the most important end point may even be different! A treatment may have very large benefits on the scale of tumour control or even a chance of curation but may have much smaller benefits on the scale of overall quality of life or physical function. Deciding—together with the patient—what is the actual preferred outcome is the first step in making the balance between benefits and harms.

The magnitude of the benefits and harms for a certain treatment in an individual older patient is very complex: the validity of available clinical research (especially clinical trials) for the older patient population is low, as studies usually do not take into account the older patient in general, let alone the heterogeneity of older patients with respect to their physical, mental and social function. In the absence of clinical evidence of certain treatments, physicians should make the best effort of understanding the typical biology of older patient as well as their individual situation and needs and incorporate this in their decision making. Furthermore, patients should be informed about the lack of solid evidence and the meaning of their individual situation for the magnitude of the benefits and harms. In a shared decision-making model, patients contribute to such by balancing the benefits and harms in light of their own frame of reference.

References

1. Boyd CM, Darer J, Boult C, Fried LP, Boult L, Wu AW (2005) Clinical practice guidelines and quality of care for older patients with multiple comorbid diseases: implications for pay for performance. JAMA 294(6):716–724
2. Sackett DL, Rosenberg WM, Gray JA, Haynes RB, Richardson WS (1996) Evidence based medicine: what it is and what it isn't. BMJ 312(7023):71–72
3. Mooijaart SP, Broekhuizen K, Trompet S, de Craen AJ, Gussekloo J, Oleksik A et al (2015) Evidence-based medicine in older patients: how can we do better? Neth J Med 73(5):211–218
4. López-Otín C, Blasco MA, Partridge L, Serrano M, Kroemer G (2013) The hallmarks of aging. Cell 153(6):1194–1217
5. Fielding RA, Vellas B, Evans WJ, Bhasin S, Morley JE, Newman AB et al (2011) Sarcopenia: an undiagnosed condition in older adults. Current consensus definition: prevalence, etiology, and consequences. International working group on sarcopenia. J Am Med Dir Assoc 12(4):249–256
6. Rockwood K, Mitnitski A (2007) Frailty in relation to the accumulation of deficits. J Gerontol A Biol Sci Med Sci 62(7):722–727
7. Fried LP, Tangen CM, Walston J, Newman AB, Hirsch C, Gottdiener J et al (2001) Frailty in older adults: evidence for a phenotype. J Gerontol A Biol Sci Med Sci 56(3):M146–M156
8. Hofman CS, Makai P, Boter H, Buurman BM, de Craen AJ, Olde Rikkert MG et al (2015) The influence of age on health valuations: the older olds prefer functional independence while the younger olds prefer less morbidity. Clin Interv Aging 10:1131–1139
9. Broekhuizen K, Pothof A, de Craen AJ, Mooijaart SP (2015) Characteristics of randomized controlled trials designed for elderly: a systematic review. PLoS One 10(5):e0126709
10. Dodd KS, Saczynski JS, Zhao Y, Goldberg RJ, Gurwitz JH (2011) Exclusion of older adults and women from recent trials of acute coronary syndromes. J Am Geriatr Soc 59(3):506–511

Prescribing for Older Patients

21

Paul Gallagher, Amanda Lavan, and Denis O'Mahony

21.1 Introduction

Prescribing for older patients presents numerous pharmacological and practical challenges, particularly in a busy emergency department where physicians have limited resources to comprehensively appraise the quality, safety and appropriateness of medication use in this heterogeneous patient group. Though the majority of older people are physically and cognitively well, emergency departments (EDs) worldwide are treating ever-increasing numbers of older patients who present with complex co-morbid illnesses, multiple concurrent medications, cognitive impairments and functional dependence, all of which increase the risk of adverse drug events (ADEs) [1–4]. Indeed, ADEs are a frequent cause of presentation to emergency departments amongst older people, common examples being falls (± injury such as hip fracture) because of sedative hypnotic drugs, gastrointestinal or intracranial haemorrhage because of anticoagulant or antiplatelet drugs, acute confusional states because of drugs with anticholinergic properties, hypoglycaemia because of antidiabetic medications and drug toxicity because of drugs with narrow therapeutic indices, e.g. digoxin [5, 6]. Most ADEs are predictable through age-related changes in pharmacokinetic (absorption, distribution, metabolism and excretion) and pharmacodynamic response to commonly prescribed drugs [7]. Physicians who assess and treat older patients in the emergency department must be mindful of these age-related physiological changes in addition to the influence of pathological processes and polypharmacy on the risk of drug-disease and drug-drug interactions, inappropriate prescribing and suboptimal adherence.

P. Gallagher, PhD FRCPI (✉) • A. Lavan, MB MRCPI • D. O'Mahony, MD FRCPI
Department of Geriatric Medicine, Cork University Hospital, Wilton, Cork, Ireland
e-mail: paul.gallagher1@hse.ie

This chapter will describe the following key issues:

(a) Epidemiology of drug use in older patients
(b) Age-related physiological changes that affect pharmacokinetics and pharmacodynamics
(c) Commonly encountered ADEs in older people including clinically significant drug-drug and drug-disease interactions
(d) Polypharmacy and its consequences
(e) Potentially inappropriate prescribing
(f) The importance of medication reconciliation
(g) The principles of good prescribing practices for older patients

21.2 Epidemiology of Prescription and Non-prescription Drug Use in Older Patients

Older adults are the largest per capita consumers of prescription and over-the-counter drugs in most developed nations [8, 9]. In the United States, 84% of community-dwelling adults aged 65–74 years and 90% of patients aged 75–85 years regularly use at least one prescribed medication with one in three older adults regularly using ≥5 medications, almost 50% using an additional over-the-counter drug and >50% using dietary supplements [8]. Forty percent of adults aged ≥65 years take 5–9 medications and 18% take 10 or more [10]. In the United Kingdom, people over the age of 65 years comprise 12% of the population but consume 45% of total prescriptions dispensed [9]. Nursing home residents receive an average of eight regular prescription medications each month, with one in three having monthly drug regimens of ≥9 medications [11, 12].

21.3 Age-Related Changes in Pharmacokinetics and Pharmacodynamics

Ageing is associated with physiological changes that affect drug pharmacokinetics (absorption, distribution, metabolism and excretion) and pharmacodynamics (the effect of drugs on the body) [7]. Normal ageing has little effect on the rate or extent of drug absorption, most of which occurs in the small bowel. However, prokinetic drugs (e.g. domperidone and erythromycin) can increase gastric emptying, thus potentially increasing the rate at which a drug is absorbed after ingestion. Anticholinergic drugs can reduce salivary secretion, thus impeding the rate but not necessarily the extent of drug absorption through the buccal mucosa for drugs such as glyceryl trinitrate and midazolam. Theoretically, the rate of absorption of intramuscular, transdermal and subcutaneous injections may be reduced because of age-related reductions in tissue perfusion. However, the clinical effect of this is usually negligible.

Systemic bioavailability of most drugs is not affected by normal ageing, other than those which undergo substantial first-pass hepatic extraction and metabolism, e.g. morphine, buprenorphine, midazolam, propranolol, nitrates, verapamil and tricyclic antidepressants. With these drugs, age-related reductions in liver volume and blood flow (of up to 30%) can result in reduced first-pass hepatic extraction with significantly higher systemic bioavailability as a result. In the case of nitrates or verapamil, this greater systemic bioavailability can result in clinically significant first-dose hypotension in some older patients. Therefore, initial doses of such drugs should be reduced in older patients with particular attention being paid to timing and dose of first administration. In general, it is recommended that a low "test dose" be prescribed, and if tolerated, the dose can be slowly up-titrated according to treatment effect ("start low and go slow").

Ageing is associated with reduced lean body weight and muscle mass and a relative increase in total body fat, thereby increasing the volume of distribution (Vd) of lipid-soluble drugs such as morphine, benzodiazepines, antipsychotics and amitriptyline. This larger Vd results in longer elimination half-lives, prolonged drug effect, accumulation with continued use and greater potential for toxicity and adverse effects such as sedation and falls. It is recommended that the starting doses of such drugs be reduced in older patients with slow up-titration according to response. Conversely, the Vd of water-soluble drugs such as lithium, theophylline and gentamycin is reduced, resulting in higher plasma concentrations after initial administration, thereby necessitating lower doses in older patients.

Most drugs are inactive when bound to circulating plasma proteins (e.g. albumin and α-1 glycoprotein) and mediate their pharmacological effects when unbound or free. Though normal ageing does not affect plasma protein concentration, serum albumin levels can diminish with chronic disease, resulting in clinically important increases in free drug concentration and subsequently increased physiological effects for compounds that are heavily protein-bound, e.g. benzodiazepines, antipsychotics, non-steroidal anti-inflammatory drugs (NSAIDs), warfarin and phenytoin. The Vd of these drugs increases with hypoalbuminaemia, thereby increasing their elimination half-life and potential for toxicity and adversity. In the case of phenytoin, caution must be exerted when interpreting serum drug levels in the context of coexisting hypoalbuminaemia as it is usually the bound fraction that is measured by most laboratory assays and not the unbound "active" fraction.

Reduced hepatic mass and blood flow occur with ageing with consequent decline in hepatic metabolism and clearance of drugs such as propranolol and theophylline. However, liver enzyme activity is usually preserved. All prescribers should be aware of potential drug interactions involving inhibition and induction of hepatic cytochrome p450 metabolising enzymes. Cytochrome p450 enzyme inhibition can lead to a rapid reduction in drug metabolism with resultant toxic accumulation, e.g. haloperidol may impede the metabolism of amitriptyline through inhibition of cytochrome p450 2D6, thereby increasing the potential for anticholinergic side effects including orthostatic hypotension and tachyarrhythmias, all of which can result in falls with injury. Clarithromycin may impede the metabolism of simvastatin through inhibition of p450 3A4, thus increasing the risk of statin-induced myositis and hepatitis. Amiodarone as well as certain antibacterial and antifungal drugs may impede the metabolism of warfarin, thereby increasing its anticoagulant effect and

Table 21.1 Inhibitors and inducers of the hepatic cytochrome p450 enzyme system

Enzyme inhibitors	Enzyme inducers
Erythromycin, clarithromycin	Carbamazepine
Sulphonamides	Phenytoin
Ciprofloxacin	Topiramate
Fluconazole, miconazole, ketoconazole	Clotrimazole
Amiodarone	Rifampicin
Diltiazem, verapamil	Dexamethasone
Cimetidine	Primidone
Fluoxetine, paroxetine	St. John's wort

increasing the risk of haemorrhage. Conversely, drugs such as carbamazepine and phenytoin can induce cytochrome p450 enzymes which accelerate the metabolism and clearance of another drug or unrelated substrate, potentially resulting in treatment failure. Some examples of cytochrome p450 inhibitors and inducers are presented in Table 21.1. In general, these drugs predictably precipitate adverse drug reactions in older patients when they are co-prescribed with substrate drugs that are metabolised by the relevant cytochrome enzyme. Clinically relevant examples of cytochrome p450 enzyme inhibitors include antimicrobials, antiarrhythmics and some anticoagulants which are frequently used to treat acute illness in the emergency department, thereby placing older patients with polypharmacy at increased risk of ADR through interaction with their regularly prescribed existing drugs.

One of the most important age-related pharmacokinetic changes is the predictable decline in renal function. Normal ageing results in reduced renal size, perfusion and concentrating ability. Indeed, a gradual decline in glomerular filtration rates begins at the age of 30 years. This is potentiated by conditions such as hypertension and diabetes and by nephrotoxic medications such as NSAIDs, gentamicin and vancomycin. It is recommended that glomerular filtration rate (GFR) is estimated for all older patients at regular intervals using readily available formulae such as the Cockcroft and Gault [13] equation or the modified diet in renal diseases (MDRD) [14]. It must be remembered that serum creatinine concentration is not a reliable measure of renal function in older people because of age-related reductions in muscle mass. Approximately 50% of older patients have a normal serum creatinine level but a reduced creatinine clearance estimate.

Acute kidney injury (AKI) is common in older patients with acute illness and can occur for multiple reasons including hypotension, dehydration, sepsis, cardiorenal syndrome/cardiac failure or NSAID use. In this context, a regularly prescribed renally eliminated medication (e.g. digoxin, dabigatran or metformin) may need to be temporarily withheld or dose reduced in order to avoid high serum levels and toxicity. Once renal impairment has been identified (be it AKI or chronic kidney disease) and creatinine clearance (Cr Cl) estimated, the need for dose alteration of renally eliminated drugs must be determined. In general, dose adjustment is needed when the creatinine clearance is below 60 ml/min (see Table 21.2).

Drugs exert their effects by binding as agonists, partial agonists or antagonists to target molecules and receptors within the body; pharmacodynamics is the study of these effects. Receptor expression, density, activity and affinity change with age,

Table 21.2 Drugs that require dose adjustment with impaired renal function (precise dose adjustments for each drug are available in comprehensive formularies such as the British National Formulary [15])

Drug/class	Examples
Cardiac drugs	Digoxin, atenolol, sotalol
Lipid lowering drugs	Pravastatin, rosuvastatin, fibrates
Hypoglycaemic drugs	Metformin, glibenclamide, Glimepiride, gliptins, insulin
Diuretics	Thiazide diuretics have limited efficacy if CrCl is <30 ml/min
	Avoid potassium-sparing diuretics if CrCl <30 ml/min
Anticoagulants	Apixaban, rivaroxaban, dabigatran, low molecular weight heparin (enoxaparin, tinzaparin)
Drugs for gout	Allopurinol, colchicine
Bone anti-resorptive drugs	Avoid bisphosphonates if CrCl <30 ml/min
Analgesic drugs	Opioids (morphine, codeine, pethidine), NSAIDs
Anticonvulsants	Topiramate, levetiracetam, vigabatrin
Psychotropic drugs	Lithium, gabapentin, amisulpride
Antibiotics	Aminoglycosides (e.g. gentamicin), vancomycin, carbapenems (e.g. meropenem), piperacillin/tazobactam, ciprofloxacin, ceftazidime
Antifungals	Fluconazole, sulfamethoxazole
Antivirals	Acyclovir, ganciclovir, famciclovir

thus leading to altered (usually increased) pharmacodynamic effects of commonly prescribed drugs including anticoagulants, opioids and antipsychotics. In practice, this means that older patients frequently have exaggerated responses to medications at doses that are normally used in younger patients, e.g. the anticoagulant response to warfarin is often increased in older patients compared to a similar dose in a younger patient, thus increasing their bleeding risk. Older patients are particularly susceptible to the central nervous system (CNS) effects of anticholinergics, benzodiazepines, opioids and other centrally acting or psychoactive drugs because of increased blood-brain barrier permeability, reduced cholinergic neurotransmission and alterations in receptor density, affinity and intracellular responses. Clinical examples of the effect of altered pharmacodynamics sensitivity are presented in Table 21.3. It is usually recommended to start such drugs at the lowest possible dose and to slowly up-titrate according to response.

Prescribers should also be aware of age-related changes in homeostatic and thermoregulatory mechanisms. With increasing age, there is a reduction in aortic and large-vessel elasticity and compliance often resulting in systolic hypertension, lower diastolic blood pressure and a tendency towards left ventricular hypertrophy. In addition, baroreceptor sensitivity and resting heart rate are reduced, thus increasing the risk of postural hypotension and falls. Many drugs can exacerbate postural hypotension including antihypertensives, vasodilators (doxazosin and tamsulosin) and drugs with anticholinergic properties, e.g. tricyclic antidepressants and first-generation antihistamines. Falls are commonly caused by orthostatic hypotension. Drugs that contribute to reducing blood pressure in any way should be carefully reviewed and dose reduced or discontinued as appropriate.

Table 21.3 Age-related changes in pharmacodynamic response to commonly prescribed drugs

Drug type	Specific drug	Pharmacodynamic response	Potential clinical consequence
Analgesia	Morphine	↑	Excessive sedation, confusion, constipation, respiratory depression
Anticoagulant	Warfarin	↑	↑ Bleeding risk
	Dabigatran (age ≥75 years, weight <50 kg)	↑	
	Apixaban	↑	
Cardiovascular system drugs	Angiotensin-receptor blocker	↑	Hypotension (↑ acute antihypertensive effect)
	Diltiazem	↑	
	Enalapril	↑	
	Verapamil	↑	Hypotension (↑ acute antihypertensive effect), bradyarrhythmias (↑ cardiac conduction effects)
	Propranolol	↓	Less reduction in heart rate
Diuretics	Frusemide	↓	↓ Diuretic effect and size of peak of diuretic response
Psychoactive drugs	Benzodiazepines	↑	Excessive sedation, confusion, postural sway, falls
	Antipsychotics	↑	Excessive sedation, confusion
Others	Levodopa	↑	Dyskinesia, confusion, hallucinations

↑, Increased pharmacodynamic response; ↓, reduced pharmacodynamic response

21.4 Drug-Drug and Drug-Disease Interactions

Older patients often have multiple co-morbidities for which they are prescribed multiple medications. Drug-drug interactions (Table 21.4) are usually predictable through known pharmacokinetic and pharmacodynamic principles as previously described. Certain drugs may also worsen coexisting diseases in older patients. These should be minimised and safer alternatives be prescribed where possible. Table 21.5 presents some clinically important drug-disease interactions including the major geriatrics syndromes of dementia, delirium, incontinence and falls, which are often significantly exacerbated by commonly prescribed medications.

21.5 Polypharmacy

Polypharmacy refers to the use of several drugs concurrently. Though multiple medications are often clinically justifiable, it is well established that polypharmacy in older patients is associated with inappropriate prescribing (i.e. where the risk of

Table 21.4 Clinically important drug-drug interactions in older patients

Drug	Drug	Interaction	Effect
Antihypertensive agent	Vasodilator, antipsychotic, TCA	Combined hypotensive effect	Orthostatic hypotension, falls
Antihypertensive agent	NSAIDs	NSAID antagonises hypotensive effect	↓ Antihypertensive effect
Potassium sparing diuretics	ACE inhibitors, spironolactone	Combined potassium sparing effects	↓ Renal function, hyperkalaemia
Digoxin	Diuretics	Diuretic-induced hypokalaemia	↑ Effect of digoxin (arrhythmia, toxicity)
Digoxin	Amiodarone, diltiazem, verapamil	↓ Clearance of digoxin	↑ Effect of digoxin (arrhythmia, toxicity)
Phenytoin	Cytochrome p450 enzyme inhibitors[a]	↓ Clearance of phenytoin	↑ Effect of phenytoin
Thyroxine	Cytochrome p450 enzyme inducers[a]	↑ clearance of thyroxine	↓ Effect of thyroxine
Lithium	NSAIDs, diuretics	↓ Clearance of lithium	↑ Effect of lithium (arrhythmia, toxicity)
Phenothiazines	Drugs with anticholinergic properties	Combined anticholinergic effects	Confusion, constipation, urinary retention, dry mouth

TCA, tricyclic antidepressant; *NSAID*, non-steroidal anti-inflammatory drug
[a]See Table 21.1

Table 21.5 Clinically important drug-disease interactions in older patients

Disease or condition	Drug	Effect of drug on disease or condition
Hypertension	NSAIDs, high sodium content drugs	↑ Blood pressure
Orthostatic hypotension	Diuretics, anticholinergics, levodopa, vasodilators	Falls, syncope, hip fracture
Falls	Benzodiazepines, antipsychotics, opioids, anticholinergics	↑ Risk of falls, sedation, gait instability
Osteoporosis	Corticosteroids	Fracture
Poorly controlled gout	Thiazide diuretic	Hyperuricaemia, ↑ risk acute exacerbation of gout
Cognitive impairment, dementia	Anticholinergics, benzodiazepines, TCAs	↑ Confusion, delirium
Cardiac failure	Verapamil, disopyramide	Exacerbation of heart failure
Renal failure	Aminoglycoside antibiotics, NSAIDs, radiological contrast	Acute kidney injury, worsening of creatinine clearance
Peptic ulcer disease	NSAIDs, anticoagulants	Peptic ulcer, upper gastrointestinal haemorrhage
Benign prostatic hyperplasia	Anticholinergics, alpha-agonists	Urinary retention

treatment outweighs the potential clinical benefit), adverse drug reactions (ADRs) and non-specific syndromes in older people including weight loss, falls and cognitive and functional decline. The World Health Organization defines an ADR as an appreciably harmful or unpleasant reaction, resulting from an intervention related to

Table 21.6 Polypharmacy in older patients: clinical associations

1. ↑ Risk of ADR including drug-drug and drug-disease interactions
2. ↑ Likelihood of inappropriate prescribing including use of drugs without clear clinical indication
3. ↑ Likelihood of prescribing cascades, i.e. where a drug is prescribed to treat a symptom attributable to an adverse effect of another drug
4. ↑ Incidence of geriatric syndromes, i.e. cognitive and functional decline, weight loss and falls
5. ↑ Risk of non-compliance and poor adherence with medication regime
6. ↑ Healthcare costs (drug costs and resource utilisation to investigate and manage adverse outcomes)

the use of a medicinal product, which predicts hazard from future administration and warrants prevention or specific treatment, alteration of the dosage regimen or withdrawal of the product [16]. Patients taking two concurrent medications have a 13% risk of ADR, which rises to 38% for four medications and 82% for greater than seven medications prescribed simultaneously [17]. Adverse consequences of polypharmacy are summarised in Table 21.6.

21.6 Inappropriate Prescribing

In pharmacological terms, inappropriate prescribing (IP) pertains to overuse (no clinical indication, therapeutic duplication or excessive duration), misuse (increased risk of ADE including drug-drug and drug-disease interactions because of age-related changes in pharmacokinetics and pharmacodynamics) and underuse of medications (omission of a clinically indicated drug of potential therapeutic benefit) [18]. Other variables which affect prescribing appropriateness include cognitive and physical dysfunction. Cognitive deficits can lead to errors with medication administration or consumption, by virtue of a patient improperly following instructions, forgetting to take medications or taking incorrect doses. Similarly, physical deficits such as hearing loss, low vision and impaired manual dexterity can make it difficult for patients to physically adhere to medication regimes, thereby resulting in low therapeutic yield and increasing the risk of adverse outcomes. Thus, for a medication to be appropriate, it must be pharmacologically suitable in the context of co-morbid illnesses and concurrent medications, and it must be taken safely and reliably.

IP is highly prevalent in older patients. At least one potentially inappropriate medication (PIM) is seen in approximately 35% of community-dwelling older patients presenting with unselected acute illness to the ED [19] and in >50% of nursing home residents [20]. Indeed, between 10 and 20% of hospital admissions of older patients are directly related to adverse effects of inappropriately prescribed drugs [19, 21]. The principal risk factor for IP is polypharmacy [22]; older patients who attend multiple doctors and multiple dispensing pharmacies are also at increased risk [23]. IP is associated with unnecessary drug use and prescribing cascades (where a drug is prescribed to treat an adverse effect of another drug). IP also increases the risk of ADE, related morbidity and health resource utilisation [24, 25]. Healthcare costs in the United States caused by improper and unnecessary use of medications exceeded $200 billion in 2012, amounting to an estimated 10 million hospital admissions, 78 million outpatient treatments, 246 million prescriptions and 4 million emergency department visits [26].

Various sets of prescribing indicators have been designed to highlight instances of potentially inappropriate prescribing in older patients, with Beers criteria [27–30] and STOPP/START (screening tool of older people's prescriptions/screening tool to alert to right treatment) criteria [31, 32] being frequently cited in the literature. Beers criteria were devised on the basis of North American formularies and comprise lists of medications which should be avoided in older patients independent of diagnosis and considering diagnosis. STOPP criteria were validated in a European context and comprise 80 clinically relevant prescribing indicators which highlight instances where drugs should be avoided or used with caution in older people with common co-morbidities or potential for drug-drug and drug-disease interactions. STOPP is designed to be used in tandem with START (screening tool to alert to right treatment) criteria for potential prescribing omissions (PPO's), the aim being to detect common and clinically important instances of PIM's and PPO's in older patients. Clinical application of STOPP/START has been shown to improve all domains of prescribing appropriateness including the use of drugs that are indicated, effectively and correctly dosed as well, reducing the risk of potential drug-drug interactions and drug-disease interactions, with this benefit being maintained for up to 6 months after intervention [33]. Intervention with STOPP/START has also been shown to reduce the incidence of in-hospital ADEs [34]. Prescribing indicators can assist with decision-making in prescribing appropriateness. However, they are intended only as a guide and not as a substitute for informed clinical judgement.

21.7 Adverse Drug Events in Older Patients Presenting to the Emergency Department

Patients aged ≥65 years account for 12–24% of all ED attendances [35]. Adverse effects of medications contribute substantially to the reason for hospital admission in approximately 10–20% of acutely ill older patients [19, 21, 36]. Budnitz et al. reported that nearly half of hospitalisations for ADEs in North America involved adults aged 80 years and older [37]. Indeed, such hospitalisations were over three times more common in patients aged ≥85 years than those 65–69 years [37]. Nearly two thirds of hospitalisations were due to unintentional overdoses. The most commonly implicated drugs were warfarin (33.3%), insulins (13.9%), antiplatelet drugs (13.3%) and oral hypoglycaemic drugs (10.7%) [37]. Improved prescribing and monitoring of these agents have the potential to reduce ED attendances and subsequent hospitalisation for ADEs in older adults. However, it must be acknowledged that ADEs often present as vague and non-specific symptoms in older patients (see Table 21.7) rendering it difficult to detect ADEs and perhaps contributing to

Table 21.7 Clinical presentations of ADEs in older patients presenting to the emergency department

Drug class	Clinical nature of ADE
Haematological agents (anticoagulants and antiplatelets)	Gastrointestinal haemorrhage
	↑ INR, abnormal laboratory indices (e.g. ↓ haemoglobin, ↓ platelets)
	Skin or wound haemorrhage
Endocrine agents	Hypoglycaemia with altered mental status or other neurological sequelae, e.g. loss of consciousness or seizure
Cardiovascular agents	Electrolyte or fluid-volume disturbance, weakness or lethargy
	Cardiac arrhythmia or abnormality in heart rate or blood pressure
	Allergic reaction, orthostatic hypotension
Central nervous system agents	Altered mental status
	Fall or other injury
	Dizziness, syncope, weakness, dyspnoea or respiratory distress
Anti-infective agents	Allergic reaction
	Dyspnoea, weakness or abnormality in heart rate or blood pressure
	Nausea, vomiting, diarrhoea

under-reporting of same. Therefore, clinicians must have a high index of suspicion of drug-related problems in any older patient presenting with acute illness to the ED. Even if the reason for presentation to the ED is not an ADE, older adults can still be exposed while under the care of an ED physician, with a reported incidence of 0.16–6% and 36–71% of these incident ADEs being preventable [38].

21.8 Medication Reconciliation

Attendance at an ED (with or without subsequent hospital admission) represents a potentially hazardous transition of pharmaceutical care because of existing polypharmacy and the requirement for new treatments for acute illness. Older adults are often at their most vulnerable when acutely ill (particularly if they have delirium or dementia) and may not be in a position to reliably discuss their mediation regimens. Often they simply don't know what medications they are prescribed or why. They may not be taking all medications on the doctor's or pharmacist's list, even if it is an up-to-date prescription. Furthermore, they may be taking additional medications not listed on the prescription, e.g. over-the-counter or complementary/alternative medicines, which may be pharmacologically relevant to their clinical reason for presentation. Therefore, a robust process to ensure that the list of medications prescribed by an ED physician accurately reflects what the patient regularly takes at home is paramount.

Medication reconciliation (MR) is a process of creating and maintaining the most up-to-date and accurate medication list for a patient, checking for all potential discrepancies. It has the potential to identify medication inconsistencies and reduce potential harm, though its precise impact on clinical outcome and readmissions is yet to be rigorously determined [39]. Table 21.8 describes the three key steps involved in MR: collecting, checking and communicating. MR is usually performed by clinical pharmacists who have knowledge of therapeutics, pharmaceutical management and effective communication skills. However, all prescribers have an ethical duty to obtain accurate and reliable information about their patients' medication history.

21.9 Optimal Prescribing for Older Patients in the ED

Prescribing for older patient is complex. It requires good clinical acumen as well as knowledge of the fundamental principles of pharmacology as previously described. Key recommendations when prescribing for older patients in the ED are presented in Table 21.9. These can be supported by comprehensive geriatric assessment, clinical pharmacy input and application of prescribing indicators such as STOPP/START criteria.

Comprehensive geriatric assessment (CGA) provides a global assessment of an older patient's co-morbidities, medication use, cognition, functional status and

Table 21.8 Stages of medication reconciliation

Collecting	Gathering all information available on current medication regimens
Checking	Checking and verifying information for any discrepancies
Communicating	New list of medications communicated to the patient and/or their carer

Table 21.9 Key recommendations when prescribing for older patients

1. Obtain an accurate and up-to-date medication list including over-the-counter and complementary/alternative medicines. Confirm adherence to this list by asking the patient and carer where appropriate. Perform structured medication reconciliation where available
2. Ensure each medication has an appropriate indication and a clear therapeutic goal. This involves careful clinical assessment and appreciation of time to obtain treatment effect and life expectancy. Clinical prescribing indicators such as STOPP/START criteria are useful when evaluating prescribing appropriateness
3. Review medications in the context of coexisting disease states, concurrent medications, functional and cognitive status and therapeutic expectation
4. Be aware that new presenting symptoms may be due to an existing medication, drug-drug interaction or drug-disease interaction. Avoid prescribing cascades to treat adverse effects of exiting medications
5. In general, start a new medication at the smallest dose and titrate slowly according to response and efficacy (except for drugs in which steady state concentration must be achieved quickly, e.g. antibiotics)
6. Use the simplest dosing regimen (e.g. once a day preferable to three times per day) and most appropriate formulation
7. Provide verbal and written instructions on indication, time and route of administration and potential adverse effects of each medication. Administer medications via a pre-prepared blister pack if available. Inform patient, carer and GP of any change to medications
8. When stopping a medication, check that it can be stopped abruptly or whether it needs to be tapered, e.g. long-term corticosteroids, benzodiazepines

social support. It can detect medication discrepancies, including IP, as it involves a detailed review of prescription and non-prescription medication at the time of consultation. Screening of high-risk older patients in the ED, followed by CGA and appropriate interventions, can improve outcomes [40]. However, CGA is time consuming and resource intensive and thus cannot be performed routinely in most EDs. Clinical pharmacists perform systematic assessments of patient's medications and can have a positive effect on the occurrence of drug-related issues and clinical outcomes [41]. However, this is a resource intensive strategy which requires pharmacists to have training and experience in geriatric pharmacotherapy. In addition, it requires co-operation of physicians and patients alike, to implement the recommendations, all of which can be challenging in the busy ED setting. Most physicians receive inadequate training in geriatric pharmacotherapy; thus many physicians are not equipped with the knowledge required to prescribe for older adults with complex illnesses and multiple medications. Therefore, educational strategies would appear to be highly relevant to improve appropriate prescribing in this group. Studies have investigated the impact of different educational approaches on prescribing quality of prescribing, with mixed results. Interactive approaches with direct feedback that target multiple disciplines are most effective. Education interventions, such as the World Health Organization guide on prescribing, can improve prescribing skills in students in a simulated environment; however further research is required to see if it has long-term benefits [42].

Computerised physician order entry (CPOE) systems have the potential to improve the appropriateness of prescribing for older adults. In the ED setting, they can reduce IP [43]. Computerised drug-lab alerts have been shown to improve surrogate clinical outcomes (e.g. time in therapeutic range for vitamin K antagonists) but have not been shown to improve clinical benefits [44]. This could be explained by the fact that physicians often over-ride the therapeutic flags generated by computerised systems because of perceived unimportance or alert fatigue, thus missing high-risk alerts. A disadvantage of these systems is that they are dependent on the quality of the computer programme, and there have been reports of them resulting in errors and related ADEs. Again they should not be used in isolation but used to enhance decision-making.

21.10 Summary

Older adults comprise an increasingly large proportion of ED attendances. They often present with multiple complex illnesses including geriatrics syndromes such as delirium, dementia, falls, immobility and incontinence. They frequently have complex medication regimens with a high prevalence of ADEs, many of which contribute to the clinical reason for presentation. Prescribing for older patients in the ED presents multiple challenges including accurate documentation of all medications (prescribed, over-the-counter and complementary/alternative) and enquiry regarding adherence with the same. Prescribers must be aware of age-related physiological changes and disease-related organ dysfunction which impact on pharmacokinetics and pharmacodynamics and increase the risk of drug-drug and drug-disease interactions. Inappropriate prescribing is highly prevalent in older adults attending the ED. Prescribing indicators such as STOPP/START criteria may be useful in identifying and reducing potentially inappropriate medications and related ADEs. Medications reconciliation, comprehensive geriatric assessment, electronic ordering systems, regular education and prescribing audit are also of benefit in optimising prescribing for older patients.

References

1. George G, Jell C, Todd BS (2006) Effect of population ageing on emergency department speed and efficiency: a historical perspective from a district general hospital in the UK. Emerg Med J 23:379–383
2. Strange GR, Chen EH, Sanders AB (1992) Use of emergency departments by elderly patients: projections from a multicentre data base. Ann Emerg Med 21:819–824
3. Aminzadeh F, Dalziel WB (2002) Older adults in the emergency department: a systematic review of patterns of use, adverse outcomes, and effectiveness of interventions. Ann Emerg Med 39:238–247
4. Salvi F, Morichi V, Grilli A, Giorgi R et al (2007) The elderly in the emergency department: a critical review of problems and solutions. Intern Emerg Med 2:292–301
5. Budnitz DS, Shehab N, Kegler SR, Richards CL (2007) Medication use leading to emergency department visits for adverse drug events in older adults. Ann Intern Med 147:755–765
6. Piromohamed M, James S, Meakin S et al (2004) Adverse drug reactions as a cause of admission to hospital: prospective analysis of 18820 patients. BMJ 329:15
7. Mangoni AA, Jackson SHD (2004) Age-related changes in pharmacokinetics and pharmacodynamics: basic principles and practical applications. Br J Clin Pharmacol 57(1):6–14
8. Qato DM, Alexander GC, Conti RM et al (2008) Use of prescription and over-the-counter medications and dietary supplements among older adults in the united states. JAMA 300:2867–2878
9. Department of Health (2004) Prescriptions dispensed in the community: statistics for 1993–2003. Department of Health, London
10. Patterns of medication use in the United States (2006) A report from the Slone survey. Slone Epidemiology Centre at Boston University, Boston
11. Doshi JA, Shaffer T, Briesacher BA (2005) National Estimates of medication use in nursing homes: findings from the 1997 medicare current beneficiary survey and the 1996 medical expenditure survey. J Am Geriatr Soc 53:438–443
12. Rousseau A, Rybarczyk-Vigouret MC, Vogel T, Lang PO, Michel B (2016) Inappropriate prescription and administration of medications in 10 nursing homes in Alsace, France. Rev Epidemiol Sante Publique 64(2):95–101
13. Cockcroft DW, Gault MH (1976) Prediction of creatinine clearance from serum creatinine. Nephron 16:31–41
14. Levey AS, Bosch JP, Lewis JB et al (1999) A more accurate method to estimate glomerular filtration rate from serum creatinine: a new prediction equation. Modification of diet in renal disease study group. Ann Intern Med 130:461–470
15. British National Formulary Mar 2015–Sept 2015. www.bnf.org
16. World Health Organisation (1972) Technical Report number 498
17. Goldberg RM, Mabee J, Chan L, Wong S (1996) Drug – drug and drug – disease interactions in the ED: analysis of a high risk population. Am J Emerg Med 14:447–450
18. Spinewine A, Schmader KE, Barber N et al (2007) Appropriate prescribing in elderly people: how well can it be measured and optimised? Lancet 370:173–184

19. Gallagher P, O'Mahony D (2008) STOPP (screening tool of older persons' potentially inappropriate prescriptions): application to acutely ill elderly patients and comparison with beers' criteria. Age Ageing 37:673–679
20. Ryan C, O'Mahony D, Kennedy J et al (2013) Potentially inappropriate prescribing in older residents in Irish nursing homes. Age Ageing 42(1):116–120
21. Hamilton H, Gallagher P, Ryan C, Byrne S, O'Mahony D (2011) Potentially inappropriate medications defined by STOPP criteria and the risk of adverse drug events in older hospitalized patients. Arch Intern Med 171(11):1013–1019
22. Maher RL, Hanlon J, Hajjar ER (2014) Clinical consequences of polypharmacy in elderly. Expert Opin Drug Saf 13:57–65
23. Frank C, Godwin M, Verma S et al (2001) What drugs are our frail elderly patients taking? Do drugs they take or fail to take put them at increased risk of interactions and inappropriate medication use? Can Fam Physician 47:1198–1204
24. Lau DT, Kasper JD, Potter DE, Lyles A, Bennett RG (2005) Hospitalization and death associated with potentially inappropriate medication prescriptions among elderly nursing home residents. Arch Intern Med 165:68–74
25. Lindley CM, Tully MP, Paramsothy V, Tallis RC (1992) Inappropriate medication is a major cause of adverse drug reactions in elderly patients. Age Ageing 21:294–300
26. IMS Institute for Healthcare Economics (2013) Available costs in U.S. Healthcare. The $200 billion opportunity from using medicines more responsibly
27. Beers MH, Ouslander JG, Rollingher I et al (1991) Explicit criteria for determining inappropriate medication use in nursing home residents. UCLA division of geriatric medicine. Arch Intern Med 151:1825–1832
28. Beers MH (1997) Explicit criteria for determining potentially inappropriate medication use by the elderly. An update. Arch Intern Med 157:1531–1536
29. Fick DM, Cooper JW, Wade WE et al (2003) Updating the beers criteria for potentially inappropriate medication use in older adults: results of a US consensus panel of experts. Arch Intern Med 163:2716–2724
30. American Geriatrics Society 2012 Beers Criteria Update Expert Panel (2012) American Geriatrics Society updated beers criteria for potentially inappropriate medication use in older adults. J Am Geriatr Soc 60:616–631
31. Gallagher P, Ryan C, Byrne S, Kennedy J, O'Mahony D (2008) STOPP (screening tool of older Person's prescriptions) and START (screening tool to alert doctors to right treatment). Consensus validation. Int J Clin Pharmacol Ther 46:72–83
32. O'Mahony D, O'Sullivan D, Byrne S et al (2015) STOPP/START criteria for potentially inappropriate prescribing in older people: version 2. Age Ageing 44:213–218
33. Gallagher PF, O'Connor MN, O'Mahony D (2011) Prevention of potentially inappropriate prescribing for elderly patients: a randomized controlled trial using STOPP/START criteria. Clin Pharmacol Ther 89:845–854
34. O'Connor MN (2014) Adverse drug reactions in older people during hospitalisation: prevalence, risk factors and recognition. MD thesis. University College Cork, Cork
35. Samaras N, Chevalley T, Samaras D, Gold G (2010) Older patients in the emergency department: a review. Ann Emerg Med 56:261–269
36. Hohl CM, Dankoff J, Colacone A, Afilalo M (2001) Polypharmacy, adverse drug-related events, and potential adverse drug interactions in elderly patients presenting to an emergency department. Ann Emerg Med 38:666–671
37. Budnitz DS, Lovegrove MC, Shehab N, Richards CL (2011) Emergency hospitalisations for adverse drug events in older Americans. N Engl J Med 365:2002–2012
38. Stang AS, Wingert AS, Hartling L, Plint AC (2013) Adverse events related to emergency department care: a systematic review. PLoS One 8:e74241
39. Lehnbom EC, Stewart MJ, Manias E, Westbrook JI (2014) Impact of medication reconciliation and review on clinical outcomes. Ann Pharmacother 48:1298–1312

40. Graf CE, Zekry D, Giannelli S, Michel JP, Chevalley T (2011) Efficiency and applicability of comprehensive geriatric assessment in the emergency department: a systematic review. Aging Clin Exp Res 23:244–254
41. Alassaad A, Bertilsson M, Gillespie U et al (2014) The effects of pharmacist intervention on emergency department visits in patients 80 years and older: subgroup analyses by number of prescribed drugs and appropriate prescribing. PLoS One 9:e111797
42. Ross S, Loke YK (2009) Do educational interventions improve prescribing by medical students and junior doctors? A systematic review. Br J Clin Pharmacol 67:662–670
43. Terrell K, Perkins A, Dexter P et al (2009) Computerized decision support to reduce potentially inappropriate prescribing to older emergency department patients: a randomized, controlled trial. J Am Geriatr Soc 57:1388–1394
44. Bayoumi I, Al Balas M, Handler SM, Holbrook A et al (2014) The effectiveness of computerized drug-lab alerts: a systematic review and meta-analysis. Int J Med Inform 83:406–415

Pain in Older People Attending Emergency Departments

22

Sophie Pautex

22.1 Introduction

Acute pain is a common reason for emergency department (ED) visits among older patients [1]. Effective treatment of acute pain is important for the relief of suffering. Furthermore, unrelieved acute pain is associated with poorer outcomes during hospitalisation, including, for example, persistent pain, longer hospital length of stay and delirium [2–7]. Despite the frequency with which this problem is encountered and the importance of effective pain treatment, disparities in pain care continue to exist for older adults when compared with younger adults, evidenced by high rates of pain at the end of the ED visit and lower rates of treatment for older versus younger adults [1, 7–14]. Although increased attention to this issue has resulted in some improvement in pain care documentation and use of analgesia in older adults, older adults with acute pain are up to 20% less likely to receive treatment than younger patients and still often leave the ED with pain [15, 16]. Furthermore, cross-sectional studies of pain reporting in individuals with dementia have presented evidence that they receive fewer analgesics than noncognitively impaired older people for the same indications [17–22]. There are multiple reasons for under-treatment (Table 22.1), but the most common reason is that pain is not detected [23–27].

The optimal management of acute pain in older adults requires an iterative process of detection, assessment, explanation, reassurance and treatment. This is true for all individuals with acute pain but particularly so for older adults because of the increased risk of adverse events. Thus, reassessment of pain is as important as providing initial treatment, and failure to reassess pain is a common cause of under-treatment of pain in older adults. Following the Assessing Care of Vulnerable Elders quality indicator approach, a task force convened by the Society for Academic

S. Pautex
Department of Community Medicine, Primary Care and Emergency Medicine,
Geneva University Hospitals, University of Geneva, Geneva, Switzerland
e-mail: sophie.pautex@hcuge.ch

Table 22.1 Barriers that participate to the under-treatment of pain in older people

Patient
  Underreporting, stoicism
  Concerns about the meaning of pain, of the diagnostic tests and hospitalisation
  Difficulties to use some assessment tools
  Multiple problems making treatment more difficult
  Polypharmacy—side effects of treatments
Health care providers
  Failure to believe patient's pain
  Failure to use some validated pain assessment tools
  Mistaking ageing for reversible and treatable disorders
  Numerous myths, such as presbyalgesia, or that the prescription of analgesia leads to addiction and lack of long-term efficacy
  The belief that failure to express pain complaints means they do not exist
  Lack of education in the assessment and management of pain in older people in the curriculum of health professionals

Table 22.2 Geriatric ED pain care quality indicators, adapted from [28]

1. Formal assessment for the presence of acute pain should be documented within 1 h of ED arrival
2. If a patient remains in the ED for longer than 6 h, a second pain assessment should be documented
3. If a patient receives pain treatment, a pain reassessment should be documented before discharge from the ED
4. If a patient has moderate to severe pain, pain treatment should be initiated (or a reason documented why it was not initiated)
5. Meperidine (Pethidine or Demerol) should not be used to treat pain in older adults
6. If a patient is prescribed opioid analgesics upon discharge from the ED, a bowel regimen should also be provided

Emergency Medicine and the American College of Emergency Physicians developed the following indicators to measure the quality of geriatric pain care received in the ED setting (Table 22.2) [28].

22.2 Definition and Types of Pain

Pain is described as an unpleasant sensory and emotional experience associated with actual or potential tissue damage or described in terms of such damage [29]. Pain may be acute, lasting from seconds to weeks until complete healing, or it may be chronic, lasting for months or years, sometimes forever. Pain has a tremendous influence on peoples' quality of life and functioning.

Acute pain plays an important role in drawing attention to injured tissues and preventing further tissue damage. Acute pain should trigger an urgent search for an underlying cause that might be immediately treated. Autonomic overactivity such as tachycardia and diaphoresis is often present.

Furthermore, older people often suffer from *chronic or persistent pain* for months to years, and as a result, they may be plagued by depression and anxiety, sleep

Table 22.3 Pain classification

Nociceptive pain
  Musculoskeletal conditions: osteoarthritis, degenerative disc disease, osteoporosis and fractures
  Rheumatologic conditions: rheumatoid arthritis, temporal arteritis
  Trauma
  Cancer
  Vascular disease
Central neuropathic pain
  Ischemia, haemorrhages located in the thalamus, spinothalamic pathways or thalamocortical projections
  Spinal cord injury
  Inflammatory CNS disease (multiple sclerosis, myelitis, syringomyelia)
Peripheral neuropathic pain
  Trigeminal neuralgia
  Nerve compression
  Neuroma
  Plexus neuropathies
  Metabolic, toxic, immune-mediated polyneuropathies
  Infectious/parainfectious neuropathies: post-herpetic, syphilis

disturbance, functional disability and compromised quality of life [24, 30–36]. The psychosocial impact of chronic pain is of greater importance in older people, not least because it can lead to emergency admissions in older people.

Most older patients will present *nociceptive pain* (stimulation of nociceptive receptors by a tissue injury process) secondary, for example, from osteoarthritis, soft tissue injuries and visceral pathology (Table 22.3). But some patients will suffer from *neuropathic pain* (pain initiated or caused by primary lesion or dysfunction in the nervous system) [29]. It is typically described as a sharp, tingling, burning or electric sensation that often radiates. Pain of neuropathic origin may be associated with dysesthesias (unpleasant abnormal sensations), hyperalgesia (mildly painful stimuli perceived as very painful) or allodynia (non-painful stimuli perceived as painful). This term encompasses a diverse range of conditions including painful peripheral neuropathies, post-herpetic neuralgia and central post-stroke pain. Neuropathic pain needs to be detected in the ED, because the management tends to be more difficult and requires a multimodal approach therapy.

Finally, patients in the ED are at a high risk of *procedural pain* related to different investigations or interventions. This type of pain must be anticipated and adequately prevented.

22.3 Pain Assessment

Pain is a subjective, complex and multidimensional experience, for which there are no objective biological markers. Despite decades of effort, there is no neurophysiologic or chemical test that can measure pain in individual patients. Self-report is considered the most accurate and appropriate pain assessment method, as health care professionals often underestimate a patient's pain [37–39]. Although sensory or cognitive impairment might affect patients' ability to report pain, self-report should always be sought as first step in any assessment [40–43]. However, it should not be assumed that older patients will automatically report their pain. A careful patient history is also essential for discriminating neuropathic pain from nociceptive pain descriptors, to identify the underlying cause, to evaluate the impact of pain and the efficacy of our treatments. It is also crucial to acknowledge that the patient's pain is real and that it will be addressed.

There are several self-report pain assessment scales, among which the visual analogue scale (VAS), the numeric rating scale (NRS), the verbal rating scale or verbal descriptor scale (VRS, VDS), the pain thermometer (PT) and the Faces Pain Scale (FPS) are the most frequently used [68]. Most of these scales have demonstrated an acceptable reliability and validity in older patients in different settings (acute care, pain clinic, nursing home, community dwelling) [29]. For example, in Herr study, intercorrelations between the scales (visual analogue scale, 21-point numeric rating scale, verbal descriptor scale, 11-point verbal numeric rating scale and Faces Pain Scale) were all statistically significant with correlations averaged between each scale pairing ranging from 0.78 to 0.94{Herr, 2004 #16}. It is important to choose the most adequate scale for each individual patient.

Patients need also to be asked when and how pain occurred, as well as the location and radiation. Duration and variation of pain should be assessed with questions such as 'is your pain always there, or does it come and go?' The presence of transitory exacerbations of pain (breakthrough pain) should be assessed. Asking the patient to describe the factors that aggravate or alleviate the pain helps to plan interventions. The impact of pain in daily life activities is very important in this population.

22.3.1 Dementia and Pain Assessment

The assessment of pain in older adults with cognitive impairment generally should combine information from multiple sources: patient self-report, searches for causes of pain, observations of the patient's facial expressions and behaviours, observational pain scales, surrogate reports and a trial of analgesic therapy. The ability to comprehend and use a self-report scale is closely related to the severity of dementia and, in particular, to the communication ability of the patient [39]. During the early to middle stages of dementia, the patient communicative abilities tend to remain sufficient for the verbal communication of pain experience [27, 35, 44–50]. A structured pain interview that includes simple questions related to the presence or absence of pain or discomfort, pain intensity, frequency, location and impact on daily activities is a feasible approach to pain assessment even in the cognitively impaired [51–53]. It may be particularly difficult to identify in severely cognitively impaired individuals as it can manifest itself atypically as agitation, increased confusion and decreased mobility [54, 55]. The American Geriatrics Society described six pain behaviours that must be assessed in older people with dementia that can no longer communicate [40] (Table 22.4).

Table 22.4 The American Geriatrics Society described six pain behaviours that must be assessed in older patients with dementia that can't communicate anymore (adapted) [40]

- Facial expressions: slight frown, sad, frightened face, grimacing, wrinkled forehead, closed or tightened eyes, any distorted expression, rapid blinking
- Verbalisations, vocalisations: sighing, moaning, groaning, grunting, chanting, calling out, noisy breathing, asking for help
- Body movements: rigid, tense body posture, guarding, fidgeting, increased pacing, rocking, restricted movement, gait or mobility changes
- Changes in interpersonal interactions: aggressive, combative, resisting care, decreased social interactions, socially inappropriate, disruptive, withdrawn, verbally abusive
- Changes in activity patterns or routines: refusing food, appetite change, increase in rest periods or sleep, changes in rest pattern, sudden cessation of common routines, increased wandering
- Mental status changes: crying or tears, increased confusion, irritability or distress

Thirty-five observational pain scales have been developed these last years [56]. However, most of the scales are not feasible in the busy ED environment. This particular setting needs an ease quickly administering pain scale. Probably the most appropriate observational scale is the 5-item ALGOPLUS developed by the 'French Doloplus collectif' in France to detect acute pain. The scale has now been translated in six different languages. Pain should be suspected if the score is greater than 2 [57].

22.4 Pain Management

22.4.1 General Principles

- A patient in the ED can be very anxious about the diagnosis and management, so a clear explanation about the origin of the pain, the nature of analgesia and the expected effects can be reassuring.
- Pain management protocols should be available for the management of pain by paramedics before ED presentation.
- Depending on the setting and the intensity of pain, some treatment can be administered in the emergency waiting room, following strict protocols.
- Early analgesia is very important in preventing delirium—e.g. fascio-iliac block for hip fracture.
- Oral forms are usually preferred, but according to expectations and perceptions of the patient, other modes of administration may be justified.
- Any possible drug interactions must be detected, especially for treatments likely to be prescribed for several days; there are particular issues about the risks of renal toxicity, e.g. from NSAIDs.
- Because of the increased risk of adverse drug events, the principle 'start low and go slow' is recommended when dosing analgesics for older adults. Careful titration with frequent reassessment allows for optimal and safe acute pain care.
- Pain should be reassessed regularly.

- If patients are discharged at home, an action plan should be provided for the continued analgesic management at home (medication dosages and schedules, rescue doses, medical contact).
- If opioids are prescribed, precautions and adverse effects should be explained to the patient; attention to the need for co-prescription of anti-emetics and laxatives is necessary.

22.4.2 Treatment

Paracetamol: It is perhaps the safest analgesic in older ED patients. Mechanism is not clearly identified but may inhibit the CNS COX and activate serotonin and cannabinoid systems, which is an analgesic and antipyretic centrally acting devoid of anti-inflammatory effect, unlike NSAIDs [58]. Effective for musculoskeletal pain, paracetamol is recommended by the American Geriatrics Society as a first-line agent for mild ongoing and persistent pain, with increased dosing if pain relief is not satisfactory (up to 3 mg/24 h) before moving onto a stronger alternative [59]. Risks of hepatic toxicity with paracetamol have primarily been observed with long-term use. In case of abuse of alcohol, paracetamol administration should not exceed 2 g daily [60].

NSAIDs: Potentially inappropriate prescription criteria have been devised and validated, called screening tool of older persons' prescriptions (STOPP) and screening tool to alert to right treatment (START) for detection of potential errors of prescribing commission and omission. According to these criteria, long-term use of NSAID (>3 months) for relief of mild joint pain in osteoarthritis should not be used, and NSAIDs should not be used in patients with history of peptic ulcer disease or gastrointestinal bleeding, unless with concurrent histamine H2 receptor antagonist, proton pump inhibitor or misoprostol (risk of peptic ulcer relapse), with moderate to severe hypertension and finally with heart failure or risk of exacerbation of heart failure [61]. Short-term use of NSAIDs, for example, ibuprofen and naproxen sodium, may be prescribed judiciously in the acute setting for older patients (without contraindications), for example, for an inflammatory process such as acute arthritis. Key issues in the selection of NSAID therapy are cardiovascular risk, nephrotoxicity, drug interactions and gastrointestinal toxicity [62–64]. When NSAIDs are administered, patients should be informed of the risks and warning signs of adverse effects (e.g., decreased urine output, abdominal pain, nausea) and initially started on lowest doses available. Finally, some studies have in recent years questioned the use of NSAIDs in patients with bone or tendon injury due to delayed healing or scarring [65, 66].

Opioids: For older adults with acute moderate to severe pain (4–10 on a 0–10 scale), opioids remain the standard treatment. When starting a treatment in older people, opioids should be prescribed at low doses and titrated to the patient's response and adverse effects ('start low, go slow'). However, a careful approach to opioid administration does not mean that time should be wasted as, in patients with severe pain, management should be aggressive and up-titration quite intensive. Changes in drug metabolism, protein binding, distribution and clearance that are associated with ageing may result in a diminished rate of elimination, thus amplifying drug effects and side effects. Careful dosing and administration will limit these risks [67, 68]; for example, because of higher fat to lean body mass ratios, older adults should have starting doses of 25–50% lower than those used in young adults [59]. The decision to use a specific opioid preparation should be based on a combination of the pain characteristics (onset, duration), the product characteristics (pharmacokinetics, pharmacodynamics), the patient's previous response to opioids (efficacy, tolerability) and above all the patient's preference for a given preparation. The common adverse effects of opioids are nausea and vomiting, constipation, sedation, confusion and, very rarely, respiratory depression in opioid-naive patients [69]. Opioids commonly used in the ED include codeine, tramadol, morphine, hydromorphone and oxycodone [70–72]; none are ideal and all should be used with caution and careful monitoring. In the ED, oral formulations are usually preferred, with topical treatments being reserved for longer-term pain control. Intravenous morphine should be used cautiously in older people unless patients are already receiving continuous intravenous morphine. The subcutaneous route is preferred because it has less side effects and the advantage to be easily manageable at home or in nursing homes. Occasionally, for unpredictable acute pain, buccal or intranasal fentanyl such as oral transmucosal fentanyl citrate (OFTC) preparations can be used [73–75]. Administration of opioids via the nasal or oral mucosa provides a non-invasive mechanism for immediate drug absorption and rapid onset of pain relief compared with oral dosing [73], although such drugs tend to be more expensive. Furthermore, they should not be used without precaution in opioid-naive patients. Health professionals should anticipate breakthrough pain and prescribe immediate-release formulations of opioids with short half-lives as required, for example, to pre-emptively treat predictable pain during a painful manoeuvre. Although opioid addiction rarely develops in unwell older patients, caution should be exercised when prescribing opioids in patients with known personality disorders or an addiction to alcohol or benzodiazepines.

22.4.3 Topical Use of Analgesics

There are many advantages to using local rather than systemic treatment. The active agent is delivered directly to the affected area, bypassing the systemic circulation, and the dose needed for pain reduction is lower, minimising the risk of side effects [76, 77]. Topical NSAIDs have been shown to be effective in patients with soft tissue injury or related with inflammatory arthritis [78].

22.4.4 Nitrous Oxide-Oxygen Gas Mixture (N_2O/O^2)

This can be a valuable tool for the management of acute procedural pain in patients in the ED, as this mixture is easy to use, has a rapid effect and is safe with limited contraindications.

22.4.5 Interventional Techniques

For example, femoral nerve blocks are a feasible and effective option for acute pain due to hip fractures. Usually, this involves administration of a long-acting local anaesthetic (e.g. bupivacaine) under ultrasound guidance [79]. Regional anaesthesia may provide excellent pain relief without exposing the patient to side effects from systemic analgesics. A combination of regional and systemic anaesthesia may also be appropriate (Fig. 22.1, Table 22.5).

22.4.6 Specific Scenarios

22.4.6.1 Exacerbation of Chronic Pain

In exacerbation of chronic pain situations, the relational aspect of care is a particularly important dimension. This support includes listening to the complaint, the search for psycho-social destabilising factors, acknowledgment of the patient's suffering, reassurance, verification of concordance of patient goals and care, the reminder that there is no miracle drug and possibly the making of minor changes to the pre-existing treatment (e.g. change a dosage). In this scenario it is important to avoid major changes and liaise with the general practitioner and the patient's usual

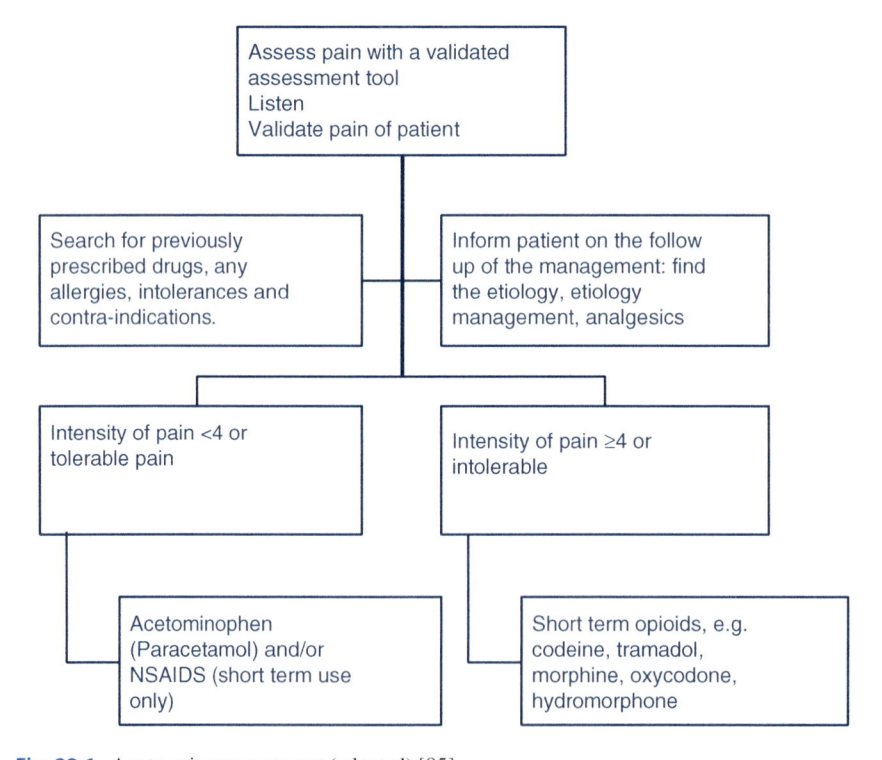

Fig. 22.1 Acute pain management (adapted) [85]

Table 22.5 Main drugs used in ED (adapted) [84]

	Onset of action min	Duration action min	Adverse effects	Precautions
Paracetamol	30–45	150	Liver or kidney damage If dose > 4 g	Well tolerated Elimination is not affected by age Lower doses should be used in older patients
NSAIDs (ibuprofen)	20–30	150	Gastric damage, renal or cardiac failure and coagulation disorders	Older people are at increased risk of developing toxicity from
Tramadol	60	150	See text adverse effect opioids	Inhibition of monoamine uptake, elimination half-life of tramadol is increased approximately twofold in patients with impaired hepatic or renal function Lower doses should be used in older patients Drugs interactions CYP 2B6- 2D6-3A4
Codeine	67	150	See text adverse effect opioids	Demethylation to morphine (offers most analgesic effects) constitutes a minor pathway accounting for less than 10% of the dose administered
Morphine oral	30–45	150	See text adverse effect opioids	Morphine and its metabolites (M3G-M6G) accumulate in renal failure making opioid toxicity more likely
Morphine sc, iv	20	90		
Hydromorphone	30–45	150	See text adverse effect opioids	Hydromorphone and its metabolites (H3G-H6G) accumulate in renal failure making opioid toxicity more likely
Buprenorphine oral	45	150	See text adverse effect opioids	Pharmacokinetics of buprenorphine change little in patients with renal failure, patients with renal impairment may benefit from use of buprenorphine
Oxycodone	30–45	150	See text adverse effect opioids	Drugs interactions CYP 2D6-3A4

network, giving priority to nondrug approaches such as physiotherapy, heat treatment, hypnosis or relaxation [80].

22.4.6.2 Neuropathic Pain

If the evaluation suggests neuropathic pain, some other treatments should be introduced. These treatments include the introduction of tricyclic or mixed antidepressants or antiepileptics (e.g. gabapentin or pregabalin). Topical lidocaine patches can be effective in patients with neuropathic pain such as post-herpetic neuralgia or diabetic neuropathy. Assessment and management of pain, with particular emphasis on central neuropathic pain, in moderate to severe dementia [81, 82].

> **Conclusion**
>
> Acute pain management in older adults is a common challenge in the ED. Because of the consequences of pain on the health and function of older adults, quality pain management is an important priority in this population. Understanding the limitations, contraindications and risks of these medications are necessary in selecting the appropriate analgesic for both ED and early outpatient treatment in older patients. Communication about risks and close outpatient follow-up with a primary physician is essential to optimise the safe and effective treatment of pain in older adults [83].

References

1. Platts-Mills TF, Esserman DA, Brown DL, Bortsov AV, Sloane PD, McLean SA (2012) Older US emergency department patients are less likely to receive pain medication than younger patients: results from a national survey. Ann Emerg Med 60:199–206
2. Desbiens NA, Mueller-Rizner N, Connors AF Jr, Hamel MB, Wenger NS (1997) Pain in the oldest-old during hospitalization and up to one year later. HELP investigators. Hospitalized elderly longitudinal project. J Am Geriatr Soc 45:1167–1172
3. Katz J, Jackson M, Kavanagh BP, Sandler AN (1996) Acute pain after thoracic surgery predicts long-term post-thoracotomy pain. Clin J Pain 12:50–55
4. Morrison RS, Magaziner J, McLaughlin MA et al (2003) The impact of post-operative pain on outcomes following hip fracture. Pain 103:303–311
5. Duggleby W, Lander J (1994) Cognitive status and postoperative pain: older adults. J Pain Symptom Manag 9:19–27
6. Lynch EP, Lazor MA, Gellis JE, Orav J, Goldman L, Marcantonio ER (1998) The impact of postoperative pain on the development of postoperative delirium. Anesth Analg 86:781–785
7. Hwang U, Baumlin K, Berman J et al (2010) Emergency department patient volume and troponin laboratory turnaround time. Acad Emerg Med 17:501–507
8. Terrell KM, Hui SL, Castelluccio P, Kroenke K, McGrath RB, Miller DK (2010) Analgesic prescribing for patients who are discharged from an emergency department. Pain Med 11:1072–1077
9. Jones JS, Johnson K, McNinch M (1996) Age as a risk factor for inadequate emergency department analgesia. Am J Emerg Med 14:157–160
10. Heins JK, Heins A, Grammas M, Costello M, Huang K, Mishra S (2006) Disparities in analgesia and opioid prescribing practices for patients with musculoskeletal pain in the emergency department. J Emerg Nurs 32:219–224
11. Heins A, Grammas M, Heins JK, Costello MW, Huang K, Mishra S (2006) Determinants of variation in analgesic and opioid prescribing practice in an emergency department. J Opioid Manag 2:335–340
12. Iyer RG (2011) Pain documentation and predictors of analgesic prescribing for elderly patients during emergency department visits. J Pain Symptom Manag 41:367–373
13. Arendts G, Fry M (2006) Factors associated with delay to opiate analgesia in emergency departments. J Pain 7:682–686
14. Mills AM, Edwards JM, Shofer FS, Holena DN, Abbuhl SB (2011) Analgesia for older adults with abdominal or back pain in emergency department. West J Emerg Med 12:43–50

15. Herr K, Titler M (2009) Acute pain assessment and pharmacological management practices for the older adult with a hip fracture: review of ED trends. J Emerg Nurs 35:312–320
16. Cinar O, Ernst R, Fosnocht D et al (2012) Geriatric patients may not experience increased risk of oligoanalgesia in the emergency department. Ann Emerg Med 60:207–211
17. Feldt KS, Ryden MB, Miles S (1998) Treatment of pain in cognitively impaired compared with cognitively intact older patients with hip-fracture. J Am Geriatr Soc 46:1079–1085
18. Scherder E, Bouma A, Borkent M, Rahman O (1999) Alzheimer patients report less pain intensity and pain affect than non-demented elderly. Psychiatry 62:265–272
19. Herr KA, Mobily PR, Kohout FJ, Wagenaar D (1998) Evaluation of the faces pain scale for use with the elderly. Clin J Pain 14:29–38
20. Morrison RS, Siu AL (2000) A comparison of pain and its treatment in advanced dementia and cognitively intact patients with hip fracture. J Pain Symptom Manag 19:240–248
21. Scherder EJ (2000) Low use of analgesics in Alzheimer's disease: possible mechanisms. Psychiatry 63:1–12
22. Pickering G, Jourdan D, Dubray C (2006) Acute versus chronic pain treatment in Alzheimer's disease. Eur J Pain 10:379–384
23. Bernabei R, Gambassi G, Lapane K et al (1998) Management of pain in elderly patients with cancer. SAGE study group. Systematic assessment of geriatric drug use via epidemiology. JAMA 279:1877–1882
24. Sengstaken EA, King SA (1993) The problems of pain and its detection among geriatric nursing home residents. J Am Geriatr Soc 41:541–544
25. Marzinski LR (1991) The tragedy of dementia: clinically assessing pain in the confused nonverbal elderly. J Gerontol Nurs 17:25–28
26. Brockopp D, Warden S, Colclough G, Brockopp G (1996) Elderly people's knowledge of and attitudes to pain management. Br J Nurs 5:556–558. 60-2
27. Cook AK, Niven CA, Downs MG (1999) Assessing the pain of people with cognitive impairment. Int J Geriatr Psychiatry 14:421–425
28. Terrell KM, Hustey FM, Hwang U, Gerson LW, Wenger NS, Miller DK (2009) Quality indicators for geriatric emergency care. Acad Emerg Med 16:441–449
29. Merkey HB, Bogduk N (1994) Classification of chronic pain. International Association for the Study of Pain Press, Seattle
30. Casten RJ, Parmelee PA, Kleban MH, Lawton MP, Katz IR (1995) The relationships among anxiety, depression, and pain in a geriatric institutionalized sample. Pain 61:271–276
31. Cohen-Mansfield J, Marx MS (1993) Pain and depression in the nursing home: corroborating results. J Gerontol 48:P96–P97
32. Scudds RJ, Mc DRJ (1998) Empirical evidence of the association between the presence of musculoskeletal pain and physical disability in community-dwelling senior citizens. Pain 75:229–235
33. Skevington SM (1998) Investigating the relationship between pain and discomfort and quality of life, using the WHOQOL. Pain 76:395–406
34. Wilson KG, Watson ST, Currie SR (1998) Daily diary and ambulatory activity monitoring of sleep in patients with insomnia associated with chronic musculoskeletal pain. Pain 75:75–84
35. Parmelee PA, Smith B, Katz IR (1993) Pain complaints and cognitive status among elderly institution residents. J Am Geriatr Soc 41:517–522
36. Giron MS, Forsell Y, Bernsten C, Thorslund M, Winblad B, Fastbom J (2002) Sleep problems in a very old population: drug use and clinical correlates. J Gerontol A Biol Sci Med Sci 57:M236–M240
37. Nekolaichuk CL, Bruera E, Spachynski K, MacEachern T, Hanson J, Maguire TO (1999) A comparison of patient and proxy symptom assessments in advanced cancer patients. Palliat Med 13:311–323
38. Pautex S, Berger A, Chatelain C, Herrmann F, Zulian GB (2003) Symptom assessment in elderly cancer patients receiving palliative care. Crit Rev Oncol Hematol 47:281–286
39. Weiner D, Peterson B, Keefe F (1999) Chronic pain-associated behaviors in the nursing home: resident versus caregiver perceptions. Pain 80:577–588

40. AGS Panel on Persistent Pain in Older Persons (2002) The management of persistent pain in older persons. J Am Geriatr Soc 50:S205–S224
41. Faries JE, Mills DS, Goldsmith KW, Phillips KD, Orr J (1991) Systematic pain records and their impact on pain control. A pilot study. Cancer Nurs 14:306–313
42. Simons W, Malabar R (1995) Assessing pain in elderly patients who cannot respond verbally. J Adv Nurs 22:663–669
43. Kamel HK, Phlavan M, Malekgoudarzi B, Gogel P, Morley JE (2001) Utilizing pain assessment scales increases the frequency of diagnosing pain among elderly nursing home residents. J Pain Symptom Manag 21:450–455
44. Ferrell BA, Ferrell BR, Rivera L (1995) Pain in cognitively impaired nursing home patients. J Pain Symptom Manage 10:591–598
45. Scherder E, Oosterman J, Swaab D et al (2005) Recent developments in pain in dementia. BMJ 330:461–464
46. Krulewitch H, London MR, Skakel VJ, Lundstedt GJ, Thomason H, Brummel-Smith K (2000) Assessment of pain in cognitively impaired older adults: a comparison of pain assessment tools and their use by nonprofessional caregivers. J Am Geriatr Soc 48:1607–1611
47. Closs SJ, Barr B, Briggs M, Cash K, Seers K (2004) A comparison of five pain assessment scales for nursing home residents with varying degrees of cognitive impairment. J Pain Symptom Manag 27:196–205
48. Scherder EJ, Bouma A (2000) Visual analogue scales for pain assessment in Alzheimer's disease. Gerontology 46:47–53
49. Pautex S, Herrmann F, Le Lous P, Fabjan M, Michel JP, Gold G (2005) Feasibility and reliability of four pain self-assessment scales and correlation with an observational rating scale in hospitalized elderly demented patients. J Gerontol A Biol Sci Med Sci 60:524–529
50. Pautex S, Michon A, Guedira M et al (2006) Pain in severe dementia: self-assessment or observational scales? J Am Geriatr Soc 54:1040–1045
51. Weiner D, Peterson B, Ladd K, McConnell E, Keefe F (1999) Pain in nursing home residents: an exploration of prevalence, staff perspectives, and practical aspects of measurement. Clin J Pain 15:92–101
52. Ferrell BA, Ferrell BR, Osterweil D (1990) Pain in the nursing home. J Am Geriatr Soc 38:409–414
53. Parmelee PA (1996) Pain in cognitively impaired older persons. Clin Geriatr Med 12:473–487
54. Ferrell BA (1995) Pain evaluation and management in the nursing home. Ann Intern Med 123:681–687
55. Buffum MD, Hutt E, Chang VT, Craine MH, Snow AL (2007) Cognitive impairment and pain management: review of issues and challenges. J Rehabil Res Dev 44:315–330
56. Lichtner V, Dowding D, Esterhuizen P et al (2014) Pain assessment for people with dementia: a systematic review of systematic reviews of pain assessment tools. BMC Geriatr 14:138
57. Rat P, Jouve E, Pickering G et al (2011) Validation of an acute pain-behavior scale for older persons with inability to communicate verbally: Algoplus. Eur J Pain 15:198.e1–198.e10
58. Wienecke T, Gotzsche PC (2004) Paracetamol versus nonsteroidal anti-inflammatory drugs for rheumatoid arthritis. Cochrane Database Syst Rev:CD003789
59. Persons O (2009) Pharmacological management of persistent pain in older persons. J Am Geriatr Soc 57:1331–1346
60. Watkins PB, Kaplowitz N, Slattery JT et al (2006) Aminotransferase elevations in healthy adults receiving 4 grams of acetaminophen daily: a randomized controlled trial. JAMA 296:87–93
61. O'Mahony D, O'Sullivan D, Byrne S, O'Connor MN, Ryan C, Gallagher P (2015) STOPP/START criteria for potentially inappropriate prescribing in older people: version 2. Age Ageing 44:213–218
62. Campanelli CM (2012) American Geriatrics Society updated beers criteria for potentially inappropriate medication use in older adults. J Am Geriatr Soc 60:616–631
63. Platts-Mills TF, Richmond NL, Hunold KM, Bowling CB (2013) Life-threatening hyperkalemia after 2 days of ibuprofen. Am J Emerg Med 31:465 e1–465 e2

64. Whelton A, Stout RL, Spilman PS, Klassen DK (1990) Renal effects of ibuprofen, piroxicam, and sulindac in patients with asymptomatic renal failure. A prospective, randomized, crossover comparison. Ann Intern Med 112:568–576
65. Taylor IC, Lindblad AJ, Kolber MR (2014) Fracture healing and NSAIDs. Can Fam Physician 60:817. e439-40
66. Li J, Waugh LJ, Hui SL, Burr DB, Warden SJ (2007) Low-intensity pulsed ultrasound and non-steroidal anti-inflammatory drugs have opposing effects during stress fracture repair. J Orthop Res 25:1559–1567
67. Cleeland CS (1998) Undertreatment of cancer pain in elderly patients. JAMA 279:1914–1915
68. Denny DL, Guido GW (2012) Undertreatment of pain in older adults: an application of beneficence. Nurs Ethics 19:800–809
69. Mercadante S, Arcuri E (2007) Pharmacological management of cancer pain in the elderly. Drugs Aging 24:761–776
70. Bijur PE, Esses D, Chang AK, Gallagher EJ (2012) Dosing and titration of intravenous opioid analgesics administered to ED patients in acute severe pain. Am J Emerg Med 30:1241–1244
71. Chang AK, Bijur PE, Gallagher EJ (2011) Randomized clinical trial comparing the safety and efficacy of a hydromorphone titration protocol to usual care in the management of adult emergency department patients with acute severe pain. Ann Emerg Med 58:352–359
72. Chang AK, Bijur PE, Meyer RH, Kenny MK, Solorzano C, Gallagher EJ (2006) Safety and efficacy of hydromorphone as an analgesic alternative to morphine in acute pain: a randomized clinical trial. Ann Emerg Med 48:164–172
73. Zeppetella G, Ribeiro MD (2006) Opioids for the management of breakthrough (episodic) pain in cancer patients. Cochrane Database Syst Rev:CD004311
74. Zeppetella G (2011) Opioids for the management of breakthrough cancer pain in adults: a systematic review undertaken as part of an EPCRC opioid guidelines project. Palliat Med 25:516–524
75. McCarberg BH (2007) The treatment of breakthrough pain. Pain Med 8(Suppl 1):S8–13
76. Woo KY, Abbott LK, Librach L (2013) Evidence-based approach to manage persistent wound-related pain. Curr Opin Support Palliat Care 7:86–94
77. Farley P (2011) Should topical opioid analgesics be regarded as effective and safe when applied to chronic cutaneous lesions? J Pharm Pharmacol 63:747–756
78. Altman RD, Barthel HR (2011) Topical therapies for osteoarthritis. Drugs 71:1259–1279
79. Mittal R, Vermani E (2014) Femoral nerve blocks in fractures of femur: variation in the current UK practice and a review of the literature. Emerg Med J 31:143–147
80. Tracy B, Morrison SR (2013) Pain management in older adults. Clin Ther 35:1659–1668
81. Schmid T, Pautex S, Lang PO (2012) Acute and postherpetic neuralgia in the elderly: analysis of evidence for therapeutic options. Rev Med Suisse 8:1374–1378. 80-2
82. Scherder EJ, Plooij B (2012) Assessment and management of pain, with particular emphasis on central neuropathic pain, in moderate to severe dementia. Drugs Aging 29:701–706
83. Hwang U, Richardson LD, Harris B, Morrison RS (2010) The quality of emergency department pain care for older adult patients. J Am Geriatr Soc 58:2122–2128
84. Pautex S, Vogt Ferrier N, Zulian GB (2014) Breakthrough pain in elderly patients with cancer: treatment options. Drugs Aging 31:405–411
85. Higgins R, Cavendish S (2006) Modernising medical careers foundation programme curriculum competencies: will all rotations allow the necessary skills to be acquired? The consultants' predictions. Postgrad Med J 82:684–687

Transitions of Care and Disposition

23

Sarah Turpin and Sarah Vince

Abbreviations

23.1 Introduction

This chapter will address the important area of care transitions for older people in the emergency department (ED).

Transitions of care can be a fraught time for both frail older people and the professionals responsible for their care. When handled smoothly, a successful transition of care can be personally satisfying for the people involved and also contribute to a safer and more efficient patient journey, which can result in better outcomes. When transitions of care are suboptimal, it can make a patient's experience in the ED even more distressing, make care less efficient and result in patient safety incidents and dangerous or even fatal errors in clinical decision making.

This chapter will describe the different types of care transition at work in a busy ED at any moment in time and discuss the barriers to these transitions occurring optimally. We will suggest some techniques and structures to provide professionals with an approach to optimise care transitions within their area of practice, be that primary care, prehospital, ED or acute hospital practice.

S. Turpin (✉)
University Hospitals of Leicester NHS Foundation Trust, Leicester, UK
e-mail: sarahturpin@nhs.net

S. Vince
Northampton General Hospital NHS Trust, Northampton, UK

© Springer International Publishing Switzerland 2018
C. Nickel et al. (eds.), *Geriatric Emergency Medicine*,
https://doi.org/10.1007/978-3-319-19318-2_23

23.2 What Is a Transition of Care?

Transition of care is, broadly speaking, defined as when the responsibility for a patient's care passes from one team to another. This can occur when a patient's physical location changes (e.g. on admission to hospital from the ED) or when the team looking after the patient changes (e.g. a shift change). Often, a transition of care results in the simultaneous change of both the location in which a patient is cared for and the team responsible for delivering care.

Frail older people who present as an emergency to secondary care are particularly vulnerable to poor care transitions. Partly, this is due to increased use of health services and longer periods of time in hospital than their younger counterparts. Additionally, the wide-ranging nature of management considerations in an older patient with frailty, which involves balancing complex comorbidity with social and environmental challenges, creates many more opportunities for communication to fall short in any single transition of care.

Frail older patients are so complex, and their dynamic and variable management approaches are so individualised, that it seems obvious that they can be at risk in sometimes chaotic and frequently pressurised environments. For emergency department staff, it may feel as though a smooth and organised transition for every complex patient is an unobtainable goal—despite this, efforts to optimise practice must prevail.

For the purposes of this chapter, we will consider various care transitions in the context of a patient, Mrs. Smith.

23.3 Mrs. Smith: A Case Description

> Mrs. Smith is an 85-year-old care home resident; she has a background of vascular dementia, hypertension and depression but is normally able to enjoy conversing with other residents in the home and can mobilise short distances with a Zimmer frame. She requires full assistance with her personal care but remains able to feed herself and suffers from intermittent urinary incontinence.
>
> Her medication list includes
>
> Lisinopril 10 mg
> Amlodipine 5 mg
> Fluoxetine 20 mg
>
> Mrs. Smith does not have insight into her dementia and is not able to take part in decisions relating to her care. She has a daughter who visits regularly and has Lasting Power of Attorney for welfare decisions. Mrs. Smith has not needed to see the GP since her admission to home last year, although at that point, after discussion with her daughter, a DNACPR (Do not attempt cardiopulmonary resuscitation) form was completed.
>
> The carers dialled 999 this morning because when they attended Mrs. Smith to assist her getting washed and dressed, she was too drowsy to converse with them,

and during an attempt to get her standing out of bed, she nearly fell to the floor. She has not eaten or drunk anything since yesterday afternoon, when she seemed unusually withdrawn and tired, but went to bed early and had a settled night.

23.4 Prehospital Care Transitions: Into the Care of the Paramedics

23.4.1 Paramedic and Technician Staff

Paramedics are responsible for obtaining the initial information relating to the reason emergency services have been called, the stabilisation of the patient at the scene and the safe transfer of the patient to the emergency department.

23.4.2 Care Home Teams

For patients who are residents in a care home, it is the responsibility of the care home team to provide the paramedic crew with adequate handover. However, studies have shown that there are commonly significant gaps in the information provided from nursing homes to the emergency medical services.

> Mrs. Smith's carers attended her at 7:10 am to get her out of bed. Following the events described above, an ambulance was called at 07:25 am, and paramedics arrived at 7:45 am. This is in the middle of shift changeover, and the carer available to speak to the paramedics had only been told that Mrs. Smith 'collapsed' by her colleagues as they ended their shift. Mrs. Smith is too drowsy to speak with the paramedics. Her observations are the scenes which are as follows:

Saturations, 94–95% (intermittent trace); HR, 80–100; BP, 112/50; temp, 35.1; RR, 20 she is drowsy but responds to voice.

23.4.3 Barriers to Clear Transitions Between Care Homes and Emergency Medical Services

There are often gaps in the information provided between care homes and emergency medical services. The reasons for this are manifold. Paramedics are often working under great pressure, and their care transitions occur in urgent or emergent circumstances. Even if there is adequate information and well-informed staff available, coordination of the transition between a care home and the ED can be challenging due to constraints on time and in the face of a patient who may be seriously unwell but challenging to assess due to frailty or immobility. Additionally, the patient may be in a state where they are unable to contribute any significant history themselves due to cognitive impairment or acute illness.

Care home staff can be transient employees, and in some settings they may have only basic training to support them in the care of the many frail complex patients under their care. A simple lack of understanding relating to what type of information is important on transfer can contribute to a paucity of useful information provided during handover to paramedics. Shift change within a care home can also result in no staff being available to handover who was present at the time the initial emergency call was made.

23.4.4 Ways to Optimise Care Transition Between Care Homes and Paramedics

23.4.4.1 The Use of a 'Grab Sheet'
Most care homes have patient profiles, which state the background conditions of the patient, their normal medications and their usual behaviour and level of function. These sheets are easily photocopied and can provide a wealth of information for the receiving team.

23.4.4.2 The Use of a Standardised Handover Tool
There have been some pilots of the use of a one-page 'transfer form' for use by paramedics when transferring patients from care homes to the emergency department. The use of such forms is not widespread although as the population of patients living in care homes with complex conditions rises, the use of such a tool to try to standardise and optimise communication during this transition seems an important strategy to explore.

23.4.4.3 Educating and Supporting Care Home Staff
A carer from the care home should ideally accompany the patient during transfer and throughout their ED stay. This provides a comforting presence for the patient, a direct source of collateral information and also a direct point of contact for communicating discharge information should the patient later be discharged. Unfortunately, many care homes run at minimum staffing levels, which means that it is not always possible for them to release a carer to accompany the patient to hospital.

During the transfer of an unwell patient from a care home to paramedics, care staff is often placed in a challenging situation and is responsible for the welfare of many frail older people simultaneously. To help support them during the handover of care to paramedics, the development of clear documentation that is succinct but comprehensive within each care home is an important step. That this information be accessible at all times and easy to photocopy/electronically transfer is an essential component of enabling the care home staff to provide objective written information about complex patients in a pressurised situation.

> The carer handing over to the paramedics this morning is an agency worker, she does not know Mrs. Smith, and she does not know her daughter's phone number. Fortunately, she was shown where the patient profiles are filed and gives the paramedics a photocopy of Mrs. Smith's patient profile, which contains a succinct description of her usual state of health and well-being and her daughter's name and number.

Patients and their carers: A patient moving from their own, self-managed environment to the apparently chaotic world of the ED is also a vulnerable transition of care. Educating patients and their carers, particularly those who are known to attend frequently or who have a chronic illness, of the importance of keeping basic medical information close at hand for use in future admissions, can be a useful intervention. Such information should include a medication list, any advance directives ('living wills') and recent hospital discharge letters.

23.5 Prehospital Care Transitions: What Information Is Needed Between Care Home and Paramedics?

- Presenting illness and cause for concern (recent history): why did they call the ambulance?
- List of comorbid conditions.
- List of current medications.
- Cognitive status: does the patient have dementia? Can the patient contribute to decisions relating to their medical treatment?
- Functional status: can they transfer/walk/toilet/feed?
- Anticipatory care plans: has the patient/family or primary care provider documented any plans/pathways or wishes relating to transfer to hospital/invasive treatments/limits of care as do not resuscitate (DNR)?
- Resuscitation status: does this patient have any resuscitation instructions in place?
- Key contacts: who is the patient's next of kin, and is there a Lasting Power of Attorney in place?

23.6 Prehospital Care Transitions: Out of the Care of the Paramedics

23.6.1 The Emergency Department Receiving Team

The transition of care from the prehospital team to the receiving team in the ED is the next important step. Any information provided by a care home must be successfully communicated to the receiving team within the ED, alongside all the paperwork and medications that may have accompanied a patient into the hospital. If a patient has been transferred directly from their own home, the paramedics have the unique position of being able to provide a direct account of any safeguarding concerns or problems relating the patient's home environment, including valuable information about the general state of the house, cleanliness, heating and the presence of any dependent or potentially abusive family members.

In addition to information provided by the care home relating to the patient's clinical complaint and the background information discussed above, there is now an additional set of information to hand over that relate to assessments made by the paramedics during the transfer to hospital: an optimal handover at this point would include (in this order):

The patients current clinical state including:

- Current clinical status:
  - Physiological parameters, Early Warning Score, etc.
- Clinical progress and change between initial assessment and arrival in the ED
- Details of any treatment given prehospital

> 'This is Mrs. Smith, an 85-year-old care home resident. Carers called the ambulance this morning after she collapsed. Observations at the scene were normal except for a slightly high heart rate although we have had difficulty maintaining a tracing on transfer. NEWS (National Early Warning Score) 5, scoring mostly on drowsiness. She's been quite drowsy on route, GCS 12-13, although she is waking up a bit now. She has a background history of dementia the carers think she might have a UTI since she was soiled this morning; she's been incontinent of urine in the ambulance. We haven't given any IV medications or fluids. Here is her grab sheet from the home—they haven't managed to contact her daughter. In her paperwork there is a form stating she is not for CPR in the event of cardiac arrest. A copy of her medications has come with the paperwork from the home'.

23.7 Barriers to Good Transition Between Prehospital Teams and the ED Team

23.7.1 Nonspecific Presentation

Frail older people often present with nonspecific problems such as delirium or reduced mobility; these clinical syndromes do not naturally lend themselves to a succinct handover. This can be a challenge for clinical staff and can lead to a vague account of the clinical story and can contribute to the beginnings of cognitive bias (see sect. 23.7.2) within the ED due to triage cueing.

Potential solutions to this include a conscious decision by both the paramedics and receiving team to acknowledge diagnostic uncertainty in a frail person rather than trying to offer an early guess based on limited or nonspecific information. The deliberate use of objective language to describe the patient's symptoms and clinical status should be encouraged to avoid unnecessary ambiguity in the context of what is already a challenging clinical syndrome to assess.

23.7.2 Under Triage Due to Different Physiological Parameters

Standardised triage tools have been shown to frequently miss critical illness in older patients. Baseline hypertension can mask shock: a large American study of older trauma patients showed that the mortality rate in older patients with a systolic blood pressure (SBP) of 110 mm Hg was comparable to that of younger adults with a SBP of 95 mm Hg. Beta blockers or other rate–limiting medication can mask tachycardia, and a third of older patients with sepsis do not mount a temperature. A patient may not trigger on any of the normal alarm boxes and can therefore be handed over with an unknowingly incorrect statement regarding their level of acuity.

A recently developed set of guidelines (HECTOR) suggests the following: age adjusted parameters should trigger immediate senior review:

SBP 110 mm Hg
Heart rate >90/min
GCS <15

Potential solutions to under-triage include focussing on trends in observations (e.g. a falling SBP) rather than on individual readings and taking a careful note of a patient's past medical history and medications to identify issues that may contribute to under-triage.

23.7.3 Technology

Correct transfer of prehospital information varies depending on the methods available. Information such as the timing and details of the 999 call, initial observations at the scene, timings of treatments and interventions such as cannulation and CPR can be miscommunicated or lost if there is a delay between verbal handover and the completion of the ambulance paperwork. Some departments are using an electronic system to more accurately transfer the objective information gained prehospital, but these systems are patchy.

Potential solutions to this involve collaborative working between prehospital providers and the ED, with support from the relevant technology services available.

23.7.4 Inter-professional Communication and Behaviour During Handover

There have been a variety of studies exploring different standardised handover proformas to aid communication between prehospital and ED staff. Standardised proformas are not widely used, and not all paramedics are formally trained in specific handover techniques but instead learn from observing colleagues. A suggested and established handover tool which is already in use by many paramedic crews is AMIST.

A—age and name
M—mechanism of injury or how it happened or what has been happening
I—injuries or complaints
S—sign and symptoms: pulse rate, breathing rate, skin colour, etc.
T—treatment and what you have done

Frustration (real or perceived) of receiving staff at an account of nonspecific clinical presentations or time pressure and the challenge of a chaotic environment where receiving staff may appear distracted by other aspects of patient care and less engaged in active listening can all contribute to less effective care transitions in this setting. An awareness of the interpersonal challenges that can reduce the quality of handover at this juncture can be addressed using a combination of staff education, environmental modification and the development of locally agreed handover protocols.

23.8 Care Transitions Within the Emergency Department

23.8.1 From Initial Assessment to the Main Department

After a patient has undergone their initial rapid assessment by the ED receiving team, they will usually move to another area within the ED. This is a common point for valuable information relating to the initial presentation to be lost. Unless the receiving team have meticulously documented all the background information provided by the paramedics, this wealth of information may not be readily available to the clinicians who are now responsible for performing a more detailed assessment. It is important that, after the patient has been transferred into the main assessment area of the department, the clinicians responsible proactively seek out this information which may have been lost. This can be done by carefully scrutinising the ambulance paperwork or logging onto the electronic prehospital database to gather information recorded by the paramedics. Online databases can provide background information on a patient's social care needs and recent healthcare encounters and is a useful source of collateral information when face to face or telephone collateral is unavailable. Unfortunately these systems are not available to all clinicians and not applicable to all localities.

23.8.2 Handover Between ED Team Members

Frail older people in the emergency department often stay longer in the department, undergo a greater number of diagnostic tests and can wait a longer time before a decision is made regarding their disposition—often due to waiting for a variety of diagnostic test results to become available.

Staff responsible for these patients are at high risk of cognitive bias, and during care transitions, this can be the result of 'inheriting someone else's thinking'.

23 Transitions of Care and Disposition

Cognitive bias in the emergency department during care transitions

Type of cognitive bias	What it means	Example
Triage cueing	A predisposition towards a certain decision as a result of a judgement made by caregivers early in the patient care process	Care home patient with intermittent drowsiness and SBP 112 mm Hg triaged as low priority when actually in established shock from pneumonia
Diagnosis momentum	The tendency for a particular diagnosis to become embedded in spite of other evidence	A delirious 85-year-old lady labelled as 'UTI' despite no urinary symptoms and no markers of infection
Framing effect	A decision being influenced by the way in which the scenario is presented or 'framed'	'This 85-year-old lady with dementia, bilateral consolidation and a 90% chance of death in the ITU'
Ascertainment effect	When thinking is preshaped by expectations	Not expecting to be able to obtain a useful history from a patient with dementia, so not attempting to take one

An awareness of these risks of cognitive bias, coupled with the use of objective, non-judgemental language, and a conscious avoidance of offering early diagnosis in the face of medical uncertainty are ways to try to reduce harm to your patients by keeping an open mind regarding the clinical situation until more information is available.

Regular review of frail older patients and clear documentation of changing clinical status, including checking vital signs, reassessing in the event of deterioration and keeping a close track of the diagnostic tests that have been requested and returned, are important aspects of maintaining their safety in the emergency department.

Mrs. Smith was initially reviewed in the rapid assessment area by a consultant who took the handover detailed above from the paramedics. The documentation in the initial assessment notes was as follows:

Presenting complaint: Collapse? Cause?

No history available from patient.

On examination: Confused and drowsy. Incontinent of urine. Off legs. Poor air entry on chest examination and reduced skin turgor. Soft abdomen. Moving all four limbs.

Impression: UTI.

Plan: Bloods, IV fluids, chest X-ray and reassess in the main assessment area

Mrs. Smith was reassessed by a junior doctor later on in the main assessment area of the department. By this point, blood results returned showing acute kidney injury and a raised white cell count. CXR (Chest X-Ray) was a poor-quality film but showed clear right basal consolidation. He reviewed her BP again and noted it had fallen from 112 to 105 mm Hg. He commenced IV antibiotics and increased the rate of her IV fluids.

On reviewing Mrs. Smith's grab sheet, he telephoned her daughter who was able to attend the ED immediately and take part in conversations about her mother's usual level of function and participate in discussions regarding her goals of care. It was decided that since Mrs. Smith normally functioned quite well within the home and there was a clearly reversible cause for her relatively sudden decline in function, an acute hospital admission for IV treatment was appropriate; however in the event of further deterioration, escalation to intensive care unit or CPR would not be appropriate.

Mrs. Smith's daughter was very upset that the home had not contacted her directly and angrily stated that they were 'on thin ice' and that 'mum's losing weight, and her skin is so dry today, I don't think they're feeding her properly—they just don't know what they're doing'.

23.9 Disposition from the Emergency Department

When discharging a patient from the ED, there are a variety of possible destinations—they could be admitted to a medical or surgical ward, transferred to a community hospital, returned to their care home or returned to their own home.

23.9.1 Transferring to an Inpatient Ward (an Acute Admission)

Handover to the admitting team is an important step—the aim should be an accurate account of the patient's clinical status and events so far, with relevant but concise information relating to their background, function and potential to deteriorate. It is good practice to commence discharge planning at the point of admission, and so any thoughts or information that are available from the ED assessment should be offered as well.

A suggested structure is as follows:

Based on the case progress detailed above, here is a suggested outline for handover, encompassing some of the things you should specifically consider when handing over a frail older patient.

Clinical narrative including communication needs and key informants	'This is Mrs. Smith; she is an 85-year-old nursing home resident. She was transferred by ambulance with reduced oral intake and drowsiness. On assessment we have found her to have a right lower lobe pneumonia with blood results suggesting acute kidney injury; she also has a hypoactive delirium. Mrs. Smith has a background of vascular dementia, and hypertension. She can normally converse but has no insight into her medical issues and lacks capacity relating to decisions about medical treatment. She usually walks with a Zimmer frame but is currently hoisted, and she is unable to communicate verbally. She is accompanied by her daughter who has Lasting Power of Attorney for welfare decisions'
Physiological parameters with individualised clinical interpretations	'Mrs. Smith's oxygen saturations are stable at 95%, and her pulse is currently 90 bpm. Her BP is 105 systolic which suggests shock in view of her background hypertension'
Medication and any changes	'We have commenced Mrs. Smith on IV antibiotics and IV fluids and withheld her ACE inhibitor and calcium channel blocker. There are no allergies'
Thoughts about discharge planning and the home environment	'Mrs. Smith's daughter has raised concerns about standards of care in the home due to some recent weight loss. We do not know whether these concerns are justified; however, this will need to be highlighted to the social worker for investigation whilst Mrs. Smith is an inpatient. We have completed a safeguarding form'
Escalation status including advance care plans	'Mrs. Smith has come with a DNACPR form which is in her notes. This can travel with her. There is no documentation from the care home about a ceiling of care or any advanced care plan; however following discussion with her daughter in the ED, we have placed a limit of ward-level treatment on Mrs. Smith's care due to her background frailty and poor functional reserve. This has been documented in her case notes, and her power of attorney is in full agreement'

23.10 Discharging a Patient

23.10.1 Back to Their Care Home or to a Cared-for Environment

Let's now consider a different scenario. For the purposes of continuity, we have moved forward in time. Mrs. Smith returned to her care home after a 4-day hospital admission where she was successfully treated for an aspiration pneumonia. It is now 6 months later; during this time period, Mrs. Smith's mobility has deteriorated to the extent that she is now in bed for long periods and requires a hoist to transfer. She has lost a further 2.5 kilos and is no longer able to converse—only opening her eyes to the sound of a familiar voice or during personal care. She now requires feeding, although her oral intake is poor. She has returned to the ED with drowsiness, reduced oral intake and another aspiration pneumonia.

> After discussion with Mrs. Smith's daughter, it is decided by the team in the emergency department that in view of Mrs. Smith's increasing frailty and significantly reduced functional abilities in the context of her advanced dementia, that rather than admitting her for further treatment, it would be in keeping with her best interests to return to the care home for palliative care. Mrs. Smith's daughter is in agreement with this, stating that her mother had frequently commented in the past that if she ever got to the point where she needed to be 'fed like a baby' then she would rather be dead. She feels sure that her mother would rather die peacefully in her own environment than spend time in the hospital, which was very stressful for her last time.

Decision making such as the return of a dying patient to a nursing home to die peacefully of an aspiration pneumonia can be rewarding and directly contribute to a good death; however, it depends ultimately on the quality of the care transition back to the nursing home. If the transition of care is poor, and the nursing home does not understand the purpose of return—to die, with symptom support from primary care—they may call an ambulance when the patient continues to deteriorate. A good transition of care back to the nursing home can stop this from happening.

A locally developed document can be a helpful way of providing structured information and handover to a care home or community hospital. This should also be supplemented by a phone call to handover the patient before their arrival and to ensure the care home or community hospital is equipped to deal with the plans that have been made. Such practice should extend to all transitions of care between the ED and care homes/community hospitals, not just cases where a patient is dying or particularly complex.

23.10.2 Transferring a Patient Back to Their Own Home

The decision to discharge a frail older person from the ED back to their own home can be difficult, and attempts have been made to develop screening tools to identify those patients who are particularly at risk of an adverse event occurring following an emergency presentation. Due to the complex nature of frail older adults, these tools have poor predictability; some patients who are high risk will flag as low risk and vice versa. Other factors that should alert an ED doctor to a patient at increased risk of an adverse outcome are patterns such as repeated attendances to the ED, a recent discharge from hospital and concerns of family members regarding 'not coping'. These, sometimes quite informal markers, should be considered as 'red flags', and particularly close attention should be paid to the situation at home and the circumstances surrounding their attendance to the ED and plans for discharge (Table 23.1).

Table 23.1 Factors to consider when discharging a patient home from the ED

Mobility	Assess mobility and compare it to the patient's baseline. Arrange for a physiotherapy assessment if necessary
Cognition	Is the patient at baseline cognition, or is there ongoing delirium requiring further assessment? If they have dementia, are they still safe to be at home alone? It is essential to check that the patient understands the plan on discharge and can retain the necessary information; if not, identifying a relative of carer to inform is essential
Safety	There are always risks associated with discharging a frail patient, particularly one with dementia. However, these must be balanced against the risk of hospital-acquired harm from admission (delirium, nosocomial infection, etc.). Careful and honest discussion around the risks and benefits of admission versus discharge with patients and family is usually the best approach
Social support	During your assessment in the ED, you should consider whether the current social setup is adequate. If the patient requires a package of care, this will need to be arranged in order for a safe discharge. Family present at the time of discharge can help ensure a smoother transition of care
Advanced care planning	If the person has a progressive chronic disease, consider discussion about future admissions, ceilings of care and resuscitation status. Consider whether community palliative care needs to be involved. The need for further discussions can be highlighted to the primary care provider in the discharge summary
Timing	The morning, or at least during daylight hours, is usually the best time of day for a planned hospital discharge to ensure that community services are available if there are any initial problems. If discharge is delayed, consider keeping the patient overnight and arranging transport for early the next morning
Medication	Drug-related problems are associated with an increased risk of hospital readmissions, morbidity and mortality. Ensure the patient understands their medication regime and the potential drug side effects to be aware of.
Education of patients and their relatives	Provide a simple explanation of the issues that have been identified and treated in the ED. Explain the ongoing treatment plan and indicators for return. Give patients and their family time to ask questions
Discharge summary	Ensure that an adequate summary of events, investigations and treatments during ED stay is provided for the primary care physician, community care team and other doctors or agencies involved in their care. This should include any arrangements that have been made for follow-up or recommendations for treatments in the community

23.11 Communicating with Primary Care

When transferring a patient back into the care of their GP, an example summary letter is given below—when communicating with primary care, it is important to keep information succinct and make requests and recommendations as specific as possible to reduce the chance of misunderstanding.

A suggested discharge summary for a GP is shown in the table below

Diagnoses made in the ED:
1. Fall secondary to postural hypotension
2. Colle's fracture secondary to fall
3. Polypharmacy
4. Short-term memory loss identified on cognitive screening

Treatment given
1. Antihypertensive medications reduced
2. Fracture reduced and set in plaster of Paris
3. Analgesia commenced

Medication changes made:
1. Lisinopril and amlodipine stopped
2. Paracetamol and codeine started
3. Laxido one sachet co-prescribed alongside codeine

Recommended actions for the GP:
1. Please consider starting bone protection in view of the fragility fracture
2. Please review this patient's blood pressure to check for ongoing postural hypotension (24-h profile most useful)
3. Please refer this patient to the memory clinic

Follow-up arranged by the ED:
1. Falls clinic referral made
2. Fracture clinic appointment given to patient

Note: In view of this patient's memory impairment, we have also provided her husband with these appointment dates

23.12 Summary

- Older patients undergo more transitions of care than their younger counterparts.
- Poor care transitions can result in adverse patient outcomes.
- Frail patients are particularly vulnerable to suboptimal care transitions due to their complex needs, frequent use of healthcare services and multiple agencies involved in their care.
- Poor communication is the commonest reason for a poor transition of care.
- The ED environment presents many challenges to communication, which need to be specifically acknowledged and managed to avoid cognitive bias and breakdowns in communication.
- An essential component of a successful transition of care is attention to detail and the presentation of information in a clear, precise and robust way.
- The development of locally agreed handover techniques and structured documentation can help to improve communication and care transitions.
- Technology offers a potential solution to some of the difficulties in obtaining background information and in optimising inter-professional and interagency communication, but development of these systems is a major challenge.

Recommended Reading

1. Campbell SG, Croskerry P, Bond WF (2007) Profiles in patient safety: a "perfect storm" in the emergency department. Acad Emerg Med Off J Soc Acad Emerg Med 14(8):743–749
2. Kessler C, Shakeel F, Hern HG, Jones JS, Comes J, Kulstad C et al (2013) An algorithm for transition of care in the emergency department. Acad Emerg Med Off J Soc Acad Emerg Med 20(6):605–610
3. Handing over to paramedics and further medical care [Internet]. National Institute of First Aid Trainers. 2014 [cited 2016 Mar 3]. Available from: http://www.nifat.com.au/handing-paramedics-medical-care/
4. Gillespie SM, Gleason LJ, Karuza J, Shah MN (2010) Healthcare providers' opinions on communication between nursing homes and emergency departments. J Am Med Dir Assoc 11(3):204–210
5. Hot Topics in Healthcare: Transitions of care: the need for a more effective approach to continuing patient care [Internet]. The Joint Commision; 2012 [cited 2016 Feb 5]. Available from: http://www.jointcommission.org/hot_topics_toc/
6. Terrell KM, Miller DK (2011) Strategies to improve care transitions between nursing homes and emergency departments. J Am Med Dir Assoc 12(8):602–605
7. Salvi F, Morichi V, Grilli A, Giorgi R, De Tommaso G, Dessì-Fulgheri P (2007) The elderly in the emergency department: a critical review of problems and solutions. Intern Emerg Med 2(4):292–301
8. Kessler C, Williams MC, Moustoukas JN, Pappas C (2013) Transitions of care for the geriatric patient in the emergency department. Clin Geriatr Med 29(1):49–69
9. ACEP Transitions of Care Task Force. Transitions of Care Task Force Report [Internet]. American College of Emergency Physicians; 2012 [cited 2016 Feb 5]. Available from: http://www.acep.org/workarea/DownloadAsset.aspx?id=91206

Principles of Rehabilitation in Geriatric Emergency Medicine

24

Ebby Sigmund

24.1 Rehabilitation in the Development of Geriatric Medicine

Rehabilitation can be defined as to restore someone to health or normal life. The origin of the word literally means to 'make fit again'.

Until the late nineteenth and early twentieth centuries, older people who were ill were usually cared for in an unskilled manner with little or no thought to the possibility of recovery. Their care was low priority and not highly regarded as a role for physicians.

Early pioneers of geriatric medicine recognised the importance of rehabilitation and implemented it as a core part of their revolutionary methods. In the UK Marjory Warren (1897–1960) was one of the first medical practitioners to introduce a systematic approach that included rehabilitation in addition to medical assessment and treatment. Her method vastly improved outcomes for older patients and led to many being discharged home. Interest in rehabilitation and the holistic needs of older patients led to early interdisciplinary collaborations, such as Dr. Exton-Smith's work with nurse Doreen Norton. Many of these early pioneers published widely and were inspirational teachers so that the previously unpopular area of medicine for older people began to attract doctors of the highest quality [1, 2]. Their vision raised standards and expectations and emphasised the importance of what we now recognise as a holistic approach, interdisciplinary working and inclusion of active rehabilitation in the treatment and care of older people. This was instrumental in the development of geriatric medicine into the unique and fascinating speciality it is today.

E. Sigmund
Occupational Therapy Department, Castle Douglas Hospital,
Academy Street, Castle Douglas DG7 1EE, UK
e-mail: e.sigmund@nhs.net

24.2 The International Classification of Functioning, Disability and Health (ICF)

The World Health Organization (WHO) defines health as 'a state of complete physical, mental and social well-being and not merely the absence of disease or infirmity' (Constitution of the [3]). Rehabilitation is viewed as a process that aims to enable individuals to remain at or return home, live independently and participate in wider occupations such as education, work, social and civic life.

The WHO produced the ICF [4] as a framework for measuring and defining health and disability issues for individuals and across populations. This free, international resource is used in many European countries. It provides a common language and conceptual basis for the measurement of disability. It is used across health, social care and education systems and can be applied at many levels from clinical practice to research and policy development. Many national and local rehabilitation guidelines draw on its concepts.

The ICF uses a biopsychosocial model. It views an individual's functioning as a dynamic process involving the interaction between their health condition, personal and environmental factors. It takes into account the individual's subjective view of their situation, focussing on the impact of a condition on daily life, rather than the disease itself.

The ICF consists of two parts:

- *Functioning and disability*—subdivided into two components:
  - Body functions and body structures
  - Activities and participation
- *Contextual factors*—subdivided into two components:
  - Environmental factors
  - Personal factors

The ICF and supporting resources are available in several languages and can be accessed and browsed online.

24.3 World Health Organization Disability Assessment Schedule 2.0 (WHODAS 2.0)

The WHODAS 2.0 is a tool for generic assessment of health and disability grounded in the conceptual framework of the ICF. It consists of six domains:

- Cognition
- Mobility
- Self-care
- Interacting with people
- Life activities
- Participation (community)

WHODAS 2.0 offers a simpler 12-item version (estimated 5 min to complete) and a more complex 36-item version (estimated 20 min to complete).

The common language provided by these tools supports a holistic, interdisciplinary approach and places an emphasis on person-centred care. All of these factors contribute to better outcomes for patients in geriatric emergency medicine [5].

24.4 Vulnerability to Poorer Outcomes in Older People Admitted to Emergency Care

The changing population demographic of the developed world means that many more people live into late old age. The oldest old, those over 85, are ten times more likely than 20–40-year-olds to have an emergency admission to hospital. They also have the longest length of stay and the highest readmission rates and are most likely to require long-term care upon leaving hospital [6]. The oldest old are more likely to suffer some form of patient safety incident in hospital [7], thus potentially incurring further injury or loss of function.

Many older people, particularly in the oldest old group, have frailty. Frailty is related to ageing and the gradual loss of the in-built reserves of multiple body systems [8, 9]. Older people are less able to withstand the onset of a new illness or apparently minor event, especially if combined with pre-existing physical frailty and/or multiple co-morbidities, sensory impairments, cognitive impairments or acute confusion. On an emergency admission, they may present with non-specific symptoms or issues such as immobility or falls that can mask a serious underlying medical problem. All these issues occurring in the context of the unfamiliar and confusing environment of an emergency unit contribute to increasing older people's vulnerability to poor outcomes following an emergency admission to hospital.

These issues are covered in more detail elsewhere in the curriculum so we will concentrate on looking at what this means for rehabilitation.

24.5 The Importance of a Rehabilitation Approach in Geriatric Emergency Medicine

The ageing population is often viewed as a problem for society. It should be remembered that many older people remain fit and active well into old age [10] and contribute to society in many ways—economically and in terms of volunteering, unpaid care provision and many civic and community roles [11].

The oldest old are certainly more likely to experience challenges to their level of function but often develop very effective coping strategies. The use of a framework such as ICF can help us to understand how an older person may have developed routines and arrangements at home that allow them to function at a level they are happy with. If admitted to hospital however, these strategies are disrupted, and they become more disabled as a result of the unfamiliar environment and their reduced ability to adapt to it. It will also be more difficult to overcome any residual deficit post discharge.

Patients in geriatric emergency medicine are often admitted for non-specific reasons, 'social admission', 'off legs' and the like. Non-typical presentation of medical conditions is common in older people, but an emergency admission can be the result of a combination of multifactorial challenges, physical, social and psychological, that have overwhelmed a person's limited reserve, possibly but not always, in the context of an acute medical illness. Even where a patient has a clear medical diagnosis, no conclusion about their level of function, now or in future, can be drawn from diagnosis alone. Reduced reserve makes older people more vulnerable to secondary complications. Any detrimental effects around the time of admission and emergency treatment can have serious consequences, and it may not be possible to regain function lost in the context of an acute admission.

There is evidence that a thorough geriatric assessment and interdisciplinary working using a systematic approach such as the comprehensive geriatric assessment [9, 12] combined with seamless interagency care can reduce adverse consequences and improve outcomes for older people [10, 13]. The use of a holistic model of assessment and a rehabilitation approach from the start of an episode of care can ensure that any problem areas are identified and the skills of the appropriate professionals within the wider interdisciplinary team are deployed at the earliest opportunity. If a patient is not yet fit to actively engage in rehabilitation, the emphasis of rehabilitation will be on preventing avoidable further deficit, for example, providing a safe environment with easy access to the toilet to maintain mobility and reduce the risk of falls and further injury.

> Eighty-year-old Mrs. A is admitted to the emergency department after injuring herself trying to get out of the bath while staying at her daughter's home. She has had mild flu-like symptoms for a few days. Mrs. A lives alone and reports she is independent. The use of an ICF-based assessment tool shows some visual impairment due to cataracts and mild balance problems following a stroke a year ago (*body functions and structures*). She gave up driving recently but is usually able to go out using familiar public transport routes, carries on with her weekly volunteering morning at a local charity shop and can manage most everyday tasks at home (*activities and participation*). Her home is on one level and close to local shops and amenities. Her family and neighbours are supportive (*environmental factors*). She does not like to worry her family and friends, so she has not mentioned that it has been getting more difficult to get out of the bath at home recently (*personal factors*).

Mrs. A probably has reduced reserve, and the combination of being mildly unwell and the different, less suitable bath at her daughter's home has been enough to lead to an injury and hospital admission. No serious injury is found, but Mrs. A has some difficulty walking due to muscular pain. She expresses anxiety about being able to manage at home. She is now in danger of further injury or adverse outcome, e.g. increased risk factors for falls in hospital or loss of confidence leading to reduced level of function.

24.6 Interdisciplinary Working

The way that geriatric medicine services are structured varies considerably at local level, but in general there is a move away from physician-led, hierarchical models of care towards a more fluid interdisciplinary approach that can be responsive to the needs of patients admitted to geriatric emergency medicine facilities. There is an increasing emphasis on a collaborative approach with some services using nurse- or other profession-led interventions and discharges [5, 14].

The use of tools such as the ICF or WHODAS 2.0 can provide a framework for assessment that ensures a holistic and person-centred approach to effectively identify areas of concern. To address a patient's needs, the skills of the wider interdisciplinary team are required. It will be essential that some issues be addressed during admission in order for a patient to return home safely. Other issues may require intervention in the longer term, and so liaison with wider, community-based services is required [10].

A detailed description of the roles of the various professional groups likely to be part of the interdisciplinary team is beyond the scope of this chapter, but some of those typically involved are nursing, occupational therapists, physiotherapists, speech and language therapists, podiatrists, dieticians, psychiatric liaison and social work or community service staff. Titles and exact roles may vary in different locations, but collectively these professionals possess a wide variety of skills and expertise to offer the rehabilitation process. In services where they are regular members of the emergency medicine team, they will have developed particular expertise in working in the context of emergency medicine, and their input can add quality to the assessment process and early stages of rehabilitation.

When rehabilitation is successfully achieved, individuals experience better health and quality of life and are less likely to use health and social services.

> Mrs. A receives an interdisciplinary assessment. The team ensure she is encouraged to mobilise, with walking aids at first, and that pain control is addressed. Equipment for bathing at home is organised, and she is offered the services of a community-based support team until she has regained her confidence at home. The team members communicate effectively with each other to make sure the right people are involved at the right time to make sure that Mrs. A does not have to remain in hospital any longer than is necessary. Mrs. A is kept informed at every stage.

24.7 What Skills and Attributes Do Geriatricians Working in Emergency Medicine Need to Develop?

In addition to excellent clinical skills, it is essential that clinicians working in geriatric emergency medicine develop the following knowledge, skills and attributes in order that patients have every opportunity to achieve the best possible outcome.

24.7.1 Understanding of a Rehabilitation Conceptual Framework

Tools such as the ICF or WHODAS 2.0 may or may not be in use locally, but a clinician who has a clear understanding of their core concepts is in a good position to ensure that their own approach, and that of the interdisciplinary team, is person centred, takes the wider context of patients' lives into account and is able to focus clearly and explicitly on the difficulties facing the patient, rather than on medical diagnosis alone.

24.7.2 Collaborative Interdisciplinary Working

Knowledge of the roles and skills of other members of the interdisciplinary team and how to access their services is essential. Some professionals may form an integral part of a team, while others attend as required. A good general awareness of the skills of each profession is important but should be combined with more detailed knowledge about specific local services, as there is considerable variation. The use of a tool such as ICF or WHODAS 2.0 can support interdisciplinary working. The move towards collaborative working may mean that clinicians need to be willing to give up some of their traditional leadership role and support other professionals in taking the lead when appropriate.

24.7.3 Interpersonal and Communication Skills

Interpersonal and communication skills are perhaps the most important of all as they underpin every intervention with the patient and with the rehabilitation team.

When taking a history or carrying out an assessment such as ICF or WHODAS 2.0 with an older person, their relatives or carers, active listening skills are required. An older person may not follow the line of questioning, but close attention to their narrative may give clues about issues that are not explicitly stated. Clinicians must also develop a range of strategies to aid communication when barriers such as sight or hearing loss, memory impairment, confusion or speech difficulties are present.

Effective collaboration with the interdisciplinary team rests on clear, timely communication. Different professional groups have their own professional 'language' so the use of a tool such as ICF or WHODAS 2.0 can contribute to interdisciplinary communication leading to more effective rehabilitation.

> **Conclusion**
> Rehabilitation has been an integral part of geriatric medicine throughout its history and a major factor in its development into a distinct speciality. A rehabilitation approach begins the moment an older person is admitted to the care of a geriatric emergency team and continues throughout their journey of care. Older people achieve the most successful outcomes in terms of function and well-being when an interdisciplinary approach, a strong rehabilitation ethos and a systematic method of assessment are in use. Clinicians working in geriatric emergency medicine must have excellent clinical skills but also need to develop their ability to work in this model to ensure the best outcomes for their patients.

References

1. Barton A, Mulley G (2003) History of the development of geriatric medicine in the UK. Postgrad Med J 79:229–234
2. Grimley Evans J (1997) Geriatric medicine: a brief history. BMJ 315:1075–1077
3. World Health Organisation (1948) Preamble to the Constitution of the World Health Organization as adopted by the International Health Conference, New York, 19–22 June, 1946; signed on 22 July 1946 by the representatives of 61 States (Official Records of the World Health Organization, no. 2, p. 100) and entered into force on 7 April 1948. http://www.who.int/about/definition/en/print.html. Accessed 14 Feb 2015
4. World Health Organisation (2001) International classification of functioning, disability and health (ICF). http://www.who.int/classifications/icf/en/. Accessed 14 Feb 2015
5. Banerjee J et al. (2012) Quality care for older people with urgent & emergency care needs "silver book". http://www.bgs.org.uk/campaigns/silverb/silver_book_complete.pdf. Accessed 15 Feb 2015

6. College of Emergency Medicine, British Geriatrics Society, Royal College of General Practitioners, Royal College of Physicians & Royal College of Nursing (2011) Joint statement on the emergency care of older people. www.collemergencymed.ac.uk/code/document.asp?ID=5925. Accessed 15 Feb 2015
7. Healthcare Improvement Scotland (2014) Think frailty. Improving the identification and management of frailty. http://www.healthcareimprovementscotland.org/our_work/person-centred_care/opac_improvement_programme/frailty_report.aspx. Accessed 28 Feb 2015
8. British Geriatric Society (2014) Fit for frailty: consensus best practice guidance for the care of older people living with frailty in community and out-patient settings. http://www.bgs.org.uk/index.php/fit-for-frailty. Accessed 15 Feb 2015
9. Ellis G, Langhorne P (2005) Comprehensive geriatric assessment for older hospital patients. Br Med Bull 71:45–59
10. Duursma S et al (2004) European union geriatric medicine society position statement on geriatric medicine and the provision of health care services to older people. J Nutr Health Ageing 8(3):190–195
11. WRVS (2011) Gold age pensioners. Valuing the socio-economic contribution of older people in the UK. http://www.royalvoluntaryservice.org.uk/Uploads/Documents/gold_age_report_2011.pdf. Accessed 28Feb 2015
12. Stuck AE et al (1993) Comprehensive geriatric assessment: a meta-analysis of controlled trials. Lancet 342:1032–1036
13. Baztan J et al (2009) Effectiveness of acute geriatric units on functional decline, living at home and case fatality among older patients admitted to hospital for acute medical disorders: meta-analysis. BMJ 338:b50
14. Royal College of Physicians (2011) Acute care toolkit 2. High quality acute care. https://www.rcplondon.ac.uk/sites/default/files/acute-care-toolkit-2-high-quality-acute-care.pdf. Accessed 28 Feb 2015

Palliative and End of Life Care for Dementia Patients in the Emergency Department

25

Jo James

25.1 Introduction

In the United Kingdom (UK), 160,000 people with dementia die every year [1], and 40% of these will die in hospital [2]. Given the increase in prevalence of dementia in the UK, it is clear that patients with dementia who have palliative care needs will be seen with increasing frequency in emergency departments. Caring for this group at the end of life can be complex and is often poorly managed (see Death and Dying: Barriers to Care (2014), 'The death and dying phase of dementia remains the forgotten aspect of what has been referred to as a silent epidemic') [3].

It is vitally important for the emergency department clinician to be able to deliver competent and compassionate care to patients with dementia with palliative care needs. There are significant challenges to managing this in the emergency department (ED) environment, and patients with dementia are 'more likely to experience uncomfortable or aggressive interventions at the end of life, blood tests, intravenous therapy, arterial gases and feeding tubes' [4]. This is compounded by the fact that the clinician is unlikely to know the patient, has little time to develop a relationship and might not have adequate resources to meet the person's needs in this setting. In order to manage these issues, the clinician needs to adopt a structured approach to assessing and delivering care to these patients:

J. James
Lead Nurse Dementia, Imperial College NHS Trust, London, UK
e-mail: Joanna.James@imperial.nhs.uk

© Springer International Publishing Switzerland 2018
C. Nickel et al. (eds.), *Geriatric Emergency Medicine*,
https://doi.org/10.1007/978-3-319-19318-2_25

(1) Identify whether the person might be at the end of life.
(2) Make a decision:
    (a) Treatment (if any) options
    (b) Where the patients are going to go:
        Stay in the department.
        Move to an inpatient area.
        Be fast-tracked at home.
(3) Communicate the plan.
(4) Manage the patient's core needs.
(5) Maintain the person's dignity.
(6) Involve the family/carer.

There is great potential to get it wrong in this situation when families and carers are often stressed and can be suspicious of hospital staff's motives. The case of Mr. and Mrs. J, highlighted by the NHS Health and Parliamentary Ombudsman in 2010 [5], illustrates the consequences of insensitivity in the emergency department.

Excerpt from Care and Compassion: Report of the Health Service Ombudsmen (2010)

> Mrs. J was 82 years old. She had Alzheimer's disease and lived in a nursing home. Her husband visited her daily, and they enjoyed each other's company.

> Mr. J told us 'She had been like that for 9 years. And I was happy being with her'. One evening, Mr. J arrived at the home and found that his wife had breathing difficulties. An ambulance was called, and Mrs. J was taken to the hospital about 10.30 pm, accompanied by her husband. She was admitted to A&E and assessed on arrival by a senior house officer who asked Mr. J to wait in a waiting room.

> Mrs. J was very ill. She was taken to the resuscitation area but was moved later when two patients arrived who required emergency treatment. Mrs. J was then seen by a specialist registrar as she was vomiting and had become unresponsive. It was decided not to resuscitate her. She died shortly after 1.00 am.

At around 1.40 am, the nursing staff telephoned the nursing home and were told that Mr. J had accompanied his wife to the hospital. The senior house officer found him in the waiting room and informed him that his wife had died. In the 3 h or so that Mr. J had been in the waiting room, nobody spoke to him or told him what was happening to his wife. As a result he came to believe that her care had been inadequate. He thought that he had been deliberately separated from her because hospital staff had decided to stop treating her. 'They let her slip away under the cloak of "quality of life" without stopping to think of any other involved party'. He felt the hospital had denied them the chance to be together in the last moments of Mrs. J's life, and he did not know what had happened to her.

No attempt was made to contact the nursing home or a family member until after she had died. The hospital failed to involve Mr. J in the decision-making process, and nobody told Mr. J what was happening to his wife until she had died. It was crucial that Mr. J was involved in the decision-making and the move to compassionate and supportive care in his wife's last moments.

Mrs. J was denied the right to a dignified death with her husband by her side.

In Mr. J's own words, 'They decided that enough was enough without bothering to include me. It was a shabby, sad end to my poor wife's life'.

25.2 Identifying Whether a Person with Dementia Is at the End of Life

Although 'dementia' is used as an umbrella term to describe a syndrome caused by different conditions, it is accepted that dementia is a terminal illness. However, it can be difficult to predict the trajectory of deterioration in a person with dementia. In broad terms, life expectancy ranges from 8 to 12 years but is dependent on the age at diagnosis and geographical location (life expectancy is considerably shorter in developing countries) [6]. Patients with dementia do not follow the same trajectory as those with conditions such as cancer, and this makes it very difficult to prognosticate about when a person with a diagnosis of dementia might die.

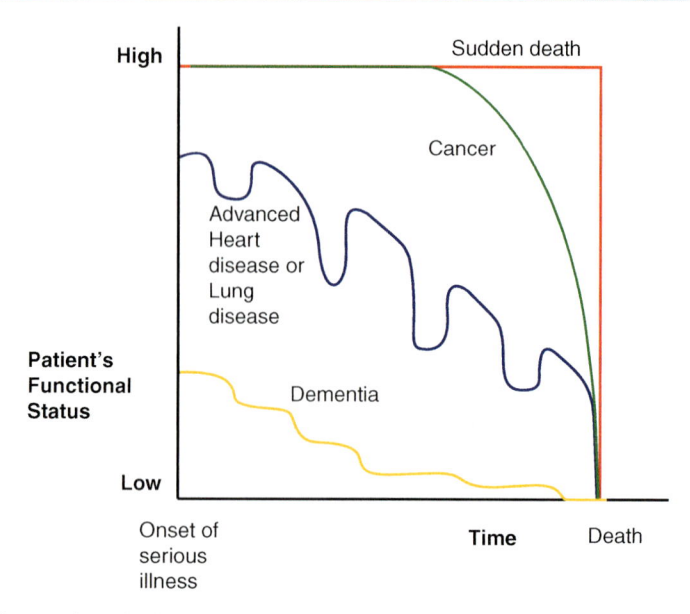

Typical illness trajectories for people with progressive chronic illness [7]

Table 25.1 The Gold Standards Framework specific clinical indicator for dementia

1. The surprise question: 'Would you be surprised if this patient were to die in the next few months, weeks, days?'
2. General indicators of decline—deterioration, increasing need or choice for no further active care
3. Specific clinical indicators related to certain conditions

There are many underlying conditions which may lead to degrees of dementia, and these should be taken into account. Triggers to consider that indicate that someone is entering a later stage are

• Unable to walk without assistance	Plus any of the following:
• Urinary and faecal incontinence	• Weight loss
• No consistently meaningful conversation	• Urinary tract Infection
• Unable to do activities of daily living (ADL)	• Severe pressures sores—stage three or four
• Barthel score <3	• Recurrent fever
	• Reduced oral intake
	• Aspiration pneumonia

The Gold Standards Framework [8] has produced guidelines to support accurate identification of end of life in the population, and this includes specific disease-related criteria. This starts with the three triggers followed by the specific clinical indicators for dementia shown in Table 25.1. Much of the information below can be obtained by getting a good collateral history from family or carers.

Considering these factors alongside the clinical presentation of the patient will help the clinician to identify whether the patient is approaching the end of life. However, it is vitally important for the ED clinician to be aware of the need for caution when using this tool.

Patients with dementia will often have a catastrophic decline in function and cognition when they are ill and might present as a picture of much more advanced dementia than they actually have. The presence of delirium will also obfuscate clinical findings around the person's dementia. This can misdirect clinical assessments and result in clinicians mistaking acute illness for end of life. The clinician must be aware of this and rely on the collateral history from family and carers which also considers the person's baseline *before* he/she was acutely ill.

25.3 Making a Decision

An unwell patient with advanced dementia will be unlikely to have capacity to make a decision about treatment options at this point. Therefore, clinical decision-making for patients with dementia will almost always be done in the person's best interests according to the Mental Capacity Act [9] (see Chap. 13). Exceptions to this will be if the person has an advance directive or a lasting power of attorney present.

> Although advance decisions can be oral or in writing, an advance refusal will only apply to life-sustaining treatment where it is in writing, is signed and witnessed and contains a statement that it is to apply even where life is at risk. Advance decisions cannot be used to refuse basic care, which includes warmth, shelter and hygiene measures to maintain body cleanliness. This also includes the offer of oral food and water but not artificial nutrition and hydration. In an emergency or where there is doubt about the existence or validity of an advance decision, doctors can provide treatment that is immediately necessary to stabilise or to prevent a deterioration in the patient until the existence, and the validity and applicability, of the advance decision can be established.
>
> BMA 2008 [10]

It is important to remember that decisions to initiate treatments (including resuscitation) always lie with the clinician and that an advance directive cannot force a clinician to initiate treatment against his/her judgement.

25.4 Transferring the Patient

A decision will need to be made whether to transfer the patient into an inpatient area. If the patient is likely to die within an hour or two, a preferable option would be to transfer to a side room in the immediate vicinity. The upheaval of a ward admission at this point can be distressing and also result in families/carers missing the opportunity to spend time with the patient.

If the clinician is aware that the person has expressed a wish to die at home, a fast-track discharge process should be initiated as soon as possible. Initiating this at the point of admission optimises the chance that the patient will get home in time to die even if it means that the patient will have to spend a short time in an inpatient bed first.

25.5 Communicating the Plan

Once the clinician has decided on a course of action for the patient, it is vitally important to clearly communicate this to the family/carer. Ideally the clinician will have sought the views of the family and will be able to have an open and honest conversation about the best course of action to take. The most effective way to keep the lines of communication open with this group is to ensure that the person with advanced dementia is never separated from the carer/family member whilst in the emergency department. If the clinician adheres to this basic principle, the situation experienced by Mr. J will never occur, and the family/carer will feel involved in the process throughout it.

25.6 Manage the Core Needs

The clinician should adopt a palliative approach to the person's needs ensuring that interventions are aimed at optimisation of comfort rather than prolonging life. If there is time, referring the patient to the palliative care team is a preferred option. The clinician should consider the following:

- *Pain*—a recent study showed that at least 50% of patients with end-stage dementia were also in pain [11] and pain in dementia patients is poorly identified and managed in the acute hospital setting [11]. Assessment of pain using a validated observational tool such as PAINAD or the Abbey pain scale should be followed by the prescription of regular analgesia via an appropriate route (oral administration of medication can often be problematic for people with advanced dementia due to impaired swallowing and also reluctance to take tablets).
- *Trolley*—ensure that the patient is moved onto a pressure relieving mattress as soon as possible to reduce discomfort and relieve pressure areas.
- *Nutrition and hydration*—encourage the family to support the patient with sips of fluid or mouthfuls of yoghurt and prescribe regular mouth care to moisturise the mouth. Ensure that the family/carers are aware that artificial nutrition and hydration will not prolong life [12, 13]. The clinician might consider subcutaneous fluids for a patient if severe dehydration is causing discomfort.
- *Environment*—if death is imminent, endeavour to move the person to a side room or a cubicle with a door in order to offer some privacy for the patient and the family. In the absence of this option, ensure that other clinical staff in the area are aware of the situation and behave accordingly.

25.7 Maintaining Dignity

Being treated with 'respect and dignity' [14] has been identified by people with dementia as one of the most important priorities at the end of life. Managing to maintain dignity, even identify what it means in practical terms, can be difficult within an acute emergency department setting. The five core factors identified by Mangset [15] offer a useful framework for the emergency department clinician. Approaching care using this framework with a patient who has advanced dementia in a time-pressured environment might seem to be an impossible expectation. However, when translated into practical terms, it becomes clear that dignified care using this framework is neither time-consuming nor impossible.

Core principle	Practical application for patient with advanced dementia
Being treated humanely	Showing kindness and consideration
	Using touch to support communication
	Adapting care to suit the needs of the patient
Being acknowledged as an individual	Knowing something about what is important to the patient (career, family, pets)
	Addressing the patient respectfully using the right form of address
	Trying to understand what the patient wants
Having autonomy respected	Asking the patient's permission before procedures
	Including the patient in the conversations about care (even if the patient cannot contribute)
Having confidence and trust in professionals	Acting professionally
Dialogue and exchange of information	Listening to the patient or patient's representative
	Explaining what is happening and what is about to happen

25.8 Involving Families and Carers

This has been referred to earlier and is illustrated by the case of Mr. and Mrs. J. People with dementia are often highly dependent on families and carers for emotional and physical support, particularly in an unfamiliar environment such as an emergency department. Carers are increasingly seen as partners in care with clinical staff and should be involved as much as possible. Unless there are safeguarding concerns, there is no reason why the patient should be separated from their family member or carer during an emergency department admission. Adopting this approach will provide the patient and carer with greater peace of mind and will result in a more effective working relationship between the staff and the family.

Conclusion
Clinicians in the emergency department are increasingly called upon to support people with dementia who are at the end of their lives. It can be difficult to distinguish between patients who are at the end of life and those whose dementia is temporarily worsened due to an acute event. The clinician must ensure that there

is a clear understanding of the patient's baseline status before making a decision that this is end of life due to dementia. Providing good palliative care in the emergency department requires consideration around when and where to transfer the patient, how to support core physical needs and also how to ensure that the person is treated with dignity and respect. It is vitally important to include the family or carers and to communicate thoughts and decisions throughout the interaction. If there is time, referral to palliative care will always be a desirable option, but if not, the emergency department clinician can optimise the quality of end of life care for people with dementia using the approaches discussed in this chapter.

References

1. Alzheimer's Society (2012) My life until the end: dying well with dementia. Alzheimer's Society, London
2. Sleeman KE, Ho YK, Verne J, Gao W, Higginson IJ (2014) Reversal of English trend towards hospital death in dementia: a population-based study of place of death and associated individual and regional factors, 2001–2010. BMC Neurol 14:59. http://tiny.cc/dementia67
3. Alzheimer's Society, Marie Curie Cancer Care (2014) Living and dying with dementia in England: barriers to care. Marie Curie Cancer Care, London
4. Harris D (2007) Forget-me-not: palliative care for people with dementia. Postgrad Med J 83(980):362–366. http://tiny.cc/dementia53
5. Parliamentary and Health Service Ombudsman (2011) Care and compassion? Report of the Health Service Ombudsman on ten investigations into NHS care of older people. The Stationary Office, London
6. Alzheimer's Disease International (2010) World report. Alzheimer's Disease International, London
7. Sachs GA, Shega JW, Cox-Hayley D (2004) Barriers to excellent end-of-life care for patients with dementia. J Gen Int Med 19(10):1057–1063
8. National Gold Standards Framework Centre for End of Life Care (2011) Prognostic indicator guidance (PIG). www.goldstandardsframework.org.uk
9. Mental Capacity Act 2005 Code of Practice (2007) Department for Constitutional Affairs. The Stationary Office, London
10. British Medical Association (2008) Mental capacity act toolkit. British Medical Association, London. www.bma.org.uk
11. Lord K, White N, Scott S, Sampson EL (2013) The behaviour and pain (bepaid) study: dementia patients who die in the Acute Hospital. http://tiny.cc/dementia87
12. Candy B, Jones L, Sampson EL (2009) Enteral tube feeding for older people with advanced dementia. Cochrane Database Syst Rev 15:CD007209. http://tiny.cc/dementia89
13. Evers MM, Purohit D, Perl D, Khan K, Marin DB (2002) Palliative and aggressive end-of-life care for patients with dementia. Psychiatr Serv 53(5):609–613
14. Dening KH, Jones L, Sampson EL (2013) Preferences for end-of-life care: a nominal group study of people with dementia and their family carers. Palliat Med 27:409–417
15. Mangset M, Erling Dahl T, Forde R, Bruun Wyller T (2008) We're just sick people, nothing else: factors contribution to elderly stroke patients' satisfaction with rehabilitation. Clin Rehabil 22:825–835

Palliative and End of Life Care for the Older Person in the Emergency Department

26

Mary Dawood

"How people die remains in the memory of those who live on"

Dame Cicely Saunders (1918–2005) founder of the modern hospice movement

26.1 Overview

Global life expectancy for both sexes increased from 65.3 years in 1990 to 71.5 years in 2013, while the number of deaths increased from 47.5 million to 54.9 million over the same interval [1]. In the developed world particularly, many deaths occur in the emergency department. In a 2011 survey, 43% of bereaved people said they thought that care for their loved one in the last 3 months of life was excellent or outstanding, but 24% said it was fair or poor—these findings suggest that end of life care for many people is just not good enough [2].

Older patients account for up to 25% of emergency department (ED) attendances, and some of these will spend their last hours in the ED [3]. There is considerable palliative care needs among older people who attend EDs, but this need can be overlooked in an environment where the primary focus is resuscitation and saving lives [4, 5]. The development of major trauma centres in the developed world has seen a rise in the number of older patients who would have previously died from their injuries, surviving devastating traumatic injuries, often with a very poor prognosis. In such circumstances, decisions about palliation and end of life care need to be made in the ED. Furthermore, as people are living to a greater age with long-term conditions, the need for palliative care will increase, and clinical staff in the ED need to be equipped to care knowledgeably and with empathy for this group.

M. Dawood
Imperial College NHS Trust, London, UK
e-mail: Mary.dawood@imperial.nhs.uk, marydawood@gmail.com

© Springer International Publishing Switzerland 2018
C. Nickel et al. (eds.), *Geriatric Emergency Medicine*,
https://doi.org/10.1007/978-3-319-19318-2_26

Palliative care was defined by the World Health Organization in 2002 as "an approach that improves the quality of life of patients and their families facing the problems associated with life-threatening illness, through the prevention and relief of suffering by means of early identification and impeccable assessment and treatment of pain and other problems, physical, psychosocial and spiritual" [6].

End of life care is defined as enabling and supporting the palliative care needs of both patient and family to be identified and met throughout the last phase of life and into bereavement. It includes management of pain and other symptoms and provision of psychological, social, spiritual and practical support [7].

Older patients are for the most part a vulnerable group, and decisions about their care should be influenced by quality of life rather than age.

Many older patients present with varying problems of a medical psychosocial nature where the presence of multiple comorbidities makes their assessment and management complex. Pathologies associated with ageing make the older person different to other patients, and these differences must be recognised if their needs are to be met in an individualised and timely way.

History taking is rarely straightforward and can be even more difficult where there is sensory impairment, dementia or delirium. Additional information and collateral history which is essential to forming an accurate overall picture may not be readily accessible, and time pressures mean staff can only focus on what appears to be the immediate problem.

Thus, there is a real need for expert knowledge, advocacy and expediency for those that are sick and dying. In addition, there is a great need for clinical staff to recognise and accept that in many situations, care may be more important than cure. It is not acceptable for older people to suffer unnecessarily due to poor recognition and under treatment of their problems and lack of access to palliative care.

Palliative and end of life care in the ED calls for a multidisciplinary response. Where a patient is dying, the goal must be to preserve the dignity and humanity of the person and to relieve suffering rather than expending valiant efforts to prolong a life which holds little or no quality for the person. When cure is not attainable and end of life approaches, the boundary between palliative care and emergency care needs to be more clearly defined. Many of the competencies that are needed to deliver effective care for people in the last few days and hours of life are generic. The professional capabilities that all doctors should possess to ensure the delivery of good-quality care across all specialties should include fundamentals such as the need to communicate effectively and empathise, as well as those more related to end of life care such as partnership and team working [8].

26.2 Priorities for the Care of Dying People

Following a review of the controversial and now discredited Liverpool Care Pathway by Julia Neuberger in 2013 [9], the Leadership Alliance for the Care of Dying People in the UK published two documents in 2014, *One Chance to Get it Right* and an accompanying document for healthcare professionals, *Priorities for Care of the*

Dying Person (LACDP, 2014b) [10, 11], which set out the approach to caring for dying people that health and care organisations need to adopt.

This approach is applicable regardless of place of death and lists five priorities for the care of dying people which focus on involving and supporting patients in their final days and hours. The five priorities focus on:

1. Recognising that someone is dying
2. Communicating sensitively with them and their family
3. Involving them in decisions
4. Supporting them and their family
5. Creating an individual plan of care that includes adequate nutrition and hydration

26.2.1 Recognising that Someone Is Dying

Very ill and injured patients brought to the ED and those whose condition is deteriorating or has deteriorated unexpectedly must be assessed by a doctor competent to judge whether this change in condition is treatable or whether the person is likely to die within the next few hours or days. If resuscitation and improvement in the person's condition are judged to be possible, consent to treatment should be sought. If the clinician in consultation with his/her team judges that the person is likely to die soon, he/she she must clearly and sensitively communicate this to the dying person, if conscious. The same communication must take place with those important to the dying person. In a trauma situation where the injury is severe and not compatible with life, the clinician needs to be honest and open with the family and carers. Any decisions or interventions taken need to be regularly reviewed and revised as the situation might change. Healthcare staff must allow time to engage with dying person and their families, actively listening and responding with empathy to their distress, worries and concerns.

26.2.2 Sensitive Communication

The second priority for care focuses further on communication. As far as possible, health professionals must offer dying people the opportunity to discuss their wishes and preferences; this must be recorded and reviewed as needed. Where a dying person has chosen a friend or family member to be with them, they must be involved in planning the care. Any plan of care must consider the beliefs and values of the person and must be agreed, communicated and regularly reviewed. Assessments of a patient's condition, mental capacity and care needs must be discussed honestly, and family and important others should be provided with clear explanations. Clinicians must make every effort to answer queries or refer to colleagues if they are unable to answer concerns. All discussions should be in "simple, plain language, without using euphemisms" [10, 11]. Difficult conversations "must not be avoided or but must be carried out sensitively, recognising that communication is an ongoing process and not a one-off event" [10, 11]. Any ambiguities or disagreements about the plan of care need to be acknowledged and resolved without delay. If there are language barriers, an interpreter must be used; the temptation to "muddle through" must be avoided as poor communication and a lack of understanding will exacerbate fear and anxiety and can have detrimental ramifications on the grieving process for the family.

26.2.3 Involving the Dying Person

As far as is possible and within reason, the dying person, and those caring for them, should be involved in decisions about treatment and care. The Leadership Alliance for the Care of Dying People recognises that individuals may have different views about being involved in decisions about their own treatment, though most would want to make or influence decisions about the care they receive. The person and their family should know the name of the doctor and nurse responsible for their care.

26.2.4 Providing Support

The needs of families and others identified as important to the dying person should be actively explored, respected and met as far as possible [10, 11]. In the ED setting, this can be challenging in terms of time pressures, providing privacy and ensuring a quieter place for the family and dying person to be together. Ideally the dying person should be moved to a ward environment away from the frenetic pace and noise of the ED. If this is not possible, a quieter area of the ED should be allocated and staff made aware of the need for privacy, dignity and respect. The named nurse should regularly review the patient and address the needs of the family and those important to the dying person. If the family wishes to participate in the "hands-on" care for the dying person, they should be supported to do so [12]. This is a particularly important consideration for people from ethnic minority cultures, where caring for a dying person, especially an elder member of the family, is considered an enormous privilege. Explaining what happens and what to expect when death is imminent is important and helps to allay the fear and anxiety that so often contributes to a less than good experience for the family. Support for family immediately after the person's death and comprehensive written information about "what happens next" is also essential.

26.2.5 Individual Care Plans

Priority five is an individual plan of care, which includes nutrition, symptom control and psychological, social and spiritual support, coordinated and delivered with compassion. This again can be challenging in the ED setting where the person is not previously known to staff. For patients arriving by ambulance, the information obtained at handover is crucial as it can impact the direction of care in a positive or negative way. Poor communication or poor listening skills can render handover ineffective; this can be detrimental particularly to the older patient who may be unable to express his/her wishes. Handovers that take place in time critical areas such as the "resus" room call for "skilled listening" so that key-sensitive information such as advanced directives or palliative care plans are not overlooked or dismissed when they need to be acknowledged and facilitated by the multidisciplinary team. In most cases, the prehospital team has had a glimpse of the patient's world that we in hospital do not see, and thus, the information they share is key to informing clinical decision-making about care pathways. Where family and carers' accompany the older person to hospital, they should be listened to and allowed to stay with the patient as much as possible or as the patient desires. Subsequent handovers need to be detailed, accurate and timely so teams taking over care are fully informed of the person's wishes, and if a dying person is transferred between care settings, a clear written plan of care must be communicated.

26.3 Environment

As far as is possible, the patient who is dying should be transferred without delay into a comfortable bed in a quiet ward area; where this is not immediately achievable, the patient should be transferred into a bed in a quiet corner/cubicle in the ED. Hospital trolleys are entirely unsuitable for frail older people, especially those who are dying. Pressure-relieving mattresses and warming blankets should be used to enhance comfort.

26.4 Pain Relief and Symptom Control

Staff need to have adequate training in symptom control and to be able to access specialist advice and support from palliative care teams both in hospital and in the community. Common symptoms requiring treatment include pain, difficulty in breathing, nausea and vomiting, constipation, depression, dysphagia, insomnia, incontinence and anxiety. Assessing and managing pain is a priority, and all medications prescribed must have a rationale. The reason for any intervention particularly uncomfortable/painful procedures such as intravenous cannulas or urinary catheters must be justified for patient comfort and clearly explained to the patient, their family and important others. All medications need to be regularly reviewed and adjusted as needed to maintain comfort; moreover, likely side-effects such as drowsiness or reduced conscious level need to be explained to the patient and family.

26.5 Eating and Drinking

The dying person should be supported to eat and drink if they wish to, providing there is no serious risk of choking (unless this is an informed choice to accept the risk of aspiration in favour of enjoying food or drink). Mouth care and other personal care needs must be attended to at regular intervals to keep the person comfortable and preserve their dignity.

26.6 Religion and Spiritual Care

Where specialist spiritual or religious support is required, health and care staff must ensure that the dying person and those important to them have ready access to information about chaplaincy or spiritual care provision. It is essential that all EDs maintain up-to-date lists of chaplains and spiritual leaders of all denominations. Staff should offer to call the chaplain/priest/imam at any time if that is what the patient desires.

26.7 Hospice Care

The clinical team caring for the patient in the ED may judge that referral for hospice care may be appropriate. Hospice care places a high value on dignity, respect and the wishes of the person who is ill and aims to look after all their needs either in a hospice or at home. This option should be discussed with the patient, family and important others stressing that hospice care provides for medical, emotional, social, practical, psychological and spiritual needs, as well as the needs of the person's family and carers. Care also extends into the bereavement period after the patient has died. The clinical team in conjunction with the patients GP needs to make this referral.

26.8 Organ Donation

There continues to be a significant gap between the availability of organs for donation and patients desperately in need of transplants [13]. Age is not a contraindication to organ donation, yet this option is rarely considered in the emergency departments in relation to older patients. Many older patients, particularly those that have sustained catastrophic brain injuries (medical or traumatic) that are clearly not survivable, may have been otherwise very healthy and may be suitable donors.

In these circumstances, before having life-sustaining treatment withdrawn, the legal wishes of the patient or their closest relatives, orally or in written form, should guide the clinician to early referral of the patient to the specialist nurses for organ donation. It is in the best interests of the patient that they are cared for in a critical care environment to allow a full assessment of their donation potential.

Conclusions

There is an increasing imperative for emergency clinicians both medical and nursing to become more informed and aware of the need to deliver, when necessary, quality palliative and end of life care to the older person in the emergency department. Perhaps more importantly we need to rethink our focus so that we identify early on patients who will benefit from palliative care and work with our community partners to develop individualised care plans that will facilitate and support people to die in their own homes with those they love around them rather than in the impersonal and clinical environment that is the ED.

References

1. GBD 2013 Mortality and Causes of Death Collaborators (2015) Global, regional, and national age-sex specific all cause and cause specific mortality for 240 causes of death, 1990–2013: a systematic analysis for the global burden of disease study 2013. Lancet 385(9963): 117–171. http://www.thelancet.com/journals/lancet/article/P11S0140-6736 (14)61682-2/fulltext. Accessed Apr 2015
2. NHS Improving Quality (2014) Care in the last days of life. tinyurl.com/NHSIQ-last-days
3. Samaras N, Chevalley T, Samaras D, Gold G (2010) Older patients in the emergency department: a review. Ann Emerg Med 56(3):261–269
4. Beynon T, Gomes B, Murtagh F, Glucksman E, Parfitt A, Burman R et al (2011) How common are palliative care needs among older people who die in the emergency department? Emerg Med J 28(6):491–495
5. Grudzen CR, Richardson LD, Morrison M, Cho E, Morrison RS (2010) Palliative care needs of seriously ill, older adults presenting to the emergency department. Acad Emerg Med 17(11):1253–1257
6. WHO (2002) National cancer control programmes: policies and managerial guidelines, 2nd edn. World Health Organization, Geneva
7. http://www.endoflifecare-intelligence.org.uk/home, Aspx. Accessed March 2015
8. Securing the future of excellent patient care Shape of Training. http://www.shapeoftraining.co.uk/static/documents/content/Shape_of_training_final. Accessed March 2015
9. Neuberger J (2013) More care, less pathway: a review of the liverpool care pathway. DH, London. www.gov.uk/government/publications/review-of-liverpool-care-pathway-for-dying-patients
10. Leadership Alliance for the Care of Dying People (2014a) One chance to get it right. tinyurl.com/one-chance-right
11. Leadership Alliance for the Care of Dying People (2014b) Priorities of care for the dying person. tinyurl.com/priorities-of-care
12. https://www.mariecurie.org.uk/globalassets/media/documents/who-we-are/diversity-and-inclusion-research/palliative-care-bame_full-report.pdf
13. NHS Blood and Transplant. Organ Donation and Transplantation Activity Report 2011–2012

Bibliography

Gawande A et al (2014) Being mortal, medicine and what matters in the end. Metropolitan Books, New York

Ethical Issues of Emergency Medical Care for Older Patients

27

Helen Askitopoulou, Katrin Singler, Thomas Frühwald, and Monique Weissenberger-Leduc

27.1 Introduction

The unique nature and goals of emergency medical practice and the diversity of emergency patients pose distinctive ethical challenges for the emergency physician (EP). The emergency department (ED) is a dynamic and complex environment with unique features and many challenges. It usually operates with an unpredictable workload under time and personnel pressure. ED crowding influences informed decision-making because of the lack of available time to review the patient's medical history [1]. In this setting, EPs must make quickly the best possible diagnostic and treatment decisions with important ethical implications for patients, with whom often are not familiar. The ethical issues and problems involved, frequently, are more difficult to address in the ED environment than in other areas of medicine [2–4].

H. Askitopoulou, MD, PhD, DA, FRCA (✉)
Faculty of Medicine, University of Crete, Heraklion, Crete, Greece

European Society for Emergency Medicine (EUSEM) Ethics Committee Chair
e-mail: askitop@gmail.com

K. Singler, MD, MME
Internal Medicine, Geriatrics, Institute for Biomedicine of Aging,
Friedrich-Alexander University Erlangen-Nürnberg, Erlangen, Germany

Klinikum Nurnberg, Paracelsus Private Medical University, Nürnberg, Germany
e-mail: Katrin.singler@klinikum-nuernberg.de

T. Frühwald, MD
Austrian Society of Geriatrics and Gerontology, Laudongasse 21, 1080 Wien, Austria
e-mail: thomas.fruehwald@wienkav.at

M. Weissenberger-Leduc
Forum Palliative Praxis Geriatrie, Weißgerber Lände 40/19, 1030 Vienna, Austria
e-mail: monique.weissenberger-leduc@gmx.at

© Springer International Publishing Switzerland 2018
C. Nickel et al. (eds.), *Geriatric Emergency Medicine*,
https://doi.org/10.1007/978-3-319-19318-2_27

Older patients are proportionately the highest consumers of ED care accounting on average for up to a quarter to one-fifth of all ED attendees aged 65 or above [5, 6]. The emergency care of these patients, who have a distinct physical but also psychological and social vulnerability, presents different ethical challenges and dilemmas to EPs. The ethical questions focus on (a) the competency of older patients to understand their condition and to choose between possible options; (b) the wishes of patients not able to communicate, because of delirium, advanced dementia or unconsciousness; (c) the aims of diagnostic and/or therapeutic efforts that must meet the patients' expectations and not those of relatives, proxies, the institution or society; (d) the physicians' responsibility to limit or discontinue active treatment; (e) the benefit–risk ratio of treatment options for the individual patient; and (f) "what should be done" instead of "what can be done".

When addressing these ethical issues for every single clinical decision the EPs make, there are ethical implications to which they should respond in a manner that will provide the greatest benefit to their patients. To assure more benefit to older patients and their families and less anguish for them, EPs need to understand and implement the four basic ethical principles of Beauchamp and Childress regarding the main ethical issues relevant to emergency care such as competence, advance directives, resource allocation, end-of-life decisions, do not attempt resuscitation (DNAR) orders, older abuse and dementia [7].

27.2 Basic Ethical Principles in Emergency Care for Older Patients

Ethics is a branch of applied philosophy encompassing the different ways of examining and understanding the moral life, with its origins dating back to ancient Greece [8a]. Medical ethics is applied ethics that focus on ethical problems in the practice of medicine, with foundations in the writings of Hippocrates, the "father of medicine". In the 1970s, bioethics emerged as a subset of ethics that use ethical principles and decision-making to solve actual or anticipated moral dilemmas in health care, health sciences and medical technology [9, 10]. Eventually, bioethics has directed Hippocratic ethics and medical ethics into new pathways with cultural and political implications. Although laws differ significantly from one country to another, medical ethics do apply across national boundaries.

The four principles approach to biomedical ethics introduced by Beauchamp and Childress called *principlism* are respect for *autonomy*, *non-maleficence*, *beneficence* and *justice* [8b]. They describe the minimum moral conditions on the behaviour of health-care professionals as they interact with patients and families, the community at large and one another. They provide a set of moral commitments and common language. At the same time, they serve as a useful framework for the care of older patients. The originators of these principles claim that no one has priority over any of the others.

27.2.1 The Principle of Respect for *Patient Autonomy*

The concept of *autonomy* is tracked down to Greek antiquity to the self-governance of independent city–states. Since then, *autonomy* has evolved to denote self-governance, self-determination and self-ownership of the individuals, so that "personal autonomy encompasses, at a minimum, self-rule free from both controlling interference by others and inadequate understanding that prevents meaningful choice" [8c]. Patient autonomy places the competent patient, rather than the physician, at the centre of a medical decision [11]. Respect for patient *autonomy* is a fundamental principle for decision-making in health care, which compels the doctor to respect the patient's right to make independent choices and decisions based on personal values and beliefs [12]. This movement in medical ethics resulted in the decline of the paternalistic physician–patient relationship and encouraged the individuals to protect their personal values by making choices about their own health care [11]. However, this rapidly changing balance between paternalistic *beneficence* and patient/family-centred *autonomy* is not homogeneous between or even within countries [13].

In the environment of the ED, the principle of *autonomy* is difficult to assess, most particularly when urgent situations arise with older patients, as often is the case [11]. In old age, it is unclear whether a person is capable of making specific health-care decisions. A busy ED is a disorienting and difficult place for these patients and their families. To make autonomous decisions, older patients should have decision-making capacity pertaining to the complexity of the situation. In this case, they can provide informed consent, which they may change at any time if they so wish. Moreover, they have the right to choose actions consistent with their values and goals, even if their choices are not in agreement with the wishes of their family or the recommendations of their doctor. Another time that the issue of mental capacity and *autonomy* arises, is when an individual wants to make an advance directive or when there is doubt about his/her understanding concerning a particular treatment [14].

27.2.1.1 Informed Consent and Decision-Making Capacity of Older Patients in the ED

Informed consent is a central concept of present-day medical ethics. It is the process by which a patient receives all pertinent information necessary to make a rational autonomous choice. The main prerequisites for giving informed consent for or informed refusal of treatment are adequate patient decision-making capacity and disclosure by the doctor of information about the proposed treatment, the alternative care options and the expected consequences or side-effects [2, 15]. After being given correct and complete information, a patient is thought to be able to give informed consent if he/she can receive, can process and understand the information provided, can comprehend and appreciate the nature and consequences of a choice, can communicate that choice and can make a stable and coherent decision consistent with previously expressed goals and life values [15, 16].

To obtain informed consent in the ED is quite a challenge, as many patients may not be capable of making decisions due to an acute life-threatening condition, intoxication, language barriers or other impairments. The EP has the unconditional duty to protect patients from inappropriate health-care decisions and has been the most appropriate person to make decisions in the patient's best interests [17]. At the same time, the EP should keep in mind that the basis for all medical decisions is the presence of a meaningful medical indication for the intended diagnostic or therapeutic intervention. In most cases, both written and verbal information must be presented appropriately with opportunities for the ED personnel to repeat and clarify the content.

Patient refusal of indicated medical treatment, especially when the treatment would be life sustaining, presents EPs with the responsibility of determining whether the patient has the capacity to refuse treatment and whether the patient's refusal is informed. As at any age, older adults with decision-making capacity have the right to refuse treatment, even if such refusal hastens or results in their death. It is not necessarily irrational for old patients with decision-making capacity to refuse unwanted medical interventions, even if the EPs consider that the refusal for an intervention is wrong [18]. Doctors have the duty to respect patient *autonomy*, which is the ethical principle that underlies informed consent. It is their responsibility to assure that the patient can meaningfully participate in the decisions and can consent voluntarily without coercion.

The assessment of an aged person's competency in decision-making about consent to treatment is a common ethical dilemma facing the emergency physician. It is a dilemma often precipitated by patient's vulnerability from the stress of illness, pain, anxiety, fear and the strange environment of the ED or age-related changes such as pre-existing cognitive or mobility impairments, sensory deficits in hearing and vision or impaired ability to ask a question, as well as insufficient social support [18]. It is estimated that acute changes in the mental status, such as delirium described in approximately 10% of frail older subjects visiting an ED, make impossible the requirement for informed consent [19].

When an older patient's wishes are unknown or unclear, the patient is unable to weigh up the information and to make a decision on treatment or the ramifications of a decision are serious, then surrogate decision-making may be used. Furthermore, the assistance of advanced directives, if available, information given by relatives, proxies or close friends or a third party such as another clinician may be valuable in discerning the most appropriate action [15]. However, if a surrogate or an advance directive is not available, consent should be presumed [18]. In such situations, when an immediate intervention is necessary to prevent death or serious harm to the patient and the necessary care must be provided instantly, informed consent does not become the first ethical priority [4]. Nevertheless, it does not mean that in other ED situations, respect for *autonomy* should not be taken into account. It has been reported that among ED patients, those judged capable of participating have a strong desire for *autonomy* in medical decision-making regardless of their acuity of illness. However, old age, as well as a lesser level of formal education, is correlated with a decreasing desire for decision-making *autonomy* [20].

Informed consent is a moral as well as a legal obligation of physicians in most countries. In the UK, the recent law about informed consent requires a doctor to take "reasonable care to ensure that the patient is aware of any material risks involved in any recommended treatment and of any reasonable alternative or variant treatments" [21]. What is important for the EP is that this law now obliges "even those doctors who have less skill or inclination for communication, or who are more hurried, to pause and engage in the discussion". However, the UK law recognises three exceptions to the duty to disclose. Firstly, the patient might tell the doctor that he/she would prefer not to know the risks. Secondly, the doctor reasonably considers that telling the patient specific information would cause serious harm to the patient's health. Thirdly, no consent is needed in circumstances of necessity, such as when a patient in need of urgent treatment is unconscious or lacks capacity [21].

27.2.1.2 Communication with Older Patients in the ED

The fundamental objective of any physician–patient communication is to improve the quality of care and patient's health outcomes. Effective communication with patients, particularly the older ones, in the ED is central to informed consent and a necessary condition for difficult decision-making. It creates a good interpersonal relationship for the exchange of information and treatment-related decisions. Good physician–patient communication may help regulate patients' emotions, facilitate comprehension of medical information and allow for better identification of patients' needs, perceptions and expectations [22]. Concerns are elicited and explored, and explanations of treatment options are balanced and understood. Successful information is characterised by being clear, complete, accurate, timely and requiring verification from the parties involved.

EPs should pay particular attention to how they communicate with older patients and should try to understand non-verbal cues if the patient is unable to talk. Their duty is to treat these patients politely and considerately, to listen to and respect their views and to give them information in a way that they can understand and accept their right to be fully involved in decisions about their care. Verifying what has been communicated is important to the process with a need to ensure that the meaning of the sent message is understood and mutually agreed upon.

EPs often have to decide quickly whether their patients lack decision-making capacity. This needs a sound clinical judgement and the competency to assess an older patient's decision-making capacity, which differs from a simple mental status examination. A brief screening testing such as the MMSE is inadequate for determining capacity except at the extremes of the score [23]. EPs should be absolutely certain that an older patient, who refuses a low risk, yet life-saving intervention, has the ability to make rational decisions [18]. Disagreement with the doctor's recommendation is not by itself reason for determining that the patient is incapable of making a decision [24] nor does cognitive impairment automatically constitute incapacity.

Commonly doctors tend to overestimate their abilities in communication. Significant miscommunication may result in patients' misunderstanding of their prognosis, purpose of care, expectations and involvement in treatment [22]. To avoid miscommunications, improve physician–patient communication and provide optimal patient care, good communication skills must be developed by formal training of health-care personnel and maintained with conscious effort and periodic review. Direct observation, video recording and focus group discussions offer a structured approach for analysing and giving feedback on doctors' communication performance that encourages subsequent reflection and self-directed learning. A careful selection of challenging patients may maximise the benefit of direct observation and feedback. Alternative methods of teaching communication skills include role play and tape recording of consultations or standardised patients, as well as standardised videos using scenarios in breaking bad news to patients, a complex and challenging communication task in the practice of medicine [25].

Good communication skills are an essential component of the physician–patient relationship. Examples of skilful communication are attentive listening skills, empathy and the use of open-ended questions [22]. ED personnel should try to improve ways of communication with older patients by identifying and implementing interventions that could support communication in the emergency setting. Experience alone does not necessarily lead to good communication skills. Surveys have shown that the physician–patient relationship often causes considerable stress and anxiety because of the lack of confidence and competence in communicating well, particularly in the ED, where doctors are required to deal with a case mix relatively new to them [25].

27.2.1.3 Advance Directives to Refuse Treatment

Advance directives (ADs), also known as advance statements or advance decisions, are refusals of consent given much earlier by individuals, in case these individuals will lack decision-making capacity when the occasion arises [26]. An advance directive may be a written document, a witnessed oral statement or a note in the patient's records following a discussion with a health-care professional. They usually take two different forms, which are not necessarily exclusive of each other. The *living wills* are written documents designed to allow people to express their preferences regarding the provision or the *withholding* of specified treatments, in the event they become unable to make decisions in the future. The *lasting (or durable) power of attorney for health care* allows individuals to appoint someone as a "health-care proxy" (e.g. a trusted relative or friend) to make health-care decisions on their behalf once they lose the ability to do so [27]. An AD made by a competent adult is binding under common law in many countries without their family or health-care professionals having to predict what their best interests are and to take critical decisions [14]. Advance directives are not limited to patient's "wishes" but also include patient's "goals and values" [27].

Advance care planning (ACP) and advance directives have become increasingly important by the growing value attached to the principle of respect for patient *autonomy* in health-care decision-making, and by giving patients some control over their future treatment [28]. They are very important documents for older adults, who are more likely than younger people, to develop later impaired decision-making capacity. The ADs promote patient *autonomy*, as they allow patients to protect their best interests and maintain control over what happens to them by refusing certain treatments in advance [18, 29]. For end-of-life care, ADs have been frequently cited as important tools for communicating patient desires [30]. Although advance directives can be helpful, studies have shown that more than 70% of older and acutely ill patients, who had expressed a clear preference regarding resuscitation, said that if they did become incapacitated, they would want the family and physician to make the resuscitation decisions rather than having their own AD followed [31]. Yet the level of agreement between the surrogate's decision and the patient's preference in real and hypothetical seriously ill patients' scenarios was only 68% in a meta-analysis of 16 studies analysing this outcome [32].

A potential limitation of advance directives is the possible changes in patients' preferences over time or circumstance. People often accommodate to disabilities, and an old *living will* may become inconsistent with the patient's revised views about the quality of life or other outcomes. It is evident that *living wills* cannot cover all conceivable end-of-life decisions [27]. Some ADs are written to apply only in particular clinical situations, such as when the patient has a terminal condition or an incurable illness, or to prohibit specific interventions, such as blood transfusions or cardiopulmonary resuscitation (CPR), in specified clinical contexts. However, there is too much variability in clinical decision-making to make an all-encompassing *living will* possible. Persons, who have written or are considering writing advance directives, should be made aware of the fact that these documents are insufficient to ensure that all decisions regarding care at the end of life will be made in accordance with their written wishes. Furthermore, the legal status of advance directives varies considerably among the European countries based on the diverse legal, sociocultural, religious and philosophical traditions of each society, while in several others, there is still a reluctance to legislate in this field [27, 33].

Advance directives must meet three criteria: existence, validity and applicability, each with its own potential problems. In emergency situations, the existence of ADs is most relevant as it might not be clear whether it exists at all. If there is no clear indication that an AD exists, doctors must not delay emergency interventions or resuscitation while trying to establish whether an AD exists that prohibits the particular intervention [27]. If on the other hand an AD exists, the EP must assess its applicability to the current condition of the patient [17]. Furthermore, ADs often do not take into account acute but potentially reversible events that frequently arise in emergency care. In these cases, it is important not to focus on the specific statements of the AD but on the intentions behind it considering the personal values and goals of the patient. To enable a decision honouring the wish of the patient, the EP should obtain information from family, friends, carers and patient's charts [3]. However, an AD, even if correctly executed and appropriately activated, cannot compel individual clinicians to act in a way which is not in keeping with their own moral codes. Under these circumstances, a second opinion or referral to another service may be required.

27.2.2 The Principle of *Non-maleficence*

The principle of *non-maleficence* imposes an obligation not to inflict harm on others [8c]. In medical ethics, it expresses the duty of health-care professionals to refrain intentionally from actions that cause harm to their patients. It has been closely related to the Hippocratic axiom "help or do not harm" [34], meaning if doctors cannot benefit their patients, at least they must try not to harm them. It represents the risk side of a risk–benefit analysis. However, Beauchamp and Childress point out the difficulty in defining the nature of harm. In health care, the primary focus of harm relates to a narrower definition of physical harm especially pain, disability, suffering or death [8d].

The principle of *non-maleficence* requires that doctors act in ways that do not inflict or cause avoidable or intentional harm to their patients. This principle can be violated with or without the intention of harm. It also includes avoiding even the risk of harm. In the case of risk imposition, both law and morality recognise a standard of "due care". This standard requires that a reasonable and prudent person takes sufficient and appropriate care to avoid causing harm. The goals pursued should justify the risks to achieving these goals [8d]. EPs cannot avoid inflicting harm, as serious emergencies justify risks that many non-emergency conditions do not justify. For example, rib and sternal fractures and injuries to internal organs are justified during attempts to resuscitate a cardiac arrest victim.

The absence of "due care" is negligence. The principle of *non-maleficence* affirms the need for medical competence. It is clear that medical mistakes may occur; however, this principle articulates a fundamental commitment on the part of health-care professionals to protect from harm those patients, who cannot protect themselves. This is particularly evident in vulnerable older patients. However, the line between "due care" and inadequate care is often difficult to draw [8d].

The principle of *non-maleficence* has implications for several areas of bioethics like medical *futility* and *withholding* and *withdrawing* life-prolonging treatments.

27.2.2.1 Futile Emergency Medical Interventions

Futility in medicine is an ancient concept. The Hippocratic treatise *The Art* clearly states that physicians should "refuse to treat those who are overmastered by their disease, realising that in such cases medicine is powerless" and "rightly refuse to undertake obstinate cases" [35a,b]. Although the concept of futile medical treatment is controversial, it generally means that treatment is useless and ineffective, or unlikely to provide any significant or meaningful medical benefit to the patient, or it does not offer a reasonable chance of survival [36]. The World Medical Association defines futile medical treatment as a treatment that "offers no reasonable hope of recovery or improvement" or from which "the patient is permanently unable to experience any benefit" [37]. The term futility covers many situations of predicted unlikely outcomes, improbable success and unacceptable benefit–burden ratio. A judgement of futility may be based on a probabilistic prediction of failure or on something closer to a medical certainty. If an older patient has a 1% chance of surviving an arduous and painful regimen, some doctors may call this procedure futile. This is considered a value judgement combined with a scientific one [8e]. The difficulty in determining futile treatment arises in the context of the prognosis of the quality of life.

Two kinds of medical *futility* are distinguished. *Quantitative futility*, when the likelihood that an intervention will benefit the patient is exceedingly poor, and *qualitative futility*, when the likelihood of benefit produced by an intervention is exceedingly poor [8e]. It is therefore important for the doctor to assess the "overall benefit" to the patient, taking into account according to the Council of Europe "not only the results of the treatment of the illness or the symptoms, but also the patient's quality of life and psychological and spiritual well-being" [38]. For example, *qualitative futility* refers to patients who have survived resuscitation with a high likelihood of harm related to the resuscitation efforts and are likely to spend their last hours or days in an intensive care unit, therefore prolonging suffering without reversing the underlying disease [39]. It is important that *futility* as a non-beneficial treatment is distinguished from rationing, which is the fair distribution of beneficial but limited resources [10].

Medical *futility* as the ineffectiveness of an intervention has the greatest ethical consensus and most utility in emergency medicine. EPs have the expertise and obligation to assess each case individually so as to determine whether the treatment would be beneficial. However, when treating the most critical patients, EPs only rarely have enough information to make a judgement that an intervention would be futile. They must intervene quickly, with only limited information about their patients' past medical history and wishes, trying to save a life. Only later, when relatives arrive or medical records become available, they may discover that the patient has a terminal disease or did not want resuscitative efforts. Yet, because of the limited information available when the patient arrives in the ED, the mandate to attempt resuscitation is morally justifiable [24].

Futility is essentially a purely medical decision [8e]. Doctors must provide information about the likely chances of success or failure of an intervention but have neither the obligation nor the justification to provide clinically inappropriate medical care and to perform medical interventions they judge that are futile or lacking the likelihood of benefit to their patients. The patients and their families have no right to request futile, clinically inappropriate treatments [40]. Beauchamp and Childress point out that "respect for the autonomy of patients is not a trump that allows them alone to determine whether a required treatment is futile" [8e]. By instituting futile treatments, the medical team falsely offers hope to the family and patient that undermines the patient's ability for rational judgement and *autonomy*. However, doctors should discuss with their patients their condition, values, goals and hopes in life in order to arrive at a shared and mutual decision [40]. They should explain to older patients with life-threatening illnesses and their family that they do not want to expose the patients to interventions that are not likely to be beneficial and instead are potentially harmful. It is essential to describe in a compassionate but unambiguous way the risks and benefits of the intervention and that the *futility* concept is not used to deny care to these patients. Even terminal patients have medical emergencies that require intervention. The goal is to ease pain and suffering, depending on the patient, the medical condition causing discomfort and the value system of the patient [24].

27.2.2.2 Withholding and Withdrawing Life-Prolonging Treatment in the ED

The *withholding* and the *withdrawing* of life-prolonging treatment refer to the process by which medical interventions are either not provided or are removed from patients as futile. The *withholding* and *withdrawing* of life-prolonging therapies, such as mechanical ventilation or artificial nutrition, are ethically and medically appropriate in certain circumstances, when the treatment no longer provides a clear health benefit to the patient [41, 42], such as to cure (if possible), to palliate symptoms, to prevent disease or their complications and to improve functional status [43]. The remarkable medical progress in supportive therapies that enables organ functions to be maintained while a patient recovers from a serious illness should not be abused to sustain indefinitely "life" that is without quality or meaning. Indeed, this goes against all four ethical principles [44].

In emergency medical care, there is a fundamental moral difference between *withholding* and *withdrawing* of life-prolonging medical treatment. In this setting, the *withholding* of critical interventions started in the first few minutes of emergency care is much more problematic, than later withdrawal of unwanted or useless interventions, when more information is known. The justification for this difference stems from three reasons. First, in emergency situations, it is always necessary to start life-sustaining treatment first and then to review this when enough information is available, more experienced opinion is on hand, there is an evolution of the clinical state or there is new light from investigations carried out. Second, in the ED setting, patients and their families have high expectations from EPs to initiate resuscitative care, expectations that complicate any proposed nontreatment. Third, these actions in the emergency setting have a high emotional impact. Resuscitative efforts, once begun, can be withdrawn if evidence emerges that resuscitation is only prolonging an imminent death or that the patient did not want these efforts to take place [24].

In the last decades, the proportion of older people, considered in discussions about *withholding* and *withdrawing* life-prolonging treatment, is increasing. *Withholding* treatment from an older person of whatever age simply because he/she is old is both morally and legally impermissible. Such treatment should not be withheld or withdrawn on the basis of patients' age alone or their quality of life. Decisions need to be made on an individual basis by clear, robust and transparent procedures [41]. Older competent patients should be encouraged to participate in decision-making, taking into consideration their preferences, beliefs and wishes and having ensured that a reversible illness that impacts on decision-making, such as delirium, sensory impairment, pain and tiredness, is treated [45]. In the case of incompetent patients, such decisions should be made in their best interests having consulted (within the limits of confidentiality) friends, family, carers and advance care planning [45]. Decisions to withhold treatment should be made by experienced senior personnel after careful assessment of the benefits, risks and burdens of treatment based on the best available qualitative information [41].

Decisions to withdraw or withhold life-prolonging medical treatment are among the most difficult a doctor can make in the face of prognostic uncertainty. Decisions must be made on a case-by-case basis, keeping in mind that each case is unique, while age or race must never be used to qualify these decisions. Also *withholding* specific medical care from older patients because of financial motives is not acceptable. However, it has been argued that it may be appropriate to consider the overall costs and potential benefits to the individual patient, the family and the society [46]. EPs must use their best judgement to ensure good medical practice and evidence-based decision-making to underline decisions about life-sustaining treatment for an older patient.

Withholding or *withdrawing* life-prolonging futile medical interventions helps an already dying patient to achieve a peaceful and dignified death and must be distinguished from euthanasia and physician-assisted suicide. The primary goal of *withdrawing* life-prolonging treatment is not to bring about the death of the patient but not to prolong unnecessary suffering and death as a result of medical intervention. When certain interventions are withheld, special efforts should be made to maintain effective communication, comfort, support and counselling for the patient, family and friends [47]. *Withholding* or *withdrawing* life-prolonging treatment does not imply that the patient will receive no care. It should be clarified to patients and their families that it is a change in focus towards palliative care with the alleviation of suffering and of distressing symptoms and with supportive measures that ensure that the rest of the patient's life is as comfortable as possible. It is essential that these discussions are recorded in the medical records.

27.2.3 The Principle of *Beneficence*

The principle of *beneficence* is not simply the opposite of *non-maleficence* but a self-evident and widely accepted goal of medicine. It refers to the moral obligation to act for the benefit of others. The meaning of this principle for health-care providers is that they have a duty to take positive steps to "do good" for the benefit or well-being of patients but also to refrain from harming them [8f]. This principle has been at the very heart of medical ethics since the time of the Hippocratic *Oath*, which expresses the obligation of the oath taker to act "for the benefit of the ill in accordance with his ability and judgment" [48].

Emergency physicians have a moral obligation to attempt to provide benefits to their patients by responding promptly to acute illnesses and injuries in order to prevent or minimise pain and suffering, loss of function and loss of life [2]. During emergencies, health-care professionals are always obliged to provide the best care under the circumstances by balancing the benefits and risks of a medical intervention [38]. This action could be considered as "paternalistic", even if the doctor acts from a benevolent spirit in providing beneficent treatment that in his/her opinion is in the best interests of the patient but without consulting the patient or by overriding the patient's wishes. Nevertheless, there is a clear situation in emergency medicine where the principle of *beneficence* is given priority over the principle of patient *autonomy*. When the patient is incapacitated by the critical nature of accident or illness, the EP presumes that the reasonable person would want to be treated aggressively, and therefore he/she intervenes by stopping the bleeding, fixing the broken part or suturing the wounded.

A significant problem in the ED common in patients of all ages, but especially in those older than 70 years, is the under-treatment of pain. This is mainly because of misconceptions about the ageing process and the side-effects of pain therapy. Improvement of pain relief for older adults is the moral duty of emergency care personnel, who have the duty to benefit their patients by "doing good" through effective pain assessment and management and by preventing harm from the adverse effects of the under-treatment of pain [49].

27.2.3.1 Patient Confidentiality

Patient *confidentiality* is an important element of the physician–patient relationship since the Hippocratic *Oath* when the oath taker vowed that "whatsoever I shall see or hear in the course of my profession … I will never divulge, holding such things to be holy secrets" [48]. In health care, the term *confidentiality* refers to the protection of patient information from unauthorised disclosure to anyone not directly involved in the patient's care and treatment [50, 51]. Doctor's *confidentiality* is a promise rooted in tradition, law and medical ethics and an essential element of the patient's right to *autonomy* and the physician's duty to "do good". It is part of the personal contract between the physician and the patient and the keystone of medical as well as emergency care [50]. EPs by protecting the privacy of their patients and the *confidentiality* of patient information they respect the principle of *beneficence* [2]. A therapeutic alliance should exist between the emergency physician and the patient. There should be fidelity, trust, *confidentiality* and protection from intended harm. The patients' health and even their lives could easily be at stake without the premise of the confidential relationship. However, there may be times when this bond has to be broken when the need for *confidentiality* may conflict with the need to protect other members of society [52].

Confidentiality encompasses respect for the privacy of vulnerable older persons who cannot choose or exercise control. Sick older emergency patients are in a dependent relationship, forced to trust EPs to protect their interests through competence, informed consent, truthfulness and maintenance of *confidentiality* of the health information [2]. EDs should develop methods of ensuring *confidentiality* for all patients. In the case of a person who is legally or physically incapable of acting in his or her own interest, disclosures may be made only to the extent necessary to protect the best interests of the patient [50]. When patients have been treated in the ED after an assault or another violent incident, the EPs should ascertain that they get the patient's consent before disclosing to the police or other authorities the information sought and that they prevent unauthorised persons from viewing patient's records [51].

27.2.4 The Principle of *Justice*

The principle of *justice* is related to fairness, equality and equity. In medicine, it requires that each patient is treated fairly, respectfully and competently and that the use of resources (particularly scarce or expensive) is fair and just for all patients who may need them, without unfairly benefiting one group over another [3, 52].

Justice in emergency medicine requires that EPs are the advocates of both the individual needs of patients and the societal need for universal access. They have to balance the burdens and benefits, the obligations of society to the individual on the one hand and the obligation of the individual to society on the other. Along these lines, they must decide how to triage, whom to refer, which are the limits of technology and how to resist the demands of persistent patients regarding inappropriate tests or treatments.

27.2.4.1 Fairness of Treatment of Older Subjects

The principle of *justice* requires fair opportunity in life so that no person should be denied social benefits on the basis of undeserved disadvantageous properties [8h]. Unfortunately, there is no consensus about what constitutes a just and fair method of balancing the preferences and requirements of individual patients against the diverse needs of society [53]. Aristotle argues that "when the whole has been divided into two halves, people then say that they 'have their own', having got what is equal; this is indeed the origin of the word 'dikaion' (just)" [54].

If *justice* is a concept about treating people fairly, then it is prudent to wonder what it means to be "fair". Which are the criteria on which a morally fair decision is based? Decisions must not be made on assumptions based solely on criteria such as advanced age, unrelated to the severity of acute and chronic illness, disability or a subjective view of a person's quality of life. The decision-making process for fair treatment or care of older patients should not be emotional or subjective but should be objective and non discriminatory subsequent to careful assessment of the patient's medical needs. Although a specific treatment theoretically might offer benefit, it does not follow that it will always offer the same benefit to all patients. The effect varies according to individual circumstances. It is important when trying to form a decision, to raise the question on who is going to be affected by the decision made and whether this decision implicates a suboptimal management of other patients.

Applying *justice* within the ED is often challenging and requires constant vigilance to ensure that objectives are fair, while at the same time it is guarding patient *autonomy*, particularly, of older vulnerable patients. It is possible that a high degree of incapacity and increased vulnerability may result in a lack of *distributive justice*. Even if they are treated equally, older fragile patients can be treated unjustly. The EP's responsibility is to optimise outcomes by guarding the good of patients who are, for example, mentally ill or demented and who do not possess the capacity to know their best interest.

27.2.4.2 Equitable Allocation of Finite Resources in the ED

Justice, more specifically understood as *distributive justice*, refers broadly to the distribution of all rights and responsibilities in society [8g]. In medicine, *distributive justice* implies that health-care professionals have a duty to distribute limited health resources equally and as fairly as possible, without discrimination, with the requirement that each individual is able to obtain, in practice, the care available [38]. The principle of *justice* recognises that health-care provision is a need and that allocation of resources should be based on the best possible outcomes.

The distribution of health resources is distinguished between macro- and micro-allocation depending on the level of decision-making authority that is of the society or of the individual doctor. In the macro-allocation level, access to emergency medical care in most countries is a fundamental right that is available to all who seek it. In the micro-allocation level, EPs have the difficult duty to reconcile the increasing scarcity of resources with the goal of equitable access to health care to all patients with acute illness or injury regardless of age, gender, race, religion, nationality or other properties [2].

In the ED, a common procedure in which the principle of *distributive justice* is applied is triage. When in a crowded ED or in a disaster, many patients simultaneously need medical attention, and the medical personnel cannot attend to all at the same time, the rule is to serve persons whose condition requires immediate attention, so that they do not deteriorate, while others, whose condition is not as serious and are stable, may be deferred. Triage involves micro-allocation decisions that distribute diagnostic and treatment resources in a timescale without compromising quality and without giving priority to one patient over another. In contrast, macro-allocation involves broad policies in public health to distribute resources across populations and, hence, improve the quality of life for many emergency people.

The principle of *justice* for the allocation of emergency health-care resources towards older patients involves decisions about their needs on an individual basis. How this principle shall be applied wisely to their individual needs must be left to the prudence of each doctor. It is one of the toughest decisions EPs have to make, while at the same time, they try to optimise the outcome for individual patients. The quality of life judgements based on prejudices against age, ethnicity, mental status or socioeconomic status should not be used, explicitly or implicitly, as the basis for rationing medical services in the ED.

Some groups suggest that it makes little sense to prolong the lives of old patients with increasingly failing health and co-morbidities and deprive younger generations of resources that might actually benefit them. In this respect, advance care planning can play a significant role in avoiding costly futile medical interventions that prolong life [28]. However, the use of any age-weighting approach that gives less value to benefits for older than for younger persons is charged as unjust age discrimination. It fails to treat old people with the same concern and respect accorded to other candidates for care, and it constitutes unfair discrimination on the grounds of life expectancy, in short, ageism [55]. Age-related allocation of resources is not a moral decision. Older patients should have equal access to treatment regardless of age. Ethical decisions should be free from ageism and should be made without regard to resource constraints and discriminatory practices [14].

27.3 Ethical Issues in Emergency Care for Older Patients

27.3.1 End-of-Life Decisions for Older Patients in the ED

Patients who are approaching the end of their life need high-quality treatment and care that support them to live as well as possible until they die and to die with dignity.

The Council of Europe defines the end-of-life situations as "those in which a severe deterioration in health, due to the evolution of a disease or another cause, threatens the life of a person irreversibly in the near future" [38]. The UK General Medical Council's (GMC) definition of patients "approaching the end-of-life" is more specific and includes those "whose death is imminent from a sudden acute crisis in their existing condition or life-threatening acute conditions caused by sudden catastrophic events" or are "likely to die within the next 12 months from advanced, progressive, incurable conditions, or general frailty and coexisting conditions" [42].

It is recognised that vulnerable older patients with complex needs frequently receive a poorer standard of end-of-life care. For these patients who are approaching the end of their lives, this is an ethically unique challenge. Doctors need to be aware of the communication, legal and ethical issues around end-of-life care, including advance directives. They have a responsibility for outlining all options, informing the patient and other relevant parties and maximising the capacity of the patient to deal with the information and make their choices. When the patient lacks capacity, the doctor will work with others who may have legal authority to decide for the patient or consult the patient's advance directives, decisions or refusals. Where agreement cannot be reached, advice or a second opinion should be sought, and this may lead to a resolution. The key aspect of the treatment and care towards the end-of-life is the centrality of the patient, rather than the doctor alone, in making decisions [42]. However, relatives without the required medical knowledge and expertise should not be expected to make such end-of-life decisions. Their decision process at an already difficult time may be altered by emotional reactions and possibly even by personal interest. These final decisions must rely mostly on the doctor in charge, in consultation with members of the medical team [44].

The Royal College of Emergency Medicine (RCEM) advocates that a senior EP should be involved with and be responsible for every patient requiring end-of-life care in an emergency so that a ceiling of treatment in the ED is set that gives most overall benefit and is least restrictive of the patient's future choices. EPs should assess competence and involve patients at the end of their life and their families as much as possible with making decisions about their care wherever possible and appropriate [17]. Advance care planning assists in identifying and respecting a patient's wishes about end-of-life care and improves such care from the perspective of the patient and the family. The benefits of advance care planning for older patients include preparation for end of life care and death, avoidance of prolongation of dying, strengthening of personal relationships, relieving burdens placed on family, and the informal communication of future wishes [56]. The older like other groups of society are worthy of value, respect and basic humane and compassionate care at all times.

Any discussions EPs have with patients regarding future care, which could assist with end-of-life care planning, should be clearly documented and communicated to the patient's general practitioner, care home or admitting hospital team. Before discharged from the ED, old patients nearing end-of-life should have a resuscitation decision made. It is also considered best practice if the ED is involved in the planning and organisation of services to enable patients to be discharged for care at home [17].

27.3.2 Resuscitation of Older Patients

Ethical issues are an integral part of the resuscitation process. Many health-care providers often encounter moral adversity in situations of resuscitation of older patients because of the historical knowledge of poor outcomes [57]. The appropriateness and effectiveness of resuscitation among different age groups in the emergency medicine setting is covered by controversies. Survival rates have been reported to be highest for patients less than 60 years and to decrease in old age [58]. However, age alone is not a valid criterion to decide whether a patient is a suitable candidate for CPR and to determine its success rate. The decisive factor is the co-morbidity that may accompany advancing years [59, 60].

Old age is associated with an increasingly lower short-term survival rate after an out-of-hospital cardiac arrest. Survival to hospital discharge was 8% for those aged 65–79, 4% for those 80–89 and as low as 2% for those ≥90 years [61]. In older resuscitated comatose patients, the 30-day mortality increased with age, reaching in numbers their age in years. After out-of-hospital cardiac arrest, patients aged 80 or more had a twofold decrease in survival to hospital discharge compared with the reference group aged 50–59 years. The survival was dismal only in the age group of those older than 90 years when the rate of successful resuscitation to be alive at discharge approached zero [62]. These data support the fact that out-of-hospital resuscitation of people up to the age of 90 years is not associated with a dismal outcome, and therefore resuscitative efforts must not be withheld from the older because of concerns of ineffectiveness.

After in-hospital resuscitation, survival to discharge was about 20% in those aged 65–69 years, declining with advancing age to about 10% in those aged 90 years or more [63]. Increasing age was also associated with lower 1-year survival after in-hospital resuscitation. In a retrospective cohort study on older patients discharged alive after CPR, the 1-year survival was 63.7, 58.6 and 49.7% among patients 65–74, 75–84 and ≥85 years of age, respectively. The neurological outcome of the older survivors of cardiac arrest was good, with 95% having a cerebral performance category score of 1–2 on discharge from ICU and 72% at hospital discharge [64]. In a retrospective review that looked at the characteristics of geriatric hospitalised patients, it was determined that selected patients, as those with cardiac arrest from a primary VT or VF arrhythmia or with respiratory–hypoxic arrest, may benefit from a short resuscitation attempt [65]. The data from in-hospital cardiac arrests suggest that biological age is less important than physiology and other risk factors when estimating prognosis. The patients at increased risk of poor outcome from a pulseless cardiac arrest were those with significant morbidity or numerous chronic pre-existing conditions and/or interventions in place [66].

27.3.2.1 Family-Witnessed Resuscitation in the ED

Witnessed resuscitation is the process of cardiopulmonary resuscitation in the presence of family members. The principle of *beneficence* necessitates that ED personnel considers how they are treating the close relatives of an old patient during resuscitation or an intervention, whereas concern has been raised about a potential breach of patient *confidentiality* [24]. Since the early 1980s, when this practice first appeared, there is wide variation in hospital policies to facilitate this process in the European countries [33]. It is also an ongoing debate about the benefits, or harm, of this practice among emergency care providers [67, 68].

Studies assessing clinicians' attitudes towards family presence during resuscitation have revealed little enthusiasm and concern with this practice related to the patient's traumatic injuries, the ethics of witnessed resuscitation, its medicolegal implications as well as the resident's training [67, 69, 70]. When surveyed, a substantial number of emergency providers reported negative experiences with family presence and in addition failure to observe any positive value [69]. However, it was found that prior experience of health-care providers with family presence was a significant predictor of their support for family presence [68]. Another survey from the UK showed a wide difference in responses among nursing and medical staff, with a positive attitude to witnessed resuscitation among nursing staff, but lesser support mainly from junior medical staff [71].

More recently, accumulating evidence suggests that family presence during end-of-life resuscitative efforts could be beneficial and would contribute to an increasingly open attitude and appreciation of the *autonomy* of both patients and relatives [13]. Several surveys note positive reactions from family members who express their wish to be present during a resuscitative attempt. Family members have reported that being at a loved one's side in the course of critical end-of-life care helped them to adjust to the death of their loved one and that saying goodbye during the final moments of life was comforting [67]. They exhibited less anxiety and depression compared with family members who were absent. They also had a sense of being included rather than excluded, which helped to strengthen their relationship with the doctor. Moreover, family members observing resuscitation efforts were able to view the major efforts, organisation and skill involved and that everything possible was being done for their loved one [70]. Family presence also maintains family–patient connection and removes uncertainty regarding what is happening to the patient during the resuscitation. However, this practice does presume that an experienced member of staff should facilitate and support the bereaved relatives during the resuscitation attempt [46, 72].

Current practice in emergency medicine about witnessed resuscitation is changing, as humane considerations outweigh potential ethical concerns, influenced by education of the patient, family and caregivers, as well as better awareness of patient rights [13, 67]. Both the European Resuscitation Council and the American Heart Association recommend the presence of family members, based on the benefit gained by them and the lack of harmful effects brought about by their being present during resuscitation [46, 73]. However, a recent survey in 31 European countries of ethical practices during resuscitation including family presence revealed a wide diversity between countries, possibly attributable to country specific, differing health-care policies and caregiver attitudes [33]. There is an obvious need for harmonisation of legislations and of education-based interpretation and routine application of the principles of bioethics. Therefore, ERC emphasises the need of appropriate education of the resuscitation team of how to deal with the presence of family by communication training and simulation scenarios on organisation and determination of roles of persons dedicated to supporting the family. This will pave the way to the widest possible consensus on ethical practices, including family presence, during resuscitation [13].

27.3.2.2 Do Not Attempt Resuscitation (DNAR) Orders for Older Patients

The decision to issue an order "do not resuscitate" (DNR) or "do not attempt resuscitation" (DNAR) is a medical order, with profound ethical implications, to forgo basic cardiac life support in the out-of-hospital setting and advanced cardiac life support in the in-hospital setting [74]. Emergency physicians should honour DNAR orders and other end-of-life orders when there are appropriately executed and express the patient's treatment preferences [2]. Since the onset of a cardiac arrest does not permit deliberative decision-making, all DNAR decisions must be made in advance and discussed with the patient, his/her family or a designated representative if the patient lacks capacity [38]. However, in emergency settings, it is not always feasible to make DNAR decisions in advance. When patients entering the hospital are unconscious or incapable of expressing their own opinions, it is appropriate to make initially the decision, which appears to be in the best interest of the patient [60].

A decision not to treat or resuscitate, because the risks outweigh the benefits, should be made by a senior doctor in collaboration with members of a multiprofessional team and only after careful consideration of all the relevant factors to the patient's current situation [17, 75]. Such factors, according to the Guidance from the British Medical Association and the UK Resuscitation Council, are related to the likelihood of restarting the person's heart and breathing and restoring circulation for a sustained period, the anticipated level of recovery after successful CPR without neurological deficit or cardiac failure, the restoration of heart beat and breathing without satisfactory mental capacity or restoration of consciousness, the known or verifiable wishes and values and advance directives of persons who lack capacity, and the patient experiencing continuing and intolerable or unacceptable pain or suffering [72]. Afterwards, the doctor should proceed with a documented discussion of his decision with the patient (unless he/she refuses such discussion), or with family, or a surrogate decision-maker of the patient, who lacks capacity. Failing to involve a patient or his family at the time of writing a DNAR order, the doctor breaches Article 8 of the European Convention on Human Rights [76, 77].

The utilisation of DNAR orders involves the application of the ethical principles of patients' *autonomy* and doctors' *beneficence*. The exercise of these principles might be in conflict if doctors deny patients' *autonomy* by not asking them about CPR preferences, even though studies have demonstrated that many older patients prefer CPR [78]. When the doctor makes such a medical decision, he/she informs the patient compassionately, seeking patient understanding of that medical decision based on the limits of medicine [79]. On the other hand, a patient cannot demand CPR if the treating clinician thinks the treatment is futile. In this case, the patient should be offered a second opinion by a senior doctor [60]. The doctor should make clear that DNAR orders only apply to CPR and that not attempting CPR does not mean giving up other treatments such as pain relief, medicines or nutrition; neither this is a reason for *withdrawing* or *withholding* other treatments [60]. The patient should be reassured that he/she will not be ignored or abandoned but rather that the intent is to protect the patient from harm and to maximise comfort and quality of life [39].

A survey on EP's practices found that most EPs attempt to resuscitate patients in cardiopulmonary arrest, regardless of reported poor outcomes, with the exception of the cases with available legal advance directive. Even then, the compliance of EPs with the directives may be variable, dependent upon the clinical circumstances. The decisions of many EPs regarding resuscitation are based on concerns of litigation and criticism, rather than on professional judgement of medical benefit [30].

27.3.3 Older Abuse

Over the past decade, older abuse has been increasingly recognised as a persistent and growing global problem with serious consequences for the health and wellbeing of old vulnerable people [80]. The World Health Organization Toronto Declaration on Older Abuse defines older abuse as "a single, or repeated act, or lack of appropriate action, occurring within any relationship where there is an expectation of trust which causes harm or distress to an older person" [81]. Older abuse may take various forms such as physical abuse with the intention of causing physical pain or injury, psychological or emotional abuse with the intention of causing emotional pain, sexual assault, financial or material exploitation, and intentional or unintentional neglect [80, 81]. A systematic review of studies measuring the prevalence of older abuse or neglect among the general population found that over 6% of older people reported significant abuse in the last month; nearly a quarter reported significant psychological abuse and a fifth neglect [82]. At the same time, older abuse is independently associated with shorter survival, as well as with significant morbidity and premature mortality in older adults [23, 80].

The World Health Organization declares that "older abuse is a violation of Human Rights and a significant cause of injury, illness, lost productivity, isolation and despair" [83]. The health implications of older abuse are an increasingly important issue for both society and the ED. Detection of and intervention in older abuse is crucial to the well-being of older patients. Very often older abuse is underreported due to fear, shame, guilt or cognitive problems [84]. Therefore, detection can be difficult and the problem to remain underestimated. The ED is the first point of contact of the abused subject with formal services [85]. Older victims who have had "accidents" resulting from neglect, self-neglect or physical abuse are likely to seek care in an ED. Emergency physicians are in an ideal position to diagnose and intervene in suspected cases of older abuse. They must be alert to the possibility of older abuse and be aware of how to identify it and therefore minimise the impact on older people [82]. Older persons who have been abused are inherently vulnerable due to physical or cognitive decline or conditions imposed by the family or the community. Therefore, building up rapport with a non-judgemental, direct approach, giving particular attention to verbal and non-verbal cues, is essential to allow these persons to disclose [85].

Emergency care professionals can assist with the screening, reporting, intervention and prevention strategies. Early detection and interventions, such as effective treatment of actual underlying issues, providing community-based services and appropriately involving family, may help delay or prevent older abuse. Recognition can be improved through education and use of resources in a multidisciplinary environment. A standardised screening for frailty, cognitive or functional impairment should be instituted in the ED to help detect risk factors for older abuse. Decision-making capacity is the cornerstone for the assessment of any cases of older abuse, in addition to balancing the ethical principles of *autonomy* and *beneficence*. However, capacity is not often completely present or completely absent. It is a gradient between the issues in question and the older person's ability to make these decisions [23]. It is beyond doubt that "confronting and reducing older abuse requires a multisectoral and multidisciplinary approach" [81].

27.3.4 Dementia in Older People

Dementia gives rise to many ethical issues affecting the individuals with dementia themselves, their close family and friends providing a lot of support, as well as society as a whole [86]. The ethical issues that arise in the context of dementia are associated with the increasing numbers of people affected by dementia, primarily because of the number of people living into old age. The Nuffield Council on Bioethics defines "dementia" as a "collection of signs and symptoms such as memory and communication problems, changes in mood and behaviour, and the gradual loss of control of physical functions …as a result of the progressive degeneration of nerve cells" [86].

The ethical issues of the emergency care of vulnerable aged patients with dementia refer to both their *autonomy* and their well-being. *Autonomy* is not simply related to their ability to make rational decisions. It involves supporting them in maintaining their sense of self and expressing their values. Well-being includes more objective factors such as their level of cognitive functioning [86]. Respecting *autonomy* becomes complicated in cases of older patients with dementia presenting to the ED with an acute problem. Individuals with impaired, fluctuating or questionable cognitive status, and those with mild and moderate dementia, may retain sufficient cognitive capability to make some, but not necessarily all, health-care decisions. It is important not to assume a priori that patients with a diagnosis of dementia and other chronic cognitive disorders have limited capacity to comprehend and make decisions. The progression of cognitive functional decline varies tremendously between early and advanced stages of dementia and also between individuals. EPs should seek direct discussion and as much additional evidence on the patient's cognitive capacity and not rely on charts or mental test scores. Another moral dilemma is generated from research on highly vulnerable patients with dementia when their decision-making capacity is seriously compromised. In particular, their capacity to give valid consent to a request that they serve as research subjects is questionable, at best.

The aged frail subjects with dementia might be at risk for being assigned low priority in the allocation of services in the ED. The stigma, which still persists about dementia, may lead to difficulties and delays in the access of emergency services. When decisions about resource allocation are made, the dementias should be considered as diseases or illnesses in just the same way as are, for example, the various forms of cancer. There should be no fundamental difference between the problems that arise as a result of dementia and, for example, responding to pain in cancer or mobility difficulties in arthritis [86]. Communication by people with dementia, as well as their ability to comprehend communication, given their potential vulnerability, can be difficult. Consequently, it is particularly important that every effort should be made to provide a supportive environment in the ED that promotes communication during therapeutic interactions and helps them to maintain their *autonomy* as much as possible [85].

27.4 Ethical Considerations for Emergency Research on Older Patients

The international declarations and conventions on research emphasise the ethical principles that should govern research on human subjects [87, 88]. They include respect for the *autonomy* of the research participant—or his or her legal representative—to give a free and informed consent prior to the initiation of research, *beneficence* in maximising the benefits and protecting the welfare and privacy of subjects and patients and *non-maleficence* in avoiding harm, and *justice* in the equitable distribution of the benefits and burdens of research [2, 89].

Informed consent is the centrepiece of the protection of human subjects during research. The Nuremberg Code of research ethics—published in 1947 following the Nazi medical experiments—clearly states that "the voluntary, well-informed, understanding consent of the human subject in a full legal capacity" is absolutely essential [90]. Informed consent for research is a process by which a subject voluntarily confirms his or her willingness to participate in a particular clinical trial, after having been informed of all aspects of the trial that are relevant to the subject's decision to participate [17].

In emergency medicine, the issue of informed consent for conducting research in human subjects is a major issue. Emergency patients, including vulnerable groups, are acutely ill and commonly in a critical, life-threatening condition which appears suddenly and unexpectedly, for which often neither the patient nor the family members have been able to prepare. Recruitment in a clinical trial, providing information and asking for consent may take time, postpone the initiation of treatment and put the patient's life in jeopardy. The risk of irreversible damage, as the consequence of time delays to seek consent, is unacceptable. Not requesting consent before a clinical trial is also contradictory. A person should not be forced to participate in a trial against his or her will. Doing good and avoiding harm and respecting the *autonomy* of the patient are factors which are in conflict in the context of emergency medical research [91].

Several solutions have been adopted for meeting the requirements for informed consent for research in the ED. Legal representatives (proxies) can give consent before inclusion in the research; the patient's and/or proxy's consent can be deferred for some time or consent can even be waived. An independent physician can give his/her consent for inclusion in a clinical trial, or patient/proxy consent can be presumed [92]. The Royal College of Emergency Medicine advises that in an emergency initially no consent or an oral consent can be obtained, with full written consent obtained later [17]. However, the responsibility for the safety and welfare of research subjects ultimately rests with the principal investigator, who shares with the research institutions the responsibility to protect research subjects [2].

Patients, who are critically ill or injured and unable to provide meaningful prospective informed consent because of their current life-threatening condition, are vulnerable and not sufficiently able to comprehend information, to deliberate and to make decisions about participation in research. These patients require additional protections, beyond those for research subjects who can speak on their own behalf [2]. The Declaration of Helsinki clearly accepts that "medical research with a vulnerable group is only justified if the research is responsive to the health needs or priorities of this group and the research cannot be carried out in a non vulnerable group". In addition, this group should "stand to benefit from the knowledge, practices or interventions that result from the research" and that "vulnerable groups and individuals should receive specifically considered protection" [88]. Research in emergency care needs to be carried out in such a way that both the needs of society and the rights of the individual are protected. Emergency physicians involved in research must consider the dignity, rights, safety and well-being of research participants and must respect the diversity of human culture. They must also have a good understanding of the principles of informed consent, of adverse event reporting and of using detailed documentation [17].

To conduct ethically sound emergency research, investigators must take appropriate steps to ensure that "vulnerable populations"—persons or groups with limited or diminished *autonomy*—will not suffer undue medical, social and psychological harm in the name of research. In fact, vulnerable populations may possess adequate *autonomy* but may lack the capacity to understand or communicate opinions regarding participation in research protocols. For example, helpless older individuals are at risk of being exploited in ethically inappropriate ways in research, because of their difficulty in providing voluntary informed consent. The purpose is not to exclude these patients from research protocols but to ensure the ability of the participant to fulfil the requirements of ethical research [93].

Medical research in emergencies brings up the ethical dilemmas of patient *autonomy*, *beneficence*, *non-maleficence* and *justice* that must be weighed against the need to do scientific investigations and to provide patients with scientific advances. These concepts should be central to protecting all human research participants. Medical research in an emergency setting should always be regarded as an exceptional situation requiring special provisions. In the case of a critical emergency, the unconscious state of the patient, the emotional stress of family members or the lack of time to start life-sustaining measures may often restrict the possibilities of communicating with the patient or his/her representative [91]. If emergency medicine research is to develop and grow, these problems must be resolved and a framework developed that will make emergency research easy to perform while patients are protected.

Conclusions

Quality emergency care for older patients must promote patient-centered care consistent with patients' best interests. Decisions about the emergency treatment of older patients should be made on an individual basis, providing the greatest benefit for incompetent patients after assessment of the particular circumstances and the individual patient's wishes and values. Emergency personnel should implement the *principlism* ethical framework of *autonomy*, *non-maleficence*, *beneficence* and *justice* to confront the ethical issues and dilemmas they are likely to encounter in the care of older patients. The ethical issues regarding older patients in the ED are related to the assessment of decision-making capacity, advance directives, fairness of treatment and resource allocation, end-of-life decisions, do not attempt resuscitation (DNAR) orders, older abuse, and dementia. The human rights of this vulnerable ageing population should be protected by ensuring that treatment should not be prolonged when it has ceased to provide a clear benefit for the patient. However, such decisions should be carefully thought based on the best scientific evidence available and the patient's best interests.

References

1. Moskop JC, Sklar DP, Geiderman JM, Schears RM, Bookman KJ (2009) Emergency department crowding, part 1- concept, causes, and moral consequences. Ann Emerg Med 53: 605–611. https://doi.org/10.1016/j.annemergmed.2008.09.019
2. American College of Emergency Physicians (2008) Code of ethics for emergency physicians. Ann Emerg Med 52:581–590
3. Pauls M, Leblanc C, Campbell S (2002) Ethics in the trenches: preparing for ethical challenges in the emergency department. CJEM 4:45–48
4. Sanders AB (1995) Unique aspects of ethics in emergency medicine. In: Iserson KV, Sanders AB, Mathieu D (eds) Ethics in emergency medicine, 2nd edn. Galen Press Ltd, Tucso, pp 7–10
5. Baker C (2015) Accident and emergency statistics. House of commons. briefing paper No. 6964
6. Samaras N, Chevalley T, Samaras D, Gold G (2010) Older patients in the emergency department: a review. Ann Emerg Med 56:261–269. https://doi.org/10.1016/j.annemergmed.2010.04.015
7. Adams J, Wolfson AB (1990) Ethical issues in geriatric emergency medicine. Emerg Med Clin North Am 8(2):183–192
8. Beauchamp TL, Childress JF (2009) Principles of biomedical ethics. Oxford University Press, New York, p. (a) 1, (b) 16–25, (c) 99–105, (d) 149–155, (e) 167–168, (f) 197, (g) 240–252, (h) 248–249

9. van Potter R (1970) Bioethics, science of survival. Persp Biol Med 14:127–153
10. Schneiderman LJ (2011) Defining medical futility and improving medical care. J Bioeth Inq 8:123–131
11. Aacharya RP, Gastmans C, Denier Y (2011) Emergency department triage: an ethical analysis. BMC Emerg Med 11:16. https://doi.org/10.1186/1471-227X-11-16
12. Kaldjian LC, Weir RF, Duffy TP (2004) A clinician's approach to clinical ethical reasoning. J Gen Intern Med. 20(3):306–311
13. Bossaert LL, Perkins GD, Askitopoulou H, Raffay VI, Greif R, Haywood KL et al (2016) Reply to letter: family presence during cardiopulmonary resuscitation: evidence-based guidelines? Resuscitation 105:e7–e8. https://doi.org/10.1016/j.resuscitation.2016.05.003
14. Das AK, Mulley GP (2005) The value of an ethics history? J R Soc Med 98(6):262–266
15. Larkin GL, Marco CA, Abbott JT (2001) Emergency determination of decision-making capacity: balancing autonomy and beneficence in the emergency department. Acad Emerg Med 8(3):282–284
16. Pellegrino ED (2000) Decisions to withdraw life-sustaining treatment: a moral algorithm. JAMA 283(8):1065–1067
17. Royal College of Emergency Medicine (2015) End of life care for adults in the emergency department. Best practice guideline. Royal College of Emergency Medicine, London
18. Mueller PS, Hook CC, Fleming KC (2004) Ethical issues in geriatrics: a guide for clinicians. Mayo Clin Proc 79:554–562
19. Singler K, Thiem U, Christ M, Zenk P, Biber R, Sieber CC et al (2014) Aspects and assessment of delirium in old age. First data from a German interdisciplinary emergency department. Z Gerontol Geriatr 47:680–685. https://doi.org/10.1007/s00391-014-0615-z
20. Davis MA, Hoffman JR, Hsu J (1999) Impact of patient acuity on preference for information and autonomy in decision making. Acad Emerg Med 6(8):781–785
21. Sokol DK (2015) Update on the UK law on consent. BMJ 350:h1481
22. Ha JF, Anat DS, Longnecker N (2010) Doctor-patient communication: a review. Ochsner J 10(1):38–43
23. Dong X (2014) Elder abuse: research, practice, and health policy. The 2012 GSA Maxwell Pollack award lecture. Gerontologist 54(2):153–162
24. Iserson KV (2004) Ethical considerations in emergency care. Israeli J Emerg Med 4(2):10–17
25. Lloyd G, Skarratts D, Robinson N, Reid C (2000) Communication skills training for emergency department senior house officers—a qualitative study. J Accid Emerg Med 17:246–250
26. Johnston C, Liddle J (2007) The Mental Capacity Act 2005: a new framework for healthcare decision making. J Med Ethics 33:94–97
27. Andorno R, Biller-Andorno N, Brauer S (2009) Advance health care directives: towards a coordinated European policy? Eur J Health Law 16:207–227
28. Aw D, Hayhoe B, Smajdor A, Bowker LK, Conroy SP, Myint PK (2012) Advance care planning and the older patient. Q J Med 105:225–230. https://doi.org/10.1093/qjmed/hcr209
29. Shaw D (2012) A direct advance on advance directives. Bioethics 26(5):267–274
30. Marco CA, Bessman ES, Kelen GD (2009) Ethical issues of cardiopulmonary resuscitation: comparison of emergency physician practices from 1995 to 2007. Acad Emerg Med 16:270–273
31. Puchalski C, Zhong Z, Jacobs MM, Fox E, Lynn J, Harrold J et al (2000) Patients who want their family and physician to make resuscitation decisions for them: observations from SUPPORT and HELP. J Am Geriatr Soc 48(Suppl 5):84–90
32. Shalowitz DI, Garrett-Meyer E, Wendler D (2006) The accuracy of surrogate decision makers. A systematic review. Arch Internal Med 166:493–497
33. Mentzelopoulos S, Bossaert L, Raffay V, Askitopoulou H, Perkins GD, Greif R et al (2016) A survey of key opinion leaders on ethical resuscitation practices in 31 European countries. Resuscitation 100:11–17. https://doi.org/10.1016/j.resuscitation.2015.12.010
34. Jones WHS (2004) Hippocrates. Epidemics I. The Loeb Classical Library, I. Harvard University Press, Cambridge, XI.9–15

35. Jones WHS (1998) Hippocrates. The Art. Vol. II. The Loeb Classical Library. Harvard University Press, Cambridge. (a) Chapter III.8–10, (b) Chapter XIV.2–3
36. Mason JK, Laurie GT (2011) Mason and McCall Smith's law and medical ethics, 8th edn. Oxford University Press, Oxford, p 476
37. World Medical Association (2009) Medical ethics manual, 2nd edn. The World Medical Association, Inc, France. http://www.wma.net/en/30publications/30ethicsmanual/pdf/ethics_manual_en.pdf. Accessed 23 Mar 2015
38. Council of Europe (2014) Committee on bioethics (DH-BIO). Guide on the decision-making process regarding medical treatment in end-of-life situations. http://www.coe.int/t/dg3/healthbioethic/conferences_and_symposia/Guide%20FDV%20E.pdf. Accessed 13 Feb 2015
39. Blinderman CD, Krakauer EL, Solomon MZ (2012) Time to revise the approach to determining cardiopulmonary resuscitation status. JAMA 307(9):917–918. https://doi.org/10.1001/jama.2012.236
40. Kidd AC, Honney K, Myint PK, Holland R, Bowker LK (2014) Does medical futility matter in 'do not attempt CPR' decision-making? Int J Clin Pract 68(10):1190–1192. https://doi.org/10.1111/ijcp.12476
41. British Medical Association (2007) Withholding or withdrawing life-prolonging medical treatment. Guidance for decision making, 3rd edn. Blackwell Publishing, London
42. General Medical Council (2010) Treatment and care towards the end of life: good practice in decision making. General Medical Council, Manchester
43. Manalo MFC (2013) End-of-life decisions about withholding or withdrawing therapy: medical, ethical, and religio-cultural considerations. Palliat Care 7:1–5
44. Vincent J-L (2005) Withdrawing may be preferable to withholding. Critical Care 9:226–229
45. Conroy S, Fade P, Fraser A, Schiff R, Guideline Development Group (2009) Advance care planning: concise evidence-based guidelines. Clin Med 9:76–79
46. Bossaert LL, Perkins GD, Askitopoulou H, Raffay VI, Greif R, Haywood KL et al (2015) European resuscitation council guidelines for resuscitation 2015: section 11. The ethics of resuscitation and end-of-life decisions. Resuscitation 95:302–311. https://doi.org/10.1016/j.resuscitation.2015.07.033
47. Marco CA, Larkin GL, Moskop JC, Derse AR (2000) Determination of "futility" in emergency medicine. Ann Emerg Med 35(6):604–612
48. Jones WHS (2004) Hippocrates. The Oath. The Loeb Classical Library, vol I. Harvard University Press, Cambridge
49. Denny DL, Guido GW (2012) Under treatment of pain in older adults: an application of beneficence. Nurs Ethics 19(6):800–809
50. Larkin GL, Moskop J, Sanders A, Derse A (1994) The emergency physician and patient confidentiality: a review. Ann Emerg Med 24:1161–1167
51. Moskop JC, Marco CA, Larkin GL, Geiderman JM, Derse AR (2005) From Hippocrates to HIPAA: privacy and confidentiality in emergency medicine—part II: challenges in the emergency department. Ann Emerg Med 45:60–67
52. Schmidt TA, Beckman A, Bradley R, DiGioia N, Girod J, Hollingsworth S, et al (2005) Guide to teaching ethics in emergency medicine residency programs. SAEM Ethics Committee. http://www.saem.org/docs/default-source/education/ethics guide.pdf?sfvrsn=0. Accessed 5 Feb 2016
53. Truog RD, Brett AS, Frader J (1992) The problem with futility. N Engl J Med 326(23):1560–1564
54. Rackham H (1934) Aristotle. Nicomachean ethics. The Loeb Classical Library, vol IV. Harvard University Press, Cambridge, pp 8–11
55. Harris J, Regmi S (2012) Ageism and equality. J Med Ethics 38(5):263–266
56. Detering KM, Hancock AD, Reade MC, Silvester W (2010) The impact of advance care planning on end of life care in elderly patients: randomised controlled trial. BMJ 340:c1345. https://doi.org/10.1136/bmj.c1345
57. Huerta-Alardín AL, Guerra-Cantú M, Varon J (2007) Cardiopulmonary resuscitation in the elderly: a clinical and ethical perspective. J Geriatr Cardiol 4:117–119

58. Cooper S, Janghorbani M, Cooper G (2006) A decade of in-hospital resuscitation: outcomes and prediction of survival? Resuscitation 68(2):231–237
59. Hilberman M, Kutner J, Parsons D, Murphy DJ (1997) Marginally effective medical care: ethical analysis of issues in cardiopulmonary resuscitation (CPR). J Med Ethics 23:361–367
60. Holm S, Jørgensen EO (2001) Ethical issues in cardiopulmonary resuscitation. Resuscitation 50:135–139
61. Deasy C, Bray JE, Smith K, Harriss LR, Bernard SA, Cameron P et al (2011) Out-of-hospital cardiac arrests in the older age groups in Melbourne, Australia. Resuscitation 82:398–403. https://doi.org/10.1016/j.resuscitation.2010.12.016
62. Swor R, Jackson RE, Tintinalli JE et al (2000) Does advanced age matter in outcomes after out-of-hospital cardiac arrest in community-dwelling adults? Acad Emerg Med 7:762–768
63. Lannon R, O'Keeffe ST (2010) Cardiopulmonary resuscitation in older people—a review. Rev Clin Gerontol 20:20–29
64. Truhlár A, Deakin CD, Soar J, Khalifa GE, Alfonzo A, Bierens JJ et al (2015) European resuscitation council guidelines for resuscitation 2015: section 4. Cardiac arrest in special circumstances. Resuscitation 95:148–201. https://doi.org/10.1016/j.resuscitation.2015.07.017
65. Elshove-Bolk J, Guttormsen A, Austlid I (2007) In-hospital resuscitation of the elderly: characteristics and outcome. Resuscitation 10:1–5
66. Larkin GL, Copes WS, Nathanson BH, Kaye W (2010) Pre-resuscitation factors associated with mortality in 49,130 cases of in-hospital cardiac arrest: a report from the National Registry for Cardiopulmonary Resuscitation. Resuscitation 81(3):302–311. https://doi.org/10.1016/j.resuscitation.2009.11.021
67. Boyd R (2000) Witnessed resuscitation by relatives. Resuscitation 43:171–176
68. Engel KG, Barnosky AR, Berry-Bovia M, Desmond JS, Ubel PA (2007) Provider experience and attitudes toward family presence during resuscitation procedures. J Palliative Med 10(5):1007–1009
69. Compton S, Magdy A, Goldstein M, Sandhu J, Dunne R, Swor R (2006) Emergency medical service providers' experience with family presence during cardiopulmonary resuscitation. Resuscitation 70:223–228
70. Critchell CD, Marik PE (2007) Should family members be present during cardiopulmonary resuscitation? A review of the literature. Am J Hosp Palliat Care 24(4):311–317
71. Mitchel MH, Lynch MB (1997) Should relatives be allowed in the resuscitation room? J Accid Emerg Med 14:366–369
72. British Medical Association, Resuscitation Council (UK) and Royal College of Nursing (2014) Decisions relating to cardiopulmonary resuscitation. Guidance from the British Medical Association, the Resuscitation Council (UK) and the Royal College of Nursing. 3rd edn. https://www.resus.org.uk/dnacpr/decisions-relating-to-cpr/. Accessed 23 Mar 2015
73. Morrison LJ, Gerald K, Diekema DS, Sayre MR, Silvers SM, Idris AH et al (2010) Part 3: ethics: American Heart Association 2010 guidelines for Cardiopulmonary Resuscitation and Emergency Cardiovascular Care. Circulation 122(Suppl 3):665–675. https://doi.org/10.1161/CIRCULATIONAHA.110.970905
74. Snyder L (2012) American college of physicians ethics manual, 6th edn. American College of Physicians, Philadelphia
75. Mockford C, Fritz Z, George R, Court R, Grove A, Clarke B et al (2015) Do not attempt cardiopulmonary resuscitation (DNACPR) orders: a systematic review of the barriers and facilitators of decision-making and implementation. Resuscitation 88:99–113. https://doi.org/10.1016/j.resuscitation.2014.11.016
76. European Court of Human Rights (2016) European convention on human rights. http://www.echr.coe.int/Documents/Convention_ENG.pdf. Accessed 28 Mar 2016
77. Fritz Z, Cork N, Dodd A, Malyon A (2014) DNACPR decisions: challenging and changing practice in the wake of the Tracey judgment. Clin Med 14:571–576. https://doi.org/10.7861/clinmedicine.14-6-571
78. Cherniack EP (2002) Increasing use of DNR orders in the elderly worldwide: whose choice is it? J Med Ethics 28:303–307

79. Bishop J, Brothers K, Perry J, Ahmad A (2010) Reviving the conversation around CPR/DNR. Am J Bioeth 10(1):61–67. https://doi.org/10.1080/15265160903469328
80. Lachs MS, Pillemer K (2004) Elder abuse. Lancet 364:1263–1272
81. World Health Organisation (2002) The Toronto declaration on the global prevention of elder abuse, Geneva. http://www.who.int/ageing/projects/elder_abuse/alc_toronto_declaration_en.pdf. Accessed 3 Feb 2016
82. Cooper C, Selwood A, Livingston G (2008) The prevalence of elder abuse and neglect: a systematic review. Age and Ageing 37:151–160
83. World Health Organisation (2002) Active ageing: a policy framework. A contribution of the World Health Organization to the Second United Nations World Assembly on Ageing, Madrid, Spain. http://apps.who.int/iris/bitstream/10665/67215/1/WHO_NMH_NPH_02.8.pdf. Accessed 3 Feb 2016
84. McAlpine C (2008) Elder abuse and neglect. Age Ageing 37(2):132–133
85. Phelan A (2012) Elder abuse in the emergency department. Intern Emerg Nurs 20:214–220
86. Hope T, Askham J, Baker M, et al (2009) For the working group of the Nuffield Council on Bioethics. Dementia: ethical issues. Nuffield Council on Bioethics, London
87. Council of Europe (2009) The convention on human rights and biomedicine (Oviedo, 4.IV.1997). Treaty No 164. http://conventions.coe.int/Treaty/en/Treaties/Html/164.htm. Accessed 23 Mar 2015
88. World Medical Association (2013) Declaration of Helsinki ethical principles for medical research involving human subjects. 64th WMA general assembly, Fortaleza, Brazil. http://www.wma.net/en/30publications/10policies/b3/. Accessed 23 Mar 2015
89. Nee PA, Griffiths RD (2002) Ethical considerations in accident and emergency research. Emerg Med J 19:423–427
90. Annas GJ, Grodin MA (1992) The Nazi doctors and the Nuremberg code: human rights in human experimentation. Oxford University Press, Oxford
91. Halila R (2007) Assessing the ethics of medical research in emergency settings: how do international regulations work in practice? Sci Eng Ethics 13(3):305–313
92. Kompanje EJO, Maas AIR, Menon DK, Kesecioglu J (2014) Medical research in emergency research in the European Union member states: tensions between theory and practice. Intens Care Med 40(4):496–503. https://doi.org/10.1007/s00134-014-3243-6
93. Quest T, Marco CA (2003) Ethics seminars: vulnerable populations in emergency medicine research. Acad Emerg Med 10:1294–1298

Index

A
Abdomen, 32, 33, 59, 80, 168, 226, 229
Abdominal aortic aneurysm (AAA), 227, 228, 280
Abdominal pain, 38, 52, 60, 62, 117. *See also* Acute abdominal pain (AAP)
Abuse, 39, 40, 120, 169
Acute abdominal pain (AAP), 62, 217
    AA, 229
    AAA, 227
    age-related physiological changes, 218
    AMI, 225
    AP, 230
    bile tract diseases, 230
    differential diagnosis, 220–221
    diverticulosis, 228–229
    epidemiology, 218
    extra-abdominal diseases, 231
    history and physical examination, 218–220
    imaging studies, 222–223
    intestinal obstruction, 228
    laboratory studies, 221–222
    management, 223–224
    NSAP, 231
    PUD, 231
Acute appendicitis (AA), 229
Acute brain failure, delirium, 51
Acute care for the elderly (ACE) model
    units, 94, 95
    inhibitors, 116
Acute coronary syndrome (ACS), 52
    diagnosis, 252
    differential diagnosis, 253
    NSTE-ACS, 251
    prognosis and outcomes, 255
    STEMI, 251
    symptoms, 252
    treatment, 253–254
        cardiac catheterization, 254
        pharmacological treatment, 254
        prasugrel, 255
        ticagrelor, 255
Acute geriatric units, 9
Acute kidney injury (AKI), 302
Acute mesenteric ischemia (AMI), 225–227
Acute myocardial infarction, 231
Acute pain, 7, 278–280, 315, 316, 319, 321, 322
Acute pancreatitis (AP), 230–231
Acute respiratory failure (ARF), 34, 261, 262
Adjuvant treatments, 283
Advance care planning (ACP), 374, 383
Advanced idiopathic skeletal hyperostosis, 167
Advance directives (ADs), 374, 375
Adverse drug events (ADEs), 54, 76, 101, 120, 299, 306, 307
Ageing/aging, 24, 180, 292, 293, 300, 301
Age-related degeneration, 148
Airway, 164
    assessment, 26–27
    management, 28–31
    protective reflexes, 59
Airway, breathing, circulation (ABC)
    approach, 8, 24, 40, 56
Amiodarone, 301
Analgesics, topical use, 321
Antibiotics, 115, 117, 128, 183, 187, 229, 236, 237, 239, 242, 266, 270
Anticoagulation, 270
Antidepressants, 213–214, 283, 284
Antihypertensives, 112, 150, 152, 305
Apnea, 30, 32, 33
Appendectomy, 229
Arterial blood gas, 61, 221
Arthritis, 31, 92, 389
Asthma, 264, 265
Asymptomatic bacteriuria (ASB), 115, 237
Atrial fibrillation, 38, 154

Autonomy, patients
    delirium, 372
    diagnostic/therapeutic intervention, 372
    health care, decision-making, 371
    informed consent, 371–373
    and mental capacity, 371
    paternalistic physician–patient
        relationship, 371
    patient refusal, 372
    principle of, 371

B
Back pain, 59, 117. *See also* Low back
    pain (LBP)
Bag-valve-mask device (BVMD), 32
Basel nonspecific complaints (BANC)
    study, 128
Baseline oxygen saturation, 30
Basic activities of daily living (BADL), 55
Beneficence, rinciple of
    ethical obligation, 379
    health-care providers, 379
    paternalistic, 379
    patient confidentiality, 380
Benzodiazepines, 143, 205, 301, 321
Beta-2 agonist, 269
Bile tract diseases, 230
Bioethics, 370, 376, 388
Biomedical ethics, 370
Bisphosphonates, 283
Blood pressure, 20, 32, 37, 38, 57, 111, 112, 143,
    150, 152, 153, 220, 249, 294, 303
Blood urea nitrogen, 60
Body temperature, 113
Boerhaave's syndrome, 250
BONES mnemonic, 29
Boston Syncope Criteria, 155
Bradycardias, 149
Breathing, 32–36, 164
    assessment, 32
    management
        apnea and irregular respirations, 32–33
        respiratory distress, 33–34
        respiratory failure, 34–36
Breathlessness, 261
Brief Confusion Assessment Method
    (bCAM), 203
Bronchodilators, 269–270
B-type natriuretic peptide (BNP), 61

C
Carbamazepine, 302
Cardiac catheterization, 254

Cardiogenic shock, 37
Cardiopulmonary resuscitation (CPR), 37,
    41–43, 384, 386, 387
Cardiorespiratory system, age-related changes,
    261, 262
Cardiovascular disease, 149
Cardiovascular system, 184
Care home services, 332
Care homes, 332
Care transitions
    within emergency department
        disposition, 338–339
        initial assessment, 336
        optimization, 332–333
        patient discharge, 340–341
    pre-hospital care transitions
        care home teams, 331
        emergency department receiving team,
            333–334
        emergency medical services and care
            home, 331
        inter-professional communication,
            335–336
        non-specific presentation, 334
        paramedic and technician staff, 331
        paramedics and care home, 333
        technology, 335
        triage, 334–335
Carotid sinus hypersensitivity (CSH), 151
Carotid sinus massage (CSM), 151
Carotid sinus syndrome (CSS), 151
Cementoplasty, 284
Central venous oxygen saturation (ScvO2),
    186, 191
Central venous pressure (CVP), 186
Chest pain, 52, 247
    ACS, 251
        diagnosis, 252
        differential diagnosis, 253
        NSTE-ACS, 251
        prognosis and outcomes, 255
        STEMI, 251
        symptoms, 252
        treatment, 253–255
    differential diagnosis, 248, 250, 251
        PE, 248–249
        tension pneumothorax, 249–250
        type A aortic dissection, 249
    management, 256, 257
Cholecystitis, 230
Chronic illness, 26
Chronic pain, 276, 317, 322, 323
Circulation
    assessment, 36–37
    management, 37–38

Clarithromycin, 301
Clostridium difficile, 244
Cognition, 101
Cognitive impairment (CI), 20, 82, 101, 199, 200
    delirium diagnostic criteria, 201
        detection, 202–203
        management, 204
        prevention, 205
        risk factors, 203–204
        subtypes, 202
    dementia, 205
        diagnosis and management, 206
        subtypes, 205–206
    ED, 200
    epidemiology, 200–201
    neurocognitive disorders, 201
    service reconfiguration with, 206–207
Coma, 58
Comprehensive geriatric assessment (CGA)
    emergency department
        conduct, 100
        evidence base, 95
    evidence base, 94–95
    homeostatic reserves assessment, 55
        functional disability, 55
        indicators, 55–56
        morbid conditions, 55
    life-threatening conditions, 50–52
    practical examples, 99–100
    preadmission functional and health status assessment
        biological pitfalls, 53
        clinical pitfalls, 53
        electrocardiogram, 53–54
        medication history, 54
    secondary assessment, 56
        abdominal symptoms, 62
        care with cognitive impairment, 62–63
        context-dependent testings, 60–61
        electrocardiogram, 60, 61
        geriatric emergency health-care centers, 63–64
        head to toe examination, 58–59
        liaison service, 63
        systematically ordered, 60
        trauma, 61–62
        vital signs and general appearance, 57–58
Computed tomography (CT), 117, 222
    dyspnoea, 267
Computed tomography pulmonary angiography (CTPA), 248
Computerised physician order entry (CPOE) systems, 310
COPD exacerbations, 263, 265

Coronary artery disease, 119
C-reactive protein, 60
Creatine kinase, 60
Crystalloid fluid resuscitation, 8
Cumulative Illness Rating Scale (CIRS), 59
Cytochrome p450 enzyme, 301, 302

D
D-dimer, 61, 266
Delirium, 51, 82, 118, 199
    diagnostic criteria, 201
    detection, 202
    management, 204
    prevention, 205
    risk factors, 203
    subtypes, 202
Dementia, 82, 118, 199, 205, 318, 388, 389
    diagnosis and management, 206
    palliative and end of life care
        communications planning, 358
        decision making, 357
        families and carers involvement, 359
        Gold Standards Framework, 355–357
        maintaining dignity, 359
        management, 358
        patient transfer, 357–358
    subtypes, 205
Depression, 58, 101
    antidepressant treatment, 213–214
    diagnosis, acute and emergency care setting, 210–211
    epidemiology, 209–210
    risk assessment, 211–212
    suicide, factors, 212
    symptoms, 211
    therapeutic intervention, 212–213
Disposition, syncope, 156, 157
Distributive justice, 381
Distributive/vasodilatory shock, 37
Diuretics, 143, 269
Diverticulosis, 228, 229
Do not attempt resuscitation (DNAR), 386, 387, 391
Domino effect, 50–51
Drug-disease interactions, 304
Drug-drug interactions, 304
Dyspepsia, 52
Dyspnoea, 261–262
    aetiology, 262, 263
    diagnosis, 263–264
        arterial blood gas, 267
        biomarkers, 266–267
        chest radiography, 265
        CT, 267

Dyspnoea (cont.)
　　electrocardiogram, 265
　　laboratory tests, 265
　　symptoms and signs, 264–265
　　ultrasound, 267
　risk stratification, 271
　treatment, 268
　　algorithm, 268, 269
　　antibiotics, 270
　　anticoagulation, 270
　　bronchodilators, 269
　　comorbidities, management, 271
　　diuretics, 269
　　oxygen and NIV, 268
Dysrhythmias, 38, 149

E
Early goal-directed therapy (EGDT), 186
Echocardiography, 37
Edinburgh Postnatal Depression Scale, 210
Effective communication, 78, 373
EGSYS, 156
Electrocardiogram, 54, 265
Electroconvulsive therapy (ECT), 214
Emergency department (ED), 9
　atypical presentations
　　abdominal pain, 117
　　abuse and neglect, 120
　　ADEs, 120
　　back pain, 117
　　common fluid and electrolyte problems, 116
　　coronary artery disease, 119
　　delirium and dementia, 118–119
　　discharge planning, 121
　　falls, 117–118
　　fever and common infections, 114
　　hidden diseases, social admissions and search for, 121
　　PE, 116
　　pneumonia, 114–115
　　thyroid disease, 116
　　UTI and ASB, 115
　care plan, 103
　care transitions within
　　disposition, 338
　　initial assessment, 336
　　team members, handover, 336–338
　CGA
　　conduct, 100
　　evidence base, 95
　cognition, 101
　conduct, 100
　　problem detection

　　assessment, domains, 100
　　high-risk population, identification, 100
　depression, 101
　early discharge planning, 102
　evidence-based solutions
　　care of older people, 92
　　follow-up, 93
　　frail older people, 93
　　history of, 93
　　interdisciplinary diagnostic process, 92
　　multidimensional assessment, 92
　　treatment, coordinated and integrated plan, 93
　falls, 102
　follow-up, 103
　frail older people in, 91
　functionality, 101
　polypharmacy, 102
　receiving team, 333
　triage
　　issues, 18
　　priorities , determination, 17
　　process, 17
　　triage environment, 18–20
　vital signs
　　blood pressure, 112
　　body temperature, 113
　　HR, 112
　　RR, 113
Emergency medical services, 331–332
Emergency physicians (EPs), 24, 369, 379, 386
Emergency Severity Index (ESI), 19
Empirical antibiotic therapy, 187, 188
End of life care, 362–365
　dying people, priorities, 362
　　individual care plans, 365
　　involvement, 364
　　providing support, 364
　　recognising, 363
　　sensitive communication, 363
　eating and drinking, 366
　environment, 365
　hospice care, 366
　organ donation, 366
　pain relief and symptom control, 365
　religion and spiritual care, 366
End-tidal carbon dioxide concentration (ETCO2), 8
Enterococcus faecalis, 239
Escherichia coli, 239
Ethics, medical practice, 384, 389
　clinical decision, 370
　clinical trial, 389

cultural and political implications, 370
definition, 370
end of life decisions, 382, 383
human culture diversity, 390
informed consent, 389, 390
psychological and social
     vulnerability, 370
research, emergencies, 390
resuscitation process, 384
    biological age, 384
    informed consent, 389
    neurological outcome, 384
    survival rates, 384
    survival to discharge, 384
vulnerable populations, 390
Evidence-based medicine, 291–292
Exercise therapy, 285
Exposure, 165–166
Extra-abdominal diseases, 231
Extremities, 168

F
4 As Test (4AT), 202
Faintness, 51
Fall, 85, 102, 117, 137, 303
    environment, 143
    epidemiology, 138
    management, 141–143
    medication, 143
    multidisciplinary and holistic
         approach, 137
    multifactorial intervention, 143
    multi-factorial management programme, 144
    poor processes and lack of access, 144
    risk factors, 138–141
Family witnessed resuscitation, 384–386
Fecal impaction, 52
Fever
    and common infections, 114
    definition, 132
Foreign body aspiration, 31
Four-item geriatric depression scale, 214
Frailty, 77, 78, 165, 293
Functional decline, 9, 51
Functional disability, 55
Futility in medicine, 376–377

G
Gamma-glutamyl transferase (GGT), 60
Gangrenous cholecystitis, 230
Geriatric emergency health-care
     centers, 63

Geriatric evaluation and management (GEM)
     units, 94
Glasgow Coma Scale (GCS), 25, 165
Glomerular filtration rate (GFR), 302
Glycemic control, 188
Grab sheet, 332

H
Head computed tomography scan, 154
Head examination, 58
Head injury, 61, 166
Head-tilt-chin-lift maneuver, 29
Heart rate (HR), 112, 133
Helicobacter pylori (*H. pylori*), 231
High-sensitivity troponin, 61
Hip fracture, 50, 61, 62, 117, 143, 204
Homeostatic reserves assessment
    functional disability, 55
    morbid conditions, 55
Horton's disease, 279
Hospice care, 366
Hospital Anxiety and Depression (HAD)
     scale, 210–211
Hyperglycemia, 188
Hyperkalaemia, 116
Hypertension, 31, 111, 227
Hypoactive delirium, 200
Hypoglycemia, 188
Hyponatraemia, 116
Hypotension, 37
Hypothermia, 41, 183
Hypovolemic shock, 37, 220
Hypoxemia, 34, 35

I
Identification of seniors at risk (ISAR), 86
IL-6, 181
Impaired mental status, 36
Inappropriate prescribing (IP), 306–307
Infections
    clinical manifestation, 132
    examination, 132
    fever, 132
    pulmonary infection, 132
    urinary tract infections, 132
    working hypothesis, 132
Inflammatory low back pain, 279
Instrumental activities of daily living, 55
Interdisciplinary geriatric consultation services
     (IGCS), 94
Intestinal obstruction, 228
Intoxication, 40–41
Irregular respirations, 32

J
Jaw-thrust maneuver, 29
Justice, principle of, 381
　fairness, opportunity, 381
　finite resources, equitable allocation, 381, 382

K
Klebsiella sp., 237, 239

L
Laxatives, 283
LEMON mnemonic, 29
Lewy bodies (LBD), 206
Liaison service, 63
Lidocaine, 323
Life-threatening conditions, 23
　acute brain failure
　　delirium, 51
　　faintness/syncope and general malaise, 51
　atypical presentations, 52
　digestive symptoms, 52
　domino effect, 50
　functional decline, 51
　referred pain and symptoms, 52
　secondary assessment, CGA, 56
　　abdominal symptoms, 62
　　care with cognitive impairment, 62
　　context-dependent testings, 61
　　electrocardiogram, 60, 61
　　head to toe examination, 58
　　systematically ordered, 60
　　trauma, 61
　　vital signs and general appearance, 57
Life-threatening emergencies, 25–26
Low back pain (LBP), 275–276
　autonomy and functional performance, 282
　clinical presentation, 277
　　evaluating pain, 280–281
　　history, 277–278
　　inflammatory, 278–279
　　lumbar spinal canal stenosis, 279–280
　　older patients, behavior change, 280
　　osteoarthritis, 280
　　osteoporotic fracture, 279
　　physical examination, 278
　epidemiology, 276
　investigations, 281–282
　management, 285
　pathophysiology, 276–277
　treatment, 282
　　adjuvant treatments, 283–284
　　exercise therapy, 285
　　nonopioid analgesics, 282–283
　　opioids, 283
　　surgical treatment, 284
Lower limbs, 59
Lumbar degenerative spondylolisthesis, 283
Lumbar puncture, 61
Lumbar spinal canal stenosis, 279

M
Magnetic resonance imaging (MRI), 168, 229, 281
Manchester Triage System (MTS), 19, 79
Mean arterial blood pressure, 37
Medicine
　ageing process, 292
　clinical guidelines, 291
　Evidence-based medicine, 291
　older patients, 293–295
　physician knowledge and experience, 296–297
　reconciliation, 308
　scientific evidence, 295
Melancholic somatic symptoms, 210
Mental health disorders (MHDs), 209
Microstomia, 31
Mild cognitive impairment (MCI), 205
Morphine, 283
Multidrug-resistant organisms (MDROs), 239

N
Natriuretic peptide type B, 266
Neck examination, 59
Neck stiffness, 54
Neglect, 120, 169
Neurologic disorder, 36
Neuropathic pain, 317, 323
Nitrates, 143, 150, 242
Nitrous oxide-oxygen gas mixture (N_2O/O^2), 321
Nociceptive pain, 317
Noninvasive positive-pressure ventilation (NIPPV), 33, 34
Non-invasive ventilation (NIV), 268
Non-maleficence principle, 375, 376
　futile medical treatment, 376, 377
　implications, 376
　life-prolonging treatment, 378, 379
Non-occlusive mesenteric ischemia (NOMI), 225, 227
Nonopioid analgesics, 282, 283

Non-prescription, drug use, 300
Nonspecific abdominal pain (NSAP), 231
Nonspecific complaints (NSCs), older patients
 adverse outcomes, 127, 128
 BANC, 128
 causes, 128–129
 diagnostic approach
  diagnostic workup, 127, 129, 130
  heart failure, 133
  infections, 132
  localised vs. generalised weakness, 130
  medical history, 130–131
  physical examination, 130–131
  specific symptoms, 129
  water and electrolyte disorder, 132–133
 disease presentation, 128
 emergency department, 127
 in-hospital mortality, 127, 128
 lack of community support, 128
Non-steroidal anti-inflammatory drugs (NSAIDs), 282, 320
NSTE-ACS, 251, 254, 255

O

Obstructive shock, 37
Older abuse, 387, 388
Older patients
 care, models of, 8–9
  acute geriatric units, 9
  community and primary care, 9–10
  ED, 9
  EMS/EMT/ambulance care, 11
  hospital at home, 10–11
  out of hours' care, 10
  traditional inpatient management models, 9
 impact on services, 4
 pathologies
  pain, 7
  recognition, 6
  time critical, 6–7
 pre-hospital geriatric patient
  anatomical and physiological differences, 5
  disability and function, 5
  epidemiology, 6
 pre-hospital personnel training, 4–5
Older people, 75–86
 communication, with frailty, 82
 functional assessments, 87–88
 geriatric giants
  dementia and delirium, 82–83
  falls and syncope, 85
  injuries, 85
  medication, 86
  pain, 85–86
  sepsis, 83–84
 management
  CGA, 77
  differential challenge, 76–77
  functional decline and altered homeostasis, 76
  multiple comorbidities, 76
  non-specific presentations, 75
 older abuse, assessing for, 87
 risk assessment, 86–87
 urgent care, identifying with frailty, 77
  carers and families, communication with patients, 78–79
  history taking, 79
  physical examination, 80
  professionals, communication between, 80–81
Opioids, 283, 320, 321
Oral transmucosal fentanyl citrate (OFTC), 321
Organ donation, 366
Orthostatic hypotension (OH), 150, 151
Osservatorio Epidemiologico sulla Sincope nel Lazio (OESIL) score, 155
Osteoarthritis, 277, 280
Osteoarticular pain, 275
Osteoporotic fracture, 279, 283
Oxygen supplementation, 268
Oxygen therapy, 33, 268
Oxygenation, 32, 267

P

Pain, 7, 85, 315, 316, 319–322
 assessment, 317–318
 behaviours, 319
 care quality indicators, 316
 chronic pain, exacerbation, 322
 classification, 317
 definition and types, 316–317
 dementia and assessment, 318–319
 drugs, 323
 management, 322
  analgesics, topical use, 321
  interventional techniques, 322
  N_2O/O_2, 321
  principles, 319–320
  treatment, 320–321
 neuropathic, 323
 optimal management, 315
 under- treatment of, 316

Painful diverticular disease, 229
Palliative care, 362–365
　　dying people, priorities, 362–363
　　　　individual care plans, 364–365
　　　　involvement, 364
　　　　providing support, 364
　　　　recognising, 363
　　　　sensitive communication, 363–364
　　eating and drinking, 366
　　environment, 365
　　hospice care, 366
　　organ donation, 366
　　pain relief and symptom control, 365
　　religion and spiritual care, 366
Paracetamol, 320
Patient communication, 373–375
Patient response/mental status assessment, 25
Patient's comorbidity, 59
Patient-centred care, 95
Pelvis, 168
Peptic ulcer disease (PUD), 231
Percutaneous epidural adhesiolysis, 284
Permissive hypotension, 8
Phenytoin, 301, 302
Plain abdominal X-rays, 222
Pneumatosis intestinalis, 227
Pneumonia, 114, 180
Polypharmacy, 76, 101, 102, 304
Postural homeostasis, 150
Potentially inappropriate medication (PIM), 306
Prasugrel, 255
Prescription
　　adverse drug events, 307–308
　　CGA, 309
　　CPOE, 310
　　drug-drug and drug-disease interactions, 304–306
　　epidemiology of, 300
　　inappropriate prescribing, 306
　　medicines reconciliation (MR), 308–309
　　pharmacokinetics and pharmacodynamics, 300–303
　　recommendations, 309
Primary care, communicating with, 341
Procalcitonin (PCT), 61, 184, 266
Procedural pain, 317
Prodromes, 150, 154
Pulmonary and heart examination, 59
Pulmonary embolism (PE), 116, 248
Pulmonary Embolism Severity Index (PESI), 271
Pulmonary infection, 132
Pyuria, 240

Q
Quality emergency care, 391
quickSOFA (qSOFA), 178, 179

R
Rapid sequence intubation (RSI), 30
Rectal examination, 59
Referred pain, 52
Rehabilitation, 345
　　collaborative inter-disciplinary working, 350
　　conceptual framework, 350
　　geriatric emergency medicine, 347–349
　　ICF, 346
　　inter-disciplinary working, 349–350
　　interpersonal and communication skills, 351
　　vulnerability, to poorer outcomes, 347
　　WHODAS 2.0, 346–347
Religion care, 366
Reperfusion, 226
Respiratory distress, 33
Respiratory failure, 34, 262
Respiratory rate (RR), 113
Resuscitation, 41–43, 164
Richmond Agitation Sedation Scale (RASS), 25, 58
Rockwood Frailty Index, 55

S
San Francisco Syncope Rule (SFSR), 155
Scientific evidence, 295–296
Senescent immune remodeling, 180
Sensitive communication, 363
Sensory exam, 59
Sepsis, 83, 152, 177, 186–189
　　causes, 180
　　clinical presentation and diagnosis, 182–185
　　epidemiology of, 179–180
　　management, 184–185
　　　　glycemic control, 188
　　　　initial resuscitation, 186–187
　　　　principles, 188–189
　　　　source control and antimicrobial treatment, 187–188
　　　　treatments, 188
　　pathophysiology, 180–181
　　prognosis and outcomes, 189–190
　　risk factors, 181–182
Septic shock, 177, 178, 184, 186–188
Sequential (sepsis-related) organ failure assessment (SOFA) score, 178

Index

Serum creatinine, 53, 60
Serum electrolytes, 60
Severe low back pain, 59
Silver Code (SC), 87
Single Question in Delirium (SQiD), 202
SIRS, 179, 191
Social admissions, 82, 121
Spinal stenosis, 284
Spine fusion, 284
Spiritual care, 366
Spondylodiscitis, 279
Standard medical therapy (SMT), 34
Standardised handover tool, 332
Staphylococcus, 239
ST-elevation myocardial infarction (STEMI), 251
Steroids, 283
Stick blood glucose, 60
Superior mesenteric artery (SMA), 225
Surviving Sepsis Campaign (SSC), 184
Syncope, 51, 85, 147
    background and epidemiology, 148–149
    disposition, 156–157
    etiologies, 149–152
    evaluation, 152–153
    multidimensional geriatric assessment, 148
    scoring tools, 154–156
    testing, 153–154
Syncope units (SUs), 156

T

Tachycardias, 149
Tension pneumothorax, 249, 250
Thorax, 167
Thyroid disease, 116
Thyroid-stimulating hormone, 61
Ticagrelor, 254, 255
Traditional inpatient management models, 9
Tramadol, 283
Transaminases, 60
Trauma, 38, 39, 61, 163
    abdomen, 168
    abuse and neglect, 169
    airway and breathing, 164–165
    clinical assessment, 166
    disability, 165
    exposure, 165–166
    extremities, 168–169
    head injury, 166–167
    imaging, 166

    neck and spine, 167
    pelvis, 168
    resuscitation, 164
    thorax, 167
Trauma Audit Research Network (TARN), 143
Triage, ED
    issues, 18
    priorities , determination, 17
    process, 17
    triage environment, 18–20
Troponin, 54, 251, 266
Type A aortic dissection, 249

U

Ultrasonography (USG), 222, 228, 229
Ultrasound, dyspnoea, 267
Urinalysis, 61, 132, 222
Urinary tract infection (UTI), 115, 132
    diagnosis
        community-dwelling older adults, 240–242
        long-term care facilities, diagnostic algorithm, 243
        long-term indwelling urinary catheter, 243–244
        patients with communication barriers, 241–242
    microbiology, 239–236
    prevention, 244–245
    risk factors, 239–240
    symptoms, 236–237
        asymptomatic bacteriuria, 237–238
        symptomatic, 238–239
    treatment, 243–244

V

Vasovagal syncope, 148, 150

W

Warfarin, 120, 143, 301, 303, 307
Water and electrolyte disorder, –133, 132
World Health Organiszation Disability Assessment Schedule 2.0 (WHODAS 2.0), 346

X

X-rays, 132, 166, 204, 222, 227, 250, 264, 281

Printed by Printforce, the Netherlands